ESSENTIALS *of* CLINICAL HYPNOSIS

Dissociation, Trauma, Memory, and Hypnosis Book Series

Steven Jay Lynn, Series Editor

Believed-In Imaginings: The Narrative Construction of Reality
Joseph de Rivera and Theodore R. Sarbin, Editors

Clinical Hypnosis and Self-Regulation: Cognitive–Behavioral Perspectives
Irving Kirsch, Antonio Capafons, Etzel Cardeña-Buelna,
and Salvador Amigó, Editors

Essentials of Clinical Hypnosis: An Evidence-Based Approach
Steven Jay Lynn and Irving Kirsch, Authors

Healing From Within: The Use of Hypnosis in Women's Health Care
Lynne M. Hornyak and Joseph P. Green, Editors

Varieties of Anomalous Experience: Examining the Scientific Evidence
Etzel Cardeña, Steven Jay Lynn, and Stanley Krippner, Editors

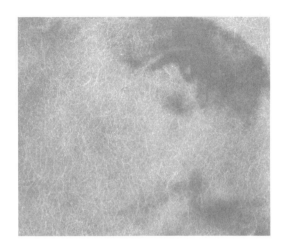

ESSENTIALS *of* CLINICAL HYPNOSIS

AN EVIDENCE-BASED APPROACH

Steven Jay Lynn and Irving Kirsch

American Psychological Association • *Washington, DC*

First Printing October 2005
Second Printing November 2011

Published by
American Psychological Association
750 First Street, NE
Washington, DC 20002
www.apa.org

To order
APA Order Department
P.O. Box 92984
Washington, DC 20090-2984
Tel: (800) 374-2721
Direct: (202) 336-5510
Fax: (202) 336-5502
TDD/TTY: (202) 336-6123
Online: www.apa.org/books/
E-mail: order@apa.org

In the U.K., Europe, Africa, and the Middle East, copies may be ordered from
American Psychological Association
3 Henrietta Street
Covent Garden, London
WC2E 8LU England

Typeset in Goudy by World Composition Services, Inc., Sterling, VA

Printer: United Book Press, Inc., Baltimore, MD
Cover Designer: Naylor Design, Washington, DC
Technical/Production Editor: Genevieve Gill

The opinions and statements published are the responsibility of the authors, and such opinions and statements do not necessarily represent the policies of the American Psychological Association.

Library of Congress Cataloging-in-Publication Data

Lynn, Steven J.
    Essentials of clinical hypnosis: an evidence-based approach / Steven Jay Lynn and Irving Kirsch.— 1st ed.
        p. cm.
    Includes bibliographical references and index.
    ISBN 1-59147-344-6
    1. Hypnotism—Therapeutic use.   2. Evidence-based medicine.   I. Kirsch, Irving, 1943- II. Title.

    RC495.L96   2006
    615.8'512—dc22   2005012320

British Library Cataloguing-in-Publication Data
A CIP record is available from the British Library.

Printed in the United States of America
First Edition

CONTENTS

PREFACE

As in the field of psychology generally, within the area of hypnosis there is often a gap between the world of the laboratory and the world of clinical practice. Many clinicians complain that most research in hypnosis fails to address the issues that they confront daily in their practices. On the other side of the divide, researchers may feel that their work is ignored by most clinicians. This book was born out of a desire to bridge the gap between research and practice.

We are best known as researchers and theorists. Between us, we have authored well over 300 journal articles, most of them focused on scientific research. But we are also clinical psychologists. Throughout our careers, we have had active clinical practices in which we have both practiced and supervised psychotherapy. We have also supervised and taught classes in psychotherapy to graduate students in the clinical psychology PhD programs at our universities. Looking at our publications alone might lead one to underestimate our professional role as clinicians. In fact, we are scientist practitioners in the tradition of the Boulder model, which shaped clinical psychology programs throughout the United States. This work represents the culmination of our individual thinking about hypnosis as well as the fruits of a 20-year collaboration.

This book is essentially clinical in nature. But it is a clinical book with a research base. The clinical strategies and techniques that we present are ones that we have used in our practice and that we have taught our graduate students to use. They are procedures with an evidential base. Many of the specific techniques we describe have been validated in clinical trials and outcome studies, and our approach to most strategic issues has been shaped by our understanding of the research literature in hypnosis, psychotherapy, and psychopathology. If there is a fundamental difference between this book and the many other guides that have been published on clinical applications of hypnosis, it is the degree to which the principles and practices we describe are evidence-based. Hence, the subtitle of this book.

We aim to bring our enthusiasm for integrating hypnosis with empirically supported methods to a wide readership and to move hypnosis more securely into the mainstream of established clinical practice. We help novices get started by presenting basic inductions and suggestive methods and describe when to use and when not to use hypnotic procedures. More advanced and specialized techniques and strategies are described for students of hypnosis at all levels. Readers will encounter fundamental information about the history of hypnosis, surveys of different theoretical perspectives on hypnosis, up-to-date literature reviews on empirically supported treatments, and discussions of thorny issues including the use of hypnosis for memory recovery. Transcripts from sessions, illustrative examples, and step-by-step procedures for treating an array of commonly encountered disorders and conditions (e.g., anxiety, depression, posttraumatic stress disorder, pain and medical conditions, smoking, and eating disorders) serve as road maps for implementing hypnotic methods. We are confident that this volume, combined with supervised experiences in using hypnotic procedures and accessible through workshops sponsored by well-established hypnosis societies (e.g., Society for Clinical and Experimental Hypnosis, American Society of Clinical Hypnosis), will provide readers with the knowledge and experience required to practice hypnosis with confidence.

As with any book, there are many people we have to thank. We owe a debt of gratitude to Susan Reynolds of the American Psychological Association for her patience and support; to Joseph Green, Linda McCarter, Sheri Oz, Fern Pritikin Lynn, Genevieve Gill, and Judith Pintar for their perceptive comments on the manuscript; to our graduate students, from whom we have learned as they have learned from us; to David Mellinger for his contributions to the chapter on anxiety; and to our patients, who, in the process of their own growth, have helped us grow as clinicians and as human beings.

ESSENTIALS *of* CLINICAL HYPNOSIS

1

INTRODUCTION:
DEFINITIONS AND EARLY HISTORY

Shrouded for centuries in mystery and myth, hypnosis has been viewed by many with suspicion. At the same time, it has attracted the interest of the most renowned scholars of human behavior. Hypnosis was given serious consideration by Sigmund Freud, Alfred Binet, William James, Wilhelm Wundt, Clark Hull, Ernest R. Hilgard, and other luminaries of psychology. Yet only recently has hypnosis begun to receive the recognition it deserves. It is a subject of intensive investigation in psychological laboratories around the world (see Fromm & Nash, 1992; Kirsch & Lynn, 1995; Lynn & Rhue, 1991a) as well as a treatment component of demonstrated efficacy. A special issue of the *International Journal of Clinical and Experimental Hypnosis* on the topic of hypnosis as an empirically supported clinical intervention has documented the effectiveness or promise of hypnosis in treating a wide variety of psychological and medical conditions ranging from acute and chronic pain to obesity (see Lynn, Kirsch, Barabasz, Cardena, & Patterson, 2000). Furthermore, meta-analytic reviews, which synthesize findings over multiple trials, have shown that hypnosis enhances the effectiveness of both psychodynamic and cognitive–behavioral psychotherapies (Kirsch, 1990; Kirsch, Montgomery, & Sapirstein, 1995).

There are a number of reasons for the slow pace of acceptance of hypnosis. One is the dramatic nature of its effects. During hypnosis, many people appear to lose control over normally voluntary behavior; some exhibit temporary, selective amnesia; and they may report seeing and hearing things that are not present and not seeing or hearing things that are present. Behavior and reported experiences of this sort seemed so extraordinary that many investigators assumed they were due to an altered state of consciousness, typically referred to as a *trance*.

The trance concept is another reason for the widespread—but diminishing—reluctance to learn and use hypnosis in clinical practice. This idea can be frightening to both clinicians and their patients. Putting someone in a trance sounds like serious business. What if the person gets stuck there and cannot come out? The accumulated data from controlled research should dispel fears of this sort. The state of consciousness produced by typical hypnotic inductions does not seem to be any different from that produced by nonhypnotic relaxation training (Edmonston, 1981; Kirsch, Mobayed, Council, & Kenny, 1992; E. Meyer & Lynn, 2004). Although most researchers have concluded that hypnotic responses are not due to a hypnotic state or trance (see Kirsch & Lynn, 1995), neither is hypnosis simply relaxation. Hypnosis can be induced with instructions to relax or feel energized. Hypnosis can even be induced while people are exercising vigorously (Bányai, 1991; Bányai & Hilgard, 1976). The issue of whether hypnosis is an altered state of consciousness or trance is still controversial and is discussed in detail in the concluding chapter.

WHAT IS HYPNOSIS?

What, then, is hypnosis? Clinicians and researchers of diverse theoretical orientations (see Kirsch, 1994a) have agreed on the following description of hypnosis, which has been officially adopted by Division 30 (Society of Psychological Hypnosis) of the American Psychological Association (APA):

> Hypnosis is a procedure during which a health professional or researcher suggests that a client, patient, or subject experience changes in sensations, perceptions, thoughts, or behavior. The hypnotic context is generally established by an induction procedure. Although there are many different hypnotic inductions, most include suggestions for relaxation, calmness, and well-being. Instructions to imagine or think about pleasant experiences are also commonly included in hypnotic inductions.
>
> People respond to hypnosis in different ways. Some describe their experience as an altered state of consciousness. Others describe hypnosis as a normal state of focused attention, in which they feel very calm and relaxed. Regardless of how and to what degree they respond, most people describe the experience as very pleasant. Some people are very responsive to hypnotic suggestions and others are less responsive. A person's ability to experience hypnotic suggestions can be inhibited by fears and concerns arising from some common misconceptions. Contrary

to some depictions of hypnosis in books, movies or on television, people who have been hypnotized do not lose control over their behavior. They typically remain aware of who they are and where they are, and unless amnesia has been specifically suggested, they usually remember what transpired during hypnosis. Hypnosis makes it easier for people to experience suggestions, but it does not force them to have these experiences. Hypnosis is not a type of therapy, like psychoanalysis or behavior therapy. Instead, it is a procedure that can be used to facilitate therapy. Because it is not a treatment in and of itself, training in hypnosis is not sufficient for the conduct of therapy. Clinical hypnosis should be used only by properly trained and credentialed health care professionals (e.g., licensed clinical psychologists), who have also been trained in the clinical use of hypnosis and are working within the areas of their professional expertise.

Hypnosis has been used in the treatment of pain, depression, anxiety, stress, habit disorders, and many other psychological and medical problems. However, it may not be useful for all psychological problems or for all patients or clients. The decision to use hypnosis as an adjunct to treatment can only be made in consultation with a qualified health care provider who has been trained in the use and limitations of clinical hypnosis. In addition to its use in clinical settings, hypnosis is used in research, with the goal of learning more about the nature of hypnosis itself, as well as its impact on sensation, perception, learning, memory, and physiology. Researchers also study the value of hypnosis in the treatment of physical and psychological problems. (Kirsch, 1994a, pp. 142–143)

A decade after the first definition was crafted, the executive committee of the APA Division 30, Society of Psychological Hypnosis (Green, Barabasz, Barrett, & Montgomery, 2005) revised the definition to encompass the widely used clinical technique of self-hypnosis, described as "the act of administering hypnotic procedures on one's own." The reformulated definition also acknowledged that "Many believe that hypnotic responses and experiences are characteristic of a hypnotic state. While some think that it is not necessary to use the word *hypnosis* as part of the hypnotic induction, others view it as essential" (p. 262). The new definition also noted that responsiveness to suggestion can be assessed by standardized scales in clinical and research settings, that scores can be grouped into low, medium, and high categories, and that "the salience of evidence for having achieved hypnosis increases with the individual's score" (p. 263). Although the definition of hypnosis has proven to be a controversial issue in general (e.g., Fellows, 1995; Hasegawa & Jamieson, 2002; Kallio & Revonsuo, 2003; Kileen & Nash, 2003; D. Spiegel, 1998; Wagstaff, 1998), the definitions of hypnosis generated by the APA constitute a useful starting place for understanding hypnosis and hypnotic phenomena.

A ROAD MAP OF THE BOOK

That said, any reasonably complete understanding of hypnosis needs to be informed by an appreciation of the historical context. Many of the current perspectives we review in this volume, as well as popular myths and misconceptions of hypnosis that abound to this day, have their roots in early conceptualizations of hypnosis. In subsequent chapters, we expand on themes we introduce in the brief history of hypnosis included in this chapter, in which we trace the history of hypnosis from healing rituals to the establishment of modern laboratories devoted to the scientific study of hypnotic phenomena. Chapter 2 presents an overview of contemporary theories and research on hypnosis, including empirical support for the principles and practices described in relation to the specific disorders and conditions we discuss. Chapters 3, 4, and 5 introduce basic and advanced techniques of hypnosis, including the decision to use hypnosis with a given patient, and inductions and suggestions for deepening the experience of hypnosis, relaxation, self-hypnosis, imaginative rehearsal, and emotional control and achieving specific posthypnotic goals. Chapters 6 through 11 illustrate how the treatment of disorders and conditions that clinicians commonly encounter, including smoking cessation, eating disorders, depression, anxiety, post-traumatic stress disorder, pain, and other medical conditions, may be combined with empirically supported clinical interventions and enhanced through the use of hypnosis. Finally, Chapter 12 addresses thorny issues and controversies surrounding hypnosis, including the following questions: Is hypnosis a special trance state? Should hypnosis be used to recover memories? Should clinicians test for suggestibility? Does hypnosis produce negative effects in patients?

A BRIEF HISTORY OF HYPNOSIS

Our use of the term *hypnosis* has its origin in the work of the 19th-century British physician James Braid (1843). However, the phenomenon to which it refers had been well known for at least a half-century earlier under the names *animal magnetism* or *mesmerism*. Believing the phenomenon to be due to magnetism, mesmerists sought its roots in ancient attempts to cure by the use of magnets (Binet & Féré, 1888). Later scholars adopted an altered state perspective and described ancient healing rituals practiced in Eastern and Western civilizations as precursors of modern hypnosis (e.g., Gravitz, 1991). The key to understanding the evolution of hypnosis, however, can be found in the intertwined histories of hysteria and demonic possession (see Spanos & Chaves, 1991).

Since the publication of the *Diagnostic and Statistical Manual of Mental Disorders* (3rd ed.; *DSM–III*; American Psychiatric Association, 1980), hysteria or hysterical neurosis ceased to exist as a recognized disorder. Its components—dissociative and conversion disorders—were regrouped, the latter as a subcategory of somatoform disorder. However, the history of these disorders and their relation to the development of hypnosis can best be understood by reverting to the earlier classification of hysteria, a disorder characterized by apparent alterations in identity, perception, and behavioral control. The symptoms once associated with hysteria are now the very behaviors elicited in standardized tests used to measure responsiveness to hypnotic suggestions.

The Wandering Womb

The history of hysteria began in ancient Egypt, where it was thought to be the result of the movement of the uterus to the affected part of the body, an explanation that was to persist for thousands of years. Hysteria was thus seen as a disorder limited to women. If a man exhibited blindness, he was blind. A woman's blindness, however, might be hysterical in nature, caused by the movement of her uterus to the area of her eyes. The Egyptians believed that the reason for the movement of the uterus was its dislike of the smell of its proper location, and the accepted treatment for hysteria was fumigation.

The ancient Greeks learned of the disorder from the Egyptians and gave it its traditional name, an adaptation of the Greek word for womb, *hysteron*. The lay meaning of the term *hysteria* to denote overly emotional and frenzied behavior is undoubtedly related to the fact that throughout history, convulsions were a frequent symptom of the disorder. This historical coincidence may be responsible for the stereotypic characterization of women as hysterical. The Greeks did not accept the Egyptian theory of the reason for the movement of the uterus. Instead, they hypothesized that the uterus moved because it desired a child. Pregnancy was thus advocated as a cure.

The association of hysteria with a wandering womb was retained in the Middle Ages, but both Egyptian and Greek accounts of why the uterus had moved were discarded. In place of fumigation and impregnation, the hysterical patient was treated with prayer, as in the following example from the 10th century:

> Oh Lord . . . stop the womb of Thy maid N [name] and heal its affliction for it is moving violently . . . . I conjure thee, oh womb, in the name of the Holy Trinity, to come back to the place . . . where the Lord has put thee originally. I conjure thee . . . to return to thy place with every possible gentleness and calm, and not to move or to inflict any molestation on that servant of God, N. . . . I conjure thee not to harm

that maid of God, N, not to occupy her head, throat, neck, chest, ears, teeth, eyes, nostrils, shoulder blades, arms, hands, heart, stomach, spleen, kidneys, back, sides, joints, navel, intestines, bladder, thighs, shins, heels, nails, but to lie down quietly in the place which God chose for thee, so that this maid of God, N, be restored to health.

The specification of these various locations was, of course, a preventive measure aimed at averting symptom substitution.

Demonic Possession and Exorcism

During the Renaissance, many people who would previously have been diagnosed as hysterical were deemed to be possessed by a demon. Earlier, in the Dark Ages, the power of the devil was proclaimed by church authorities to be limited to deluding the gullible with nightmares (Kirsch, 1978, 1980). The development of observational science in the Renaissance occasioned the publication of numerous case studies by respected physicians, in which presumably hysterical symptoms defied the constraints of physical possibility. A prominent example is the following report by Antonio Benivieni, the 15th-century "father of pathological anatomy":

> A new and extraordinary disease is nowadays rife which, though I have seen and treated it, I scarcely dare to describe. A girl in her 16th year ... broke into terrible screaming and her belly swelled up at the spot, so that it looked as if she were 8 months pregnant. . . . She flung herself about from side to side on the bed, and, sometimes touching her neck with the soles of her feet, would spring to her feet, then again falling prostrate and again springing up. . . . Investigating this disorder, I concluded that it arose from the ascent of the womb, harmful exhalations being thus carried upwards and attacking the heart and the brain. I employed suitable medicines, but found them of no avail. Yet it did not occur to me to turn aside from the beaten track until she grew more frenzied . . . and vomited up long bent nails and brass pins together with wax and hair mixed in a ball, and last of all a lump of food so large that no one could have swallowed it whole. . . . I decided she was possessed by an evil spirit who blinded the eyes of the spectators while he was doing all this. She was handed over to physicians of the soul. (Benivieni, 1954, p. 35)

Similar phenomena were described by other physicians of the period, including evidence from autopsies in which pieces of wood, iron, knives, and other large items were found in the stomachs of the deceased. In other medical reports, large solid objects were described as having been projected into and out of the bodies of patients without rupturing the skin. These reports continued well into the 17th century. Jan Batiste van Helmont, for example, the 17th-century physician and chemist who discovered the existence of gases other than air and coined the word *gas*, wrote a number of incredible firsthand accounts, including one in which a boy vomited a rack—the kind on which accused witches might be tortured—complete with base, feet, wheel, and ropes. Because the rack was too large to have passed through the boy's throat, van Helmont hypothesized that it had actually emerged through the pores of the skin, but that a demon had produced a hallucination among the spectators, causing them to misperceive the event. Reports of this sort complemented the wave of witchcraft trials that reached its peak during the midst of the scientific revolution.

The problem for medical and ecclesiastical practitioners was to make a differential diagnosis between hysteria and possession. In the earliest witch-hunting manual, by Kramer and Sprenger (1484/1971), church authorities assigned this task to physicians, who used the strategy described in the earlier quotation by Benivieni. Medicines believed effective in the treatment of hysteria were to be tried first. If these were not effective or if there was other evidence of supernatural intervention, the case would be referred to a "physician of the soul."

Later, diagnoses were made directly by priests and ministers. The procedures used by Father Johann Joseph Gassner in 18th-century Munich were typical:

> Gassner told the first [patient] to kneel before him, asked her briefly about her name, her illness, and whether she agreed that anything he would order should happen. She agreed. Gassner then pronounced solemnly in Latin: "If there be anything preternatural about this disease, I order in the name of Jesus that it manifest itself immediately." The patient started at once to have convulsions. According to Gassner, this was proof that the convulsions were caused by an evil spirit and not by a natural illness, and he now proceeded to demonstrate that he had power over the demon, whom he ordered in Latin to produce convulsions in various parts of the patient's body; he called forth in turn the exterior manifestations of grief, silliness, scrupulosity, anger, and so on, and even the appearance of death. (quoted in Ellenberger, 1970, p. 54)

The similarity of Gassner's exorcisms to modern stage hypnosis is remarkable, but not merely coincidental, as we soon shall see.

The Wizard From Vienna

During the Enlightenment in the 18th century, supernatural explanations fell out of favor, and the theories of demonic possession and the wandering womb were replaced by that of animal magnetism. The theory of animal magnetism was the brainchild of Franz Anton Mesmer (1734–1815), a flamboyant Viennese physician, who might have been the prototype for the depiction of the magician in "The Sorcerer's Apprentice" in the movie *Fantasia*. His theatrical healing methods even included the use of a magnetic wand, with which he touched the patient's body.

Mesmer believed that an invisible magnetic fluid permeated the universe. According to his theory, this fluid was the cause of gravitation, magnetism, and electricity and it also had profound effects on the human body. Imbalances in magnetic fluid caused nervous illnesses, and the restoration of balance through mesmerism was the method by which these illnesses could be cured.

The first patient to be mesmerized was Francisca Oesterline, a young Viennese woman who visited Mesmer in 1773 because of a hysterical disorder that included convulsions among its many symptoms (Mesmer, 1779). Finding orthodox medical treatment of no avail, Mesmer decided to try applying magnets to his patient's body. According to Mesmer, the effect of this procedure was to produce some painful sensations, after which her symptoms went into remission. Subsequent treatments reliably produced the convulsions from which she suffered, and Mesmer discovered that he could control the location of his patient's convulsions by touching or pointing to various parts of her body, a phenomenon that he proudly demonstrated to others.

The symptoms of hysteria appear to be culturally transmitted, as evidenced by their tendency to go in and out of fashion. Glove anesthesia was popular in one era, demonic possession in another; dissociative identity disorder has been the most recent popular disorder with symptoms of hysteria. Therefore, Fraulein Oesterline's convulsions might be ascribed to the cultural knowledge that they were typical symptoms of hysterical disorders and demonic possession. In particular, the exorcisms of Father Gassner were widely discussed in Viennese society, and it is almost certain that she knew of his work (Mesmer, 1779). This knowledge may also account for the responsiveness of Oesterline's convulsions to Mesmer's indications of specific body locations, which was also a prominent feature of Gassner's exorcisms.

Mesmer's magnetic treatment of Fraulein Oesterline gradually led to her recovery, and the story of her cure brought him new patients. Knowing the story of Fraulein Oesterline's treatment, these new patients must also have known of her convulsive response to it, and that knowledge may have led them to expect a similar response. Thus it was that convulsive crises became the hallmark of mesmerism. With wild looks in their eyes, mesmerized patients laughed, cried, shrieked, and thrashed about, eventually falling into a stupor. In the 18th century, it was this convulsive crisis, which lasted up to 3 hours, that was seen as the definitive characteristic of mesmerism. This phenomenon—mistaking a product of suggestion for the essence of hypnosis—has occurred over and over again in the history of hypnosis.

What later came to be regarded as a hypnotic trance was discovered by one of Mesmer's disciples, the Marquis de Puysegur, whose patients were the peasantry around his chateau. They were less likely than the patients of other magnetists to know that they were supposed to respond by going into a crisis; because de Puysegur had disliked the idea of the crisis from the beginning of his training, he was not likely to inform them of this characteristic. One of his early patients, a 23-year-old peasant named Victor Race, appeared to enter a sleeplike state when magnetized. His behavior in this state seemed quite remarkable; as mesmerists became more interested in what they called *artificial somnambulism*, the convulsive crisis gradually disappeared, somnambulism became more common, and another product of suggestion was mistaken for the essence of mesmerism.

Fluid or Fraud?

In 1778, Mesmer moved to Paris, where his practice became so popular that large-scale group treatments were instigated. These were facilitated by the use of a large vat of "magnetized" water, called a *baquet*. The setting was described by Binet and Féré (1888) as follows:

> A circular, oaken case, about a foot high, was placed in the middle of a large hall, hung with thick curtains, through which only a soft and subdued light was allowed to penetrate. This was the baquet. . . . The patients were ranged in several rows round the baquet, connected with each other by cords passed round their bodies, and by a second chain, formed by joining hands. As they waited, a melodious air was heard, proceeding from a pianoforte, or harmonicon, placed in the adjoining room. . . . Mesmer, wearing a coat of lilac silk, walked up and down amid this palpitating crowd. . . . [He] carried a long iron wand, with which he touched the bodies of the patients, and especially those parts which were diseased. (pp. 8–10)

Putting aside his wand, Mesmer frequently magnetized young women with his hands. As described by contemporaries, the woman sat with her knees pressed firmly between the thighs of the mesmerist, who applied pressure to her "ovarium," while stroking her body until she began to convulse. This was referred to as "making passes." According to Binet and Féré (1888, p. 11), "young women were so much gratified by the crisis, that they begged to be thrown into it anew."

The Franklin Commission

No doubt, the use of procedures of this sort contributed to the government's decision in 1784 to launch an investigation into the theory and practice of mesmerism (see Lynn & Lilienfeld, 2002; Nash, 2002). Two investigating commissions were established, one of which included among its members, Benjamin Franklin, the American ambassador to France; Antoine Lavoisier, the founder of modern chemistry; and the infamous Dr. Guillotin, best known for his mechanical solution to the mind–body problem (Franklin et al., 1785/1970).

The commissioners devised a series of experiments that included some surprisingly sophisticated expectancy control procedures. For example, a tree in Benjamin Franklin's garden was "magnetized" by one of Mesmer's disciples, but the experimental subject was intentionally brought to the wrong tree. Another subject was told that a container of water had been magnetized; in fact it had not. Yet another subject was misinformed that the mesmerist was magnetizing her from behind a closed door.

The success of these expectancy manipulations led the commissioners to conclude that the effects of mesmerism were due to imagination and belief. These 18th-century experiments are remarkable for their methodological sophistication and are the first demonstrations of the role of expectancy in the phenomenon from which modern hypnosis evolved. They effectively demonstrate that hypnotic phenomena depend on people's beliefs about the procedures being used, rather than on the procedures themselves.

In the age of enlightenment, the commission's judgment that the effects of mesmerism were due to imagination was tantamount to concluding that they were not real. One of Mesmer's disciples (quoted in Binet & Féré, 1888, p. 17) asked wisely, "If the medicine of the imagination is the most efficient, why should we not make use of it?" But this suggestion was widely ignored, and mesmerism fell into decline.

NORMAL, PARANORMAL, OR ABNORMAL?

Burdened with the justly discredited theory of animal magnetism, the phenomenon that Mesmer and de Puysegur had discovered had little chance of widespread professional acceptance. Nor was its reputation enhanced by the extravagant claims of its proponents, who professed that magnetism endowed people with supernatural powers including the ability to see without the use of the eyes and to detect disease by seeing through the skin. Although these and other outrageous claims were debunked by the mid-19th century, they no doubt contributed to the mystique of hypnosis, which persists to this day.

Early clinical reports of the apparent success of mesmeric procedures in relieving the pain of major surgery during the preanesthetic era (prior to the 1840s) also shaped the popular idea that hypnosis involves a powerful and mysterious force (T. X. Barber, Spanos, & Chaves, 1974; Chaves, 1989; Spanos, 1986). For example, James Esdaile used mesmerism to perform thousands of minor surgical procedures and several hundred major surgeries in India, including the excision of large scrotal tumors. However, even the most impressive examples of early 18th-century surgical feats with mesmerized patients can be matched with examples of awake, nonmesmerized patients who displayed an equally extraordinary lack of reactivity to surgical pain (Chaves, 1989, 2000; Chaves & Barber, 1976). Contributing to the medical establishment's widespread skepticism of painless surgery, many individuals who underwent mesmeric analgesia displayed nonverbal indications (e.g., grimacing) of felt pain (Chaves, 2000).

James Braid

By the early 1800s, the reputation of hypnosis was in need of rehabilitation. Substantial credit for the professional resurrection of hypnotic phenomena should be given to the 19th-century Scottish physician, James Braid. Initially a skeptic, Braid was impressed by a stage demonstration in which a participant was magnetized by staring at a shiny object. Braid rejected the fluid theory of magnetism and hypothesized instead that the behaviors of magnetized participants resulted from neural inhibition that flowed backward from the eyes (strained by staring) to the brain and produced a condition akin to sleep. Braid (1843) labeled this phenomenon *neurohypnosis*, and the shortened term *hypnosis* gradually replaced the term *magnetism*.

As Braid gained more experience, he realized that the behavior of hypnotized individuals was greatly influenced by ideas and expectations transmitted to them by the hypnotist. He modified his earlier theory of neural inhibition and developed the notion of monoideism. Monoideism was based on the notion of ideomotor action. According to this notion, vivid ideas or images that remain uncontradicted in the mind of a subject lead automatically to the corresponding action. Thus, if a person vividly imagines that his or her arm is light and rising in the air, and if this vivid imagining is not contradicted by other thoughts, then the vivid imagery will lead the arm to rise automatically.

Braid's early ideas about neurohypnosis strongly influenced the famous French neurologist Jean Martin Charcot. Unfortunately, Charcot was not influenced by Braid's later notion of monoideism or by his emphasis on how the hypnotist's expectations influence the subject's responses. Charcot studied patients who were diagnosed with hysteria and came to believe that both hypnosis and hysteria reflected a neurological weakness. It followed that only patients with hysteria could be hypnotized.

Early Controversies

According to Charcot, there were three stages to hypnosis: lethargy, catalepsy, and somnambulism. Each was produced by a different induction procedure, and each was associated with distinct and invariable behavioral symptoms. Lethargy was produced by eye fixation and induced a sleeplike state, in which the person did not react to stimuli. Catalepsy was induced by a sudden intense stimulus (e.g., a bright light or an oriental gong) and elicited waxy flexibility. Somnambulism, the most difficult of the three stages, was brought about by pressure applied to the head. It was only in this condition, Charcot believed, that patients were able to hear, speak, and respond to suggestion. Only the most severely disturbed hysterics exhibited all three stages, and their presence was interpreted as an indication of physical pathology.

Initially believing that hysteria resulted from physical trauma to the brain, Charcot's (1889) experience with hypnosis led him to formulate the hypothesis that there was also a dynamic form of hysteria, produced by dissociation. According to this hypothesis, psychological trauma could produce a hypnoid state in neurologically susceptible individuals, during which they might suggest conversion symptoms to themselves. They would not be aware that the symptoms were due to self-suggestion, however, because those ideas would be dissociated from the rest of consciousness. Charcot's evidence for this formulation consisted of the ability to produce conversion symptoms through posthypnotic suggestion, with the patient professing no memory of the suggestion being administered. Dissociation theory was further developed by two of Charcot's students, Pierre Janet (1889/1973) and Alfred Binet (1892). Its greatest influence, however, was on Sigmund Freud (1915/1961), whose theory of a dynamic unconscious as the source of psychopathology was inspired by Charcot's demonstrations. However, Freud's psychoanalytic theory, along with experimental studies, revealed little support for the idea that streams of awareness could operate independently with little or no interference (see Kirsch & Lynn, 1998). These developments, along with the rise of behaviorism, conspired to eclipse dissociation theory until it was revived by Ernest Hilgard in the 1970s, a development we review in the next chapter.

Braid's transformation of mesmerism into hypnosis also influenced the physician August Liebeault and his colleague, the professor of medicine, Hippolyte Bernheim, both from the French town of Nancy. According to Bernheim (1886/1887) hypnotic behavior resulted from suggestion and its occurrence was not due to physical or psychological abnormality. He noted that people differ in suggestibility and proposed that suggestions produce their effects by leading participants to develop corresponding ideas that led through ideomotor action to hypnotic behavior. Bernheim rejected Charcot's notions that hypnosis was related to hysteria and that degrees of hypnosis were associated with invariant behavioral symptoms. Instead, Bernheim argued that Charcot inadvertently suggested to his hysterical patients those very behaviors that he came to erroneously believe resulted automatically from hypnosis. This disagreement led to an intense but short-lived debate between Charcot and the Nancy School (Liebeault and Bernheim), the outcome of which was the complete rejection of Charcot's theory. Bernheim's conception of hypnosis became the dominant foundation for hypnosis theory, research, and practice in the 20th century.

The 20th Century

Freud studied briefly with both Charcot and Bernheim, and hypnosis was a prominent component of his early therapeutic work. He later rejected the therapeutic use of hypnotic procedures, and his rejection of hypnosis relegated it to the fringes of medicine and psychology for much of the first half of the 20th century, with notable exceptions including the work of Clark Hull (1933) and P. C. Young (1926), whose systematic experimental studies constituted important contributions.

One of Clark Hull's students, Milton H. Erickson, became a highly influential clinical innovator and practitioner of hypnosis. Some of Erickson's ideas about the nature of hypnosis have been disconfirmed by subsequent data (e.g., Green et al., 1990; Orne, 1959; J. Young & Cooper, 1972). However, many of his innovative techniques (e.g., reframing, paradoxical interventions) have a foundation in research in clinical, cognitive, and social psychology (e.g., Lynn & Hallquist, 2004; Sherman & Lynn, 1990). The surge of interest in Erickson's techniques (see Matthews, Lankton, & Lankton, 1993) played a role in reigniting the historical fascination with hypnosis as a transcendent methodology—one with profound implications for therapeutic intervention.

The growth of hypnosis has been facilitated by the advent of organized and increasingly influential hypnosis societies and interest groups, which have expanded the training and clinical repertoire of many individuals across a gamut of professions, including social work and dentistry. The neat fit of hypnotic methods with the movement toward brief cognitive–behavioral, strategic, and problem-focused interventions; sophisticated experimental studies of hypnotic phenomena; controversies about the use of hypnosis to recover memories and in the treatment of dissociative disorders; and the advent of the health psychology movement all have propelled hypnosis into the mainstream of clinical psychology, where it resides today (see Lynn & Fite, 1998).

2

CONTEMPORARY THEORIES
AND RESEARCH

More than 40 years ago, Sutcliffe (1960) observed that different schools of thought about hypnosis make radically different assumptions, adopt different methodologies, and accept different data as admissible evidence. This observation holds true today. Competing models vie for attention and empirical support and have stimulated vigorous research programs that have contributed immeasurably to the current understanding of hypnosis. In this chapter, we review influential perspectives on hypnosis. Our discussion provides a conceptual and empirical foundation for the strategies and tactics of clinical practice that we describe in the remainder of the volume.

PSYCHOANALYTIC THEORY AND
TOPOGRAPHIC REGRESSION

Psychoanalytic theory represents a broad and coherent model of human functioning regarding "what hypnosis is, and what hypnosis is not" (Nash, 1997, p. 291). Although Freud was impressed by the apparent submissiveness of certain hypnotized participants and likened hypnosis to being in love, there is no evidence to support the idea that hypnosis fosters an erotic or sexual therapist–patient relationship. This state of affairs (no pun intended) has led modern psychoanalytic theorists (Baker, 1981, 1987; Fromm, 1979;

Fromm & Nash, 1997; Gill & Brenman, 1959; Nash, 1991) to place less emphasis on sexual and aggressive instincts than have traditional psychoanalysts, and relatively greater emphasis on the availability of imagination, fantasy, and other expressions of primary process thinking during hypnosis.

On the basis of a review of more than 100 studies of hypnotic age regression, Nash (1987) concluded that hypnosis does not permit participants to literally reexperience the events of childhood or function in a truly childlike fashion. Rather, Nash (1991) maintained that hypnosis engenders a topographic regression with specific properties that go well beyond age-regression phenomena. These properties include an increase in primary process material, more spontaneous and intense emotion, unusual body sensations, the experience of nonvolition, and the tendency to displace core attributes of important others on the hypnotist (e.g., transference).

Many participants do report unusual perceptual and bodily experiences during and after hypnosis. However, studies indicate that hypnotized participants' reports are indistinguishable from nonhypnotized participants' reports in a variety of test conditions that involve eye closure, relaxation, imagining suggested events, and focusing on body parts that parallel body parts that are the target of hypnotic suggestions (see Coe & Ryken, 1979; Lynn, Brentar, Carlson, Kurzhals, & Green, 1992). Altered bodily experiences are apparently by no means unique or specific to hypnotic conditions.

Support for psychoanalytic concepts has come from other quarters. Several studies (see Mare, Lynn, Kvaal, Segal, & Sivec, 1994) are consistent with the proposition that hypnosis increases primary process thinking. Nevertheless, it is unclear whether increased primary process during hypnosis is attributable to suggestions for eye closure, relaxation, and attention to imagery or to unique characteristics of hypnosis. Studies that document the role of unconscious influences on hypnotic responses (Frauman, Lynn, Hardaway, & Molteni, 1984), the experience of nonvolition during hypnosis (see Lynn, Rhue, & Weekes, 1990), the importance of rapport (see Lynn et al., 1991; Sheehan, 1991), and the bond with the hypnotist (Nash & Spinler, 1989) are also generally supportive of Nash's theory. Although the findings of these studies can also be explained in nonpsychoanalytic terms, they underscore the heuristic value of psychoanalytic theory.

NEODISSOCIATION THEORIES

After a long hiatus of interest in dissociation, E. R. Hilgard (1977) published an influential book that revitalized the concept by proposing a neodissociation theory based on a contemporary cognitive model of divisions of consciousness. According to neodissociation theory (Hilgard, 1977, 1986,

1994), multiple cognitive systems or cognitive structures exist in hierarchical arrangement under some measure of control by an executive ego. The executive ego or central control structure is responsible for planning and monitoring functions of the personality. During hypnosis, relevant subsystems of control are temporarily dissociated from conscious executive control and are instead directly activated by the hypnotist's suggestions. This lack of conscious control is largely dependent on an amnesic barrier or process that relegates ideas, imaginings, and fantasies to unconsciousness. Diminished executive control, in turn, is responsible for the subjective impression of nonvolition that typically accompanies hypnotic responses.

The empirical roots of neodissociation theory can be traced to Hilgard's introduction of the metaphor of the hidden observer to describe the phenomenon by which a person registers and stores information in memory, without being aware that the information had been processed. Hilgard and his associates' initial research on the hidden observer phenomenon involved experimental studies of pain and hearing. In a typical pain study, highly hypnotizable participants are able to recover concealed experiences or memories of pain during hypnotic suggestions for analgesia when they are informed that they possess a hidden part (i.e., a hidden observer) that can experience high levels of pain during analgesia and that this part can be contacted by the hypnotist with a prearranged cue. Research in Hilgard's laboratory has demonstrated that hidden observer reports can penetrate hypnotic blindness, hypnotic deafness, and positive hallucinations (see Hilgard, 1991). For example, when a hidden observer is contacted, it might report that it actually can hear following a suggestion for hypnotic deafness, while the "hypnotized part" appears to be deaf to a particular sound.

Hidden observer studies and their interpretation have been controversial. For instance, Spanos and his associates have shown that the behavior of the hidden observer depends on cues given in the instructions used to elicit the phenomenon. In prior studies, changing instructions led to hidden observers that experienced more pain or less pain or that perceived things normally or in reverse (reviewed in Kirsch & Lynn, 1998; Spanos & Hewitt, 1980), which led Kirsch and Lynn (1998) to dub the phenomenon the *flexible observer*. In fact, in one study, two hidden observers were created, one storing memories of abstract words and the other storing memories of concrete words (Spanos, Radtke, & Bertrand, 1984). According to this perspective, the hidden observer is implicitly or explicitly suggested by the hypnotist. It therefore can be thought of as no different from any other suggested hypnotic phenomenon that is guided by the participants' expectancies and situational demand characteristics. Whether the hidden observer reflects a true or preexisting division of consciousness that is directly accessed by hypnotic suggestions or whether it is a product of suggestion continues to stimulate research and theoretical controversy.

Kihlstrom (1992, 1998a, 1998b, 2003) credits the neodissociation perspective with acknowledging the presence of common dissociations within hypnosis that occur between explicit and implicit memory in posthypnotic amnesia, posthypnotic suggestions, negative hallucinations, and hypnotic analgesia. Kihlstrom has extended neodissociation theory in interesting directions that incorporate concepts of modern cognitive psychology, including memory models and the distinctions between procedural and declarative knowledge.

Bowers, Woody, and their colleagues (Bowers & Davidson, 1991; Farvolden & Woody, 2004; Miller & Bowers, 1993; Woody & Bowers, 1994; Woody & Farvolden, 1998; Woody & Sadler, 1998) advanced the dissociated-control hypothesis as an alternative to E. R. Hilgard's neodissociation model of hypnosis. Dissociated-control theory rejects amnesia as fundamental to dissociation. Instead, hypnosis is thought to involve the direct and automatic activation of subsystems of control by the hypnotist's suggestions and a weakening of frontal-lobe brain functions responsible for the initiation and monitoring of behavior. As predicted by dissociated-control theory, Farvolden and Woody (2004) found that individuals with high hypnotic ability had more difficulty with tasks that were sensitive to frontal-lobe function (e.g., source amnesia, free recall, proactive interference) than did individuals with low hypnotic ability (see also Kallio, Revonsuo, Hamalainen, Markela, & Gruzelier, 2001). It is interesting to note that high and low suggestible participants did not differ in their responses on tasks that were not sensitive to frontal-lobe functioning. However, differences between high and low suggestible individuals were found in nonhypnotic conditions as well as in the hypnotic context. This finding implies that hypnosis per se does not engender differences in frontal-lobe functions, as predicted by the dissociated-control hypothesis. Controversies aside, the neodissociation perspective continues to be one of the dominant contemporary hypnosis perspectives and has inspired a great deal of research and provides a rationale for much clinical work (see Kihlstrom, 2003).

SOCIOCOGNITIVE PERSPECTIVE

The sociocognitive perspective rejects dissociation as an explanatory mechanism and challenges many widely held beliefs about hypnosis. Sociocognitive hypnosis theorists contend that hypnotic behavior is social behavior that can be explained without recourse to any special process or mechanism unique to hypnosis. Rather, participants' expectancies, attitudes, imaginings, and beliefs about hypnosis, as well as their interpretations of suggestions, are crucial to understanding hypnotic responding.

Sarbin and Coe's Theory

The sociocognitive perspective can be traced to attacks on the concept of hypnosis as an altered state of consciousness. In 1950, Theodore Sarbin challenged the traditional concept of hypnosis as a state. Sarbin (1950) contended that hypnosis could be conceptualized as *believed-in imaginings* and developed a role theory of hypnosis that relied heavily on the metaphor of role to capture parallels between the hypnotic interaction and a miniature drama in which both the hypnotist and the subject enact reciprocal roles to follow an unvoiced script (Sarbin, 1997). Sarbin and his colleague, W. C. Coe, developed role theory (Coe & Sarbin, 1991; Sarbin, 1999; Sarbin & Coe, 1972) and conducted research that highlighted the importance of (a) participants' knowledge of what is required in the hypnotic situation; (b) self- and role-related perceptions, expectations, and imaginative skills; and (c) situational demand characteristics that guide the way the role is enacted.

Coe and Sarbin (1991) have more recently used the constructs of self-deception, secrets, metaphors, and narratives to expand role theory. Narrative psychology holds that human actions and self-perceptions are storied. Coe and Sarbin's narrative or dramaturgical model underlines the motivated, active, and constructive nature of hypnotic experiences and performances. By inducting the patient into the role of a hypnotic subject by way of education and dispelling misconceptions about hypnosis; by ensuring that the patient's ongoing self-narrative is consistent with the shifting requirements of the hypnotic role and treatment goals; and by monitoring the patient's role-related behaviors, experiences, and expectancies throughout the hypnotic proceedings, the therapist can harness the patient's imaginative abilities to achieve therapeutic ends.

Theodore X. Barber's Model

Theodore X. Barber was influenced by Sarbin's theorizing and criticized the state concept because of its logical circularity (i.e., hypnotic responsiveness can both indicate the existence of a hypnotic state and be explained by it). In an extensive series of studies in the 1960s (T. X. Barber, 1969; T. X. Barber & Calverly, 1964) and early 1970s (T. X. Barber, Spanos, & Chaves, 1974), Barber and his associates demonstrated that attitudes, expectations, and motivations are influential determinants of hypnotic responding. Moreover, well-motivated nonhypnotized and hypnotized participants were comparably responsive to suggestions. There is therefore no need for clinicians to ensure that their patients are in a trance before meaningful therapeutic suggestions are provided (Lynn & Sherman, 2000).

T. X. Barber (1985) has forcefully argued that hypnosis can improve therapeutic outcomes by (a) generating positive treatment motivation and expectancies that serve as self-fulfilling prophecies; (b) capitalizing on patients' beliefs that therapists who use hypnosis are more highly trained, skilled, and knowledgeable; and (c) permitting the therapist to talk to the patient in a very personal and meaningful way that is ordinarily not possible in a two-way conversation.

According to T. X. Barber (1985), many suggestions (e.g., relaxation, imagery rehearsal) that are commonly used in clinical practice do not require special hypnotic ability. Rather, therapeutic suggestions can be administered to many patients, regardless of their formal level of hypnotic suggestibility. Research shows that even low hypnotizable persons can benefit from hypnotic interventions and that suggestibility is not a very good predictor of treatment success (Kirsch, 1994b; Lynn & Sherman, 2000).

T. X. Barber (1999) has advanced the intriguing hypothesis that individuals have distinct styles of responding to hypnotic suggestions. Whereas the great majority of individuals respond primarily in terms of situational demand characteristics, as predicted by sociocognitive theory, Barber contended that a much smaller percentage of individuals respond because they become imaginatively (Wilson & Barber, 1981, 1983) or dissociatively (e.g., experience spontaneous amnesia) involved with suggestions. Barber's most recent position can thus be seen as a "cautious integration" of sociocognitive and dissociation accounts of hypnotic responding (Farvolden & Woody, 2004, p. 21).

Spanos and His Colleagues' Model

Spanos and his colleagues' (Spanos, 1986, 1991; Spanos & Chaves, 1989) extensive research program has focused on the importance of social psychological processes (e.g., expectancies, attributions, and interpretations of hypnotic communications and one's own behavior) and the importance of goal-directed activities and strategic responding (e.g., imagery, fantasy, allocation of attention) to suggestions in responding to hypnotic suggestions in the laboratory and in alleviating pain in medical and dental situations (Chaves, 1997b, 2000).

Suggestions often contain strategies that facilitate an appropriate response (T. X. Barber et al., 1974; Spanos & Barber, 1974; Spanos, Cobb, & Gorassini, 1985; see also Wagstaff, 1991, 1998). Consider how the wording of suggestions can foster the sense that responses are involuntary occurrences or happenings, rather than deliberate, willful actions. To facilitate the response of hand levitation, the therapist might intone, "Your hand is getting lighter and lighter; it will rise by itself." Note that the suggestion implies that the hand will lift involuntarily. Spanos (1971) hypothesized that participants experience their response to suggestions as involuntary when they become absorbed in a pattern of imaginings that he termed *goal-directed fantasy* (GDF). GDFs are "imagined situations which, if they were to occur, would be expected to lead to the involuntary occurrence of the motor response called for by the suggestion" (Spanos, Rivers, & Ross, 1977, p. 211). For instance, persons administered a hand levitation suggestion would exhibit a GDF if they report imagining a helium balloon lifting their hand or a basketball being inflated under their hand (Lynn & Sherman, 2000).

Reports of GDF are, in fact, related to the feeling of involuntariness that accompanies the response to a particular suggestion. However, GDF does not determine how many test suggestions a person successfully passes (see Lynn & Sivec, 1992, for a review). Why is this the case? Some patients are fully absorbed in imagery, yet they passively wait for the arm to rise in response to a hand levitation suggestion. This response set virtually guarantees failure. In contrast, when patients understand that it is important to lift their arm, they are more likely to pass the suggestion. In short, how patients interpret suggestions can have a bearing on how they respond to them.

Spanos challenged the accepted wisdom that hypnotic responsivity is traitlike and can be modified only within narrow limits. He argued that social psychological processes could account for the apparent stability of hypnotic suggestibility. A study by Piccione, Hilgard, and Zimbardo (1989), using a 25-year follow-up, reported a .71 test–retest correlation. However, according to Spanos, this stability reflects nothing more than attitudes and beliefs about hypnosis and interpretations of hypnotic suggestions that remain stable over time.

Spanos and his colleagues (see Gfeller, 1993; Gorassini & Spanos, 1986) have developed a social-learning, cognitive-skills-based hypnotic suggestibility modification program. This program provides low suggestible participants with information designed to modify their attitudes about hypnosis, increase their involvement in suggestion-related imaginings, and interpret hypnotic communications in a manner consistent with passing hypnotic suggestions (Gorassini & Spanos, 1999). Studies have shown that about half of the participants who are selected for low suggestibility score in the highly suggestible range of hypnotic responsiveness when they are tested after they undergo the training. These impressive findings have been replicated in other laboratories (see Gorassini & Spanos, 1999), and the effects of training have been shown to generalize to a variety of difficult test suggestions and testing situations.

Kirsch's Response Expectancy Theory

Virtually all schools of psychotherapy acknowledge the importance of bolstering positive expectancies as a way of maximizing treatment gains (see Kirsch, 1991; Lynn & Garske, 1985; Lynn & Sherman, 2000). Kirsch (1994b) maintained that like placebos, hypnosis produces therapeutic effects by changing the patient's expectancies. But unlike placebos, hypnosis does not require deception to be effective. Kirsch's response expectancy theory (see Kirsch, 1985, 1991, 1994b) is an extension of Rotter's social learning theory and is based on the idea that expectancies can generate nonvolitional responses. Kirsch's research has shown that a wide variety of hypnotic responses covary with people's beliefs and expectancies about their occurrence. In fact, expectancy, along with waking suggestibility (Braffman & Kirsch, 1999), is one of the few stable correlates of hypnotic suggestibility (Kirsch & Lynn, 1995). It is interesting to note that expectancy remains a significant predictor of hypnotic response even with waking suggestibility controlled (Braffman & Kirsch, 1999; Kirsch, Silva, Comey, & Reed, 1995). In short, hypnotic responding is regarded as nonhypnotic responding that is bolstered by participants' enhanced readiness to respond due to enhanced motivation and positive expectancies associated with hypnosis. Successful imagining of suggestions likely lends credibility to the patients' efforts to respond and fortifies response expectancies, while rapport with the hypnotist fuels motivation to respond in keeping with the demands and cues of the situation. In chapter 3, we discuss the role of expectancies in greater detail and contend that rather than avoiding expectancy effects, clinicians should exploit them.

Lynn's Integrative Model

According to Lynn and his colleagues (e.g., Lynn & Sivec, 1992), people who respond successfully to hypnotic suggestions act as creative problem-solving agents who seek and integrate information from an array of situational, personal, and interpersonal sources. Research in Lynn's laboratory has documented the importance of affective, relational, and rapport factors (Frauman & Lynn, 1985; Lynn et al., 1991); response sets and expectancies (Lynn, Nash, Rhue, Frauman, & Sweeney, 1984); the criteria or performance standards by which participants judge the success or failure of their responses to hypnosis (Lynn, Green, Jacquith, & Gasior, 2003); how hypnotic communications, sensations, and actions are processed and interpreted (Lynn, Snodgrass, Rhue, Nash, & Frauman, 1987); the dynamic and at times unconscious motives and fantasies that come into play during hypnosis (Frauman et al., 1984); and the features of the hypnotic context that discourage awareness and analysis of the personal and situational factors that influence hypnotic behavior (see Lynn et al., 1990).

Response Set Theory

Response set theory (Kirsch & Lynn, 1998, 1999; Lynn, 1997) centers on the observation that much of human activity seems to be unplanned and automatic (e.g., formation of letters while writing). The theory makes the radical proposal that all actions, mundane or novel, planned or unplanned, hypnotic or otherwise, are at the moment of activation initiated automatically, rather than by a conscious intention.

Response sets prepare actions for automatic activation. Response sets include intentions and expectancies. Both are temporary states of readiness to respond in particular ways, to particular stimuli, under particular conditions. Expectancies and intentions differ only in the attribution the participant makes about the volitional character of the anticipated act (Kirsch, 1985, 1990); that is, people intend to perform behaviors they regard as voluntary (e.g., stop at a stop sign), but they expect to emit automatic behaviors such as crying at a wedding or responding to a hypnotic suggestion. In the case of hypnosis, a highly suggestible participant would expect to respond like an excellent subject (i.e., respond in a particular way) following a hypnotic induction (i.e., particular stimuli), in a situation defined as hypnosis (i.e., particular circumstance). Response expectancies are anticipations of automatic subjective and behavioral responses to particular situational cues, and they elicit automatic responses in the form of self-fulfilling prophecies. In short, people get what they expect. In the case of hypnosis, if people expect to be responsive, they will be. Individuals perceive their responses to hypnosis as involuntary not only because their actions are triggered automatically, just as with mundane actions, but also because of the dominant cultural view that hypnotic responses are not self-initiated. Rather, suggested responses are commonly seen as the byproduct of a trance or special altered state of consciousness that accounts for their seemingly involuntary, automatic nature.

Kirsch and Lynn contended that although hypnotic responses are triggered automatically, suggestion alone is not sufficient to trigger them. Instead, suggested physical movements are preceded by altered subjective experiences (Lynn, 1997; Silva & Kirsch, 1992). The response expectancy for arm levitation, for example, is that the arm will rise by itself. Yet a sufficiently convincing experience of lightness must be present to trigger upward movements. Subjective experiences thus have an important role in this theory of hypnosis.

THE QUESTION OF COMPLIANCE

Some workers in the field (e.g., D. Spiegel, 1998) have claimed that social–cognitive theorists reduce responding to hypnotic suggestion to mere compliance with suggestions. However, this is a misconception of the socio-cognitive position. Although intentional compliance to please a therapist or researcher may play some role in hypnotic responding (Sarbin, 1989; Spanos, 1991; Wagstaff, 1991), most hypnotized people are neither faking nor merely complying with suggestions. Unlike people who have been asked to pretend to be hypnotized (i.e., simulators), highly responsive research participants remain responsive to suggestion when they think they are alone (Kirsch, Silva, Carone, Johnston, & Simon, 1989; Spanos, Burgess, Roncon, Wallace-Capretta, & Cross, 1993).

Sociocognitive models of hypnosis have been criticized for exaggerating the extent to which hypnotic behaviors are strategic, goal-directed, and volitional. Perry and Laurence (1986), for instance, argued that purposeful-ness and nonvolition may coexist in hypnosis. Nash (1997), in turn, has suggested that sociocognitive theorists valorize agency at the expense of acknowledging unconscious influences on behavior, although this criticism cannot be applied with equal force to all sociocognitive theorists (e.g., Lynn & Rhue, 1991a). Bowers and Davidson (1991) further contended that responses to suggestions, such as for analgesia (Miller & Bowers, 1986), can occur in the absence of goal-directed activities (e.g., suggestion-related fantasy activity such as imagining that a hand and arm are made of rubber following an analgesia suggestion), which indicates that such patterns of imaginative activity are more limited in their ability to account for the experience of nonvolition and responses to suggestion than some sociocogni-tive theorists acknowledge. Finally, sociocognitive theorists grant that even though expectancies, motivation, and responsiveness to waking suggestion, for example, account for a great deal of variability in response to hypnotic suggestions, these variables cannot account entirely for individual differences in hypnotic suggestibility (Braffman & Kirsch, 1999; Kirsch, 1991; Kirsch & Lynn, 1998).

PHENOMENOLOGICAL–INTERACTIVE THEORIES

Phenomenological–interactive theories place particular emphasis on understanding hypnotic experience and the interaction of multiple variables during hypnosis (Lynn & Rhue, 1991a). Of course sociocognitive theories also highlight the potential interaction of multiple determinants of hypnotic suggestibility. However, phenomenological–interactive theorists focus more on the differences between hypnotic and waking behavior and cognitive activity than do sociocognitive theorists.

Orne's Model

In the late 1950s, Orne (1959) underscored the importance of understanding the subjective experiences and subtle cognitive changes of hypnotized participants. Although never rejecting the concept of a hypnotic state, Orne argued that participants are actively involved in interpreting and responding to the social demands of the hypnotic situation. Orne (1979) devised a simulator control methodology that he initially believed would enable the separation of those subtle cognitive characteristics that constituted the essence of hypnosis from what he considered to be behavioral artifacts produced in response to social demands. Orne contended that if a particular suggested response of highly suggestible participants (i.e., reals) could not be mimicked by low suggestible individuals (i.e., simulators) who were instructed to role-play being hypnotized, then it was a potential indicator of a genuine hypnotic response that revealed unique characteristics of hypnosis.

Lynn, Martin, and Hallquist (2004) reviewed 12 indices tested with the real–simulator methodology. Each index had been purported to characterize important features or characteristics of hypnotized participants (e.g., literal responding to questions, nonvolitional experiences, measures of emotion, writing like an adult during age regression). To date, a distinguishing feature or characteristic of hypnosis has proven elusive. Many studies indicated that simulating participants successfully mimicked the responses of hypnotized individuals. In other studies, participants who were not hypnotized but asked to imagine what was suggested, or simply given motivational instructions to do their best, responded comparably to *reals*, who received a traditional hypnotic induction.

Research using the real–simulator design has drawn attention to the pervasive influence of demand characteristics and their potential role in accounting for a wide range of hypnotic phenomena. Nevertheless, studies of simulators have the potential to reveal subtle cognitive and experiential differences between hypnotized and nonhypnotized participants.

Sheehan's Contextual Model

Sheehan's contextual model (1991) highlights the interactive reciprocal relations between an active organism and an active context, the fine-grained variation in responsiveness to suggestions that exists among very highly suggestible participants. Sheehan's research has also established the relevance of hypnotic rapport to a range of hypnotic phenomena (e.g., hypnotic dreams, hypnotically created memories). Sheehan contended that during hypnosis, highly suggestible participants displayed a striking *motivated cognitive commitment* to find ways to respond to suggestions that was not evident when they were not hypnotized.

McConkey's Model

According to McConkey (1991), to understand the essential variability that typifies participants' hypnotic responses, it is necessary to examine the meaning that participants place on the hypnotist's communications, the idiosyncratic ways in which they cognitively process suggestions, and intra-individual differences that can occur in responding across suggestions. McConkey's research (1991) has supported the hypothesis that high suggestibility reflects the ability to process information that is both consistent and inconsistent with a suggested event in such a way that facilitates the belief in the reality of the event. Sheehan and McConkey's models are related to other interactional models (Bányai, 1991; Labelle, Dixon, & Laurence, 1996; Laurence, 1997; Nadon, Laurence, & Perry, 1991) of hypnosis that consider multiple, potentially interactive determinants of hypnotic responding (e.g., person, situational variables).

CLINICAL IMPLICATIONS

So far we have identified a number of important clinical implications of contemporary models of hypnosis. Several additional examples will prove instructive. Nash's (1991) psychoanalytic model implies that clinicians should not be surprised if primary process material, intense affect, and a strong and personal connection with the clinician arise during the course of hypnosis, and they should be wary of trusting the accuracy of memories that surface during age regression. In the final chapter of this volume, we discuss how therapists can manage the emergence of unsuggested, unexpected, and at times untoward experiences during hypnosis, and provide the reader with caveats regarding the use of hypnosis for the purpose of recovering historically accurate memories. We recommend Fromm and Nash's (1997) book for its numerous illustrations of how hypnosis can be artfully integrated into psychoanalytically oriented psychotherapies.

Many clinicians accept the tenets of neodissociation theory and couch their work with patients in terms of dissociation. The appeal of neodissociation theory may arise from the fact that suggestions for hidden observers and the like have clinical utility, despite the fact that the appearance of a hidden observer in treatment in all likelihood represents a suggested phenomenon. Research indicates that suggestions for hidden observers can be used to elicit information pertaining to hypnotic dreams and experiences during age regression (see Lynn, Mare, Kvaal, Segal, & Sivec, 1994). Later in this volume, we explain how suggestions for an *inner observer*, *inner advisor*, and a *new you* can be used productively in psychotherapy. Nevertheless, we recommend that patients be informed that the hidden observer phenomenon is the by-product of suggestion, rather than the manifestation of an actual indwelling identity or part of the larger personality, and can be construed as a metaphor or imaginative creation that can be used to access and channel valuable personal resources (see Lynn, 2000).

Taken together, the sociocognitive and phenomenological interactive perspectives imply that it is possible to significantly enhance hypnotic suggestibility in clinical as well as research contexts (Gfeller, 1993) and that therapists would do well to do the following:

- Develop a positive rapport and therapeutic alliance with the patient.
- Conduct a careful assessment and understand the patient's motives and agenda (i.e., constellation of plans, intentions, wishes, and expectancies).
- Identify the personal connotations that hypnosis has for the patient, including conflict and ambivalence about experiencing hypnosis.
- Dispel myths and misconceptions about hypnosis and create positive treatment expectancies and response sets.
- Assess patients' stream of awareness and internal dialogue during hypnosis.
- Assist patients in how to interpret different suggestions and encourage patients to adopt lenient criteria for passing suggestions (e.g., "You don't have to imagine what I suggest realistically; even a faint image is fine").
- Motivate involvement in hypnosis and encourage the use of imagination and attention to subtle alterations in experiences and responses.
- Devise suggestions and hypnotic communications that are tailored to patients' psychodynamics and minimize resistance and increase perceived control during hypnosis.

Many, if not all, of these points are acknowledged as important by therapists of diverse persuasions. Clinicians of all stripes also agree that hypnosis affords the therapist immense flexibility, enlarging the boundaries of how the therapist and patient interact (Yapko, 1993). What therapists suggest is limited only by their creativity. In the mind's eye, virtually anything is possible, and what can be imagined can, at least some of the time, be realized in actuality. In subsequent chapters, we expand on themes we have introduced; illustrate how positive treatment expectancies and response sets can be created, maintained, and fortified to maximize treatment gains; and provide examples of how disorders and conditions that clinicians commonly encounter in practice can be treated through evidence-based principles and practices.

3

THE BASICS OF CLINICAL HYPNOSIS: GETTING STARTED

One of the most surprising discoveries made by hypnosis researchers is that whatever can be experienced with hypnosis can also be experienced without it (T. X. Barber, 1969; Hilgard, 1965). This is true even of the most startling hypnotic responses, such as positive and negative hallucinations. Conversely, anything that can be done without hypnosis might also be done in a hypnotic context. Given these premises, how is one to decide whether to augment an intervention by establishing a hypnotic context?

Some patients come to therapy requesting hypnosis or are referred for hypnotic treatment by another therapist. The latter occurs with increasing frequency as a therapist gains a reputation as a hypnotherapist. These patients almost invariably hold positive attitudes and expectations about hypnosis, which makes them good candidates for hypnotic interventions. The danger in these cases is that the patients' expectations may be too positive. They may think of hypnosis as a powerful procedure that will do the work for them, so little effort on their part is required. This, of course, is a setup for failure, and hypnotic treatment should not be started without first educating the patient about the real nature of hypnosis.

Although some patients come to a therapist requesting hypnosis, most come asking for help because of a particular set of problems they are facing, and they look to the therapist to suggest the treatment procedures that will be used. Therapists sometimes evaluate the suitability of patients for hypnotic treatment by assessing their hypnotic suggestibility. However, as we noted in the previous chapter, the correlation between suggestibility and treatment outcome is modest, at best, probably because most of the suggestions that are given are not particularly difficult and can be passed by most patients (Lynn, Kirsch, Barabasz, Cardena, & Patterson, 2000). Many individuals who do not score well on measures of suggestibility thus may benefit considerably from hypnotic treatment (Holroyd, 1996; Schoenberger, 2000), especially those with positive attitudes toward hypnosis and for whom the use of hypnosis makes therapy more credible. (In the final chapter, we discuss the pros and cons of administering standardized hypnotic suggestibility scales.)

Perhaps the best way of deciding whether to use hypnosis with particular patients is to ask them about their preferences. Allowing patients to choose between therapeutic alternatives enhances treatment outcome (Devine & Fernald, 1973; Kanfer & Grimm, 1978). Myers (2000) found that therapists who imposed their positions and perspectives while dismissing their patients' viewpoints and preferences were rated as less empathic than therapists who paid close attention to the details of patients' positions. Also, meta-analytic studies of therapist empathy (Bohart, Elliott, Greenberg, & Watson, 2002; Cooley & LaJoy, 1980) indicated that patients' belief that they are understood contributes to both positive therapeutic outcome and the sense of active collaboration with the therapist (Strupp, 1998). Because typical hypnotic inductions are virtually identical to relaxation training, the difference between hypnotic and nonhypnotic treatment may amount to nothing more than the choice of a label, but this label can make a substantial difference in outcome as a function of the attitudes, beliefs, and expectancies attached to it (Kirsch, Silva, Comey, & Reed, 1995; Lazarus, 1973).

THE THERAPEUTIC RATIONALE

Therapeutic rationales are important because they provide a foundation for therapeutic outcome expectancies. Research indicates that identical treatment procedures can have dramatically different effects depending on the patients' understanding of them (e.g., Southworth & Kirsch, 1988). The effective clinician will present a convincing rationale and then check to ensure that the patient has accepted it. This process can be facilitated by taking what is known of the patient's experiences and worldview into account when formulating the rationale. A particular treatment can be explained in different ways, and an explanation that is consistent with the patient's beliefs is most likely to be accepted. To help the patient make an informed choice, the therapist needs to make sure the patient knows something about hypnosis and its effects. The therapist can draw on a substantial body of knowledge about hypnotic phenomena that has been accumulated through more than a half century of careful research.

Some Facts About Hypnosis

Clinicians can now rely on the following empirically derived information to educate their patients and work toward a collaborative decision about whether to use hypnosis (Lynn, Kirsch, Neufeld, & Rhue, 1996; Nash, 2001):

- Hypnosis is not a dangerous procedure when practiced by qualified clinicians and researchers (see Lynn, Martin, & Frauman, 1996).
- The ability to experience hypnotic phenomena does not indicate gullibility or weakness (T. X. Barber, 1969).
- Hypnosis is not a sleeplike state (Bányai, 1991).
- Most hypnotized participants do not describe their experience as a trance but as focused attention on suggested events (McConkey, 1986).
- Hypnosis depends more on the efforts and abilities of the subject than on the skill of the hypnotist (Hilgard, 1965).
- Suggestions can be responded to with or without hypnosis, and the function of a formal induction is primarily to increase suggestibility to a minor degree (see T. X. Barber, 1969; Hilgard, 1965).
- A wide variety of hypnotic inductions can be effective (e.g., inductions that emphasize alertness can be just as effective as inductions that promote physical relaxation; Bányai, 1991).
- Direct, traditionally worded hypnotic techniques appear to be just as effective as permissive, open-ended, indirect suggestions (Lynn, Neufeld, & Mare, 1993).
- All of the behaviors and experiences occurring in hypnosis can also be produced by suggestions given without the prior induction of hypnosis (reviewed in Kirsch, 1997b).
- Participants retain the ability to control their behavior during hypnosis, to refuse to respond to suggestions, and even to oppose suggestions (see Lynn, Rhue, & Weekes, 1990).
- Hypnosis does not increase the reliability of memory (Lynn, Lock, Myers, & Payne, 1997) or foster a literal reexperiencing of childhood events (Nash, 1987).
- Spontaneous amnesia is relatively rare (Simon & Salzberg, 1985) and can be prevented by informing patients that they

will be able to remember everything they are comfortable remembering.

Helping the Patient Choose

Armed with this information, the therapist can present a patient who seeks treatment for a fear of public speaking, for example, with the following choice:

> There are two procedures that we can use to help you with your fear. One of these is hypnosis. Contrary to what you have learned from movies and TV shows, hypnosis is not very mysterious. It merely involves focusing your attention inward, so that you can make full use of your imaginative abilities. You don't have to go into a trance to use hypnosis, and you would remain in full control of yourself. I'll tell you much more about that if we decide to use it. We would use hypnosis here in the office, and I would teach you to use self-hypnosis at home. I would also teach you to use self-hypnosis skills when you actually make the speech you are planning.
>
> A second possibility is to use a desensitization procedure that involves relaxation training and imagery. In either case, once you achieve some initial fear reduction, either through hypnosis or through the relaxation and imagery exercises, I'll ask you to begin practicing these skills in real-life settings. We'll start with relatively easy situations and work our way up to more difficult tasks once you have mastered the easier ones.
>
> Now, both of these methods are very effective, and in fact, they are very similar to each other. Many people find hypnosis particularly helpful, and there is evidence that it can increase the effectiveness of treatment, but some people are uncomfortable about being hypnotized and prefer nonhypnotic relaxation training. As you know yourself much better than I do, you're probably the best judge of which method would work better for you. What are your thoughts about using hypnosis?

When patients have a strong preference for hypnotic or nonhypnotic treatment, that choice should be respected. Because treatment outcome depends at least partially on response expectancies, patients generally are excellent judges of what will work best for them.

However, many patients are unsure about whether to use hypnosis. They would like the most efficacious treatment, but because of misconceptions derived from fictional portrayals and the misleading performances of stage hypnotists, they are apprehensive. When this is the case, additional information about the nature of hypnosis—such as that presented in the next chapter—should be presented prior to having the patient make a choice. Mildly negative initial attitudes need not preclude the use of hypnosis. Although people with very set, negative attitudes toward hypnosis are likely to drop out of treatment if its use is insisted on, most people who have not yet experienced hypnosis have tentative and unstable expectancies that can be changed substantially by their initial experience of hypnosis. Clinical research has established that patients' attitudes toward hypnosis can be improved by the correction of mistaken preconceptions (Schoenberger, 1996).

A ROSE BY ANOTHER NAME

The similarity of hypnosis to relaxation and imagery is sometimes a concern to therapists considering using it for the first time. Indeed, a sizable body of studies (see Edmonston, 1991) indicates that relaxed participants are generally as suggestible as individuals who undergo hypnosis, and that the subjective experiences are similar during and after hypnosis as well (Meyer & Lynn, 2005). So it is no wonder that some clinicians question whether they may have been hypnotizing their patients without their knowledge all along and are concerned about whether this is ethical. Others express the opposite concern and wonder whether calling a procedure *hypnosis* is a sham.

In fact, hypnosis and relaxation training are not identical. Relaxation is only one of many methods of inducing hypnosis. For example, hypnosis can be induced with suggestions to remain wide awake and become especially alert and focused. Relaxation during hypnosis can be prevented by having patients ride stationary bicycles or engage in other forms of vigorous exercise (Bányai, 1991). The same certainly could not be said of relaxation training.

Hypnosis has a historically derived cultural context, to which particular meanings have been attached. Meanings and interpretations are what much of psychological disorder and psychological therapy are about. It is not stimuli per se that cause problems, but rather one's perceptions and interpretations of them.

Some of the meanings attached to the term *hypnosis* can make some patients—and even some therapists—needlessly apprehensive about its use. Based on sensationalized stories without factual foundation, these meanings can often be overcome by the educational messages and procedures described in the next chapter.

Other meanings attached to the term are responsible for its therapeutic efficacy. As we mentioned earlier, hypnosis can provide a disinhibiting context, allowing patients to exhibit responses that they do not realize they are capable of making. That is why people are more responsive to suggestion—including therapeutic suggestions—after a hypnotic induction than they were before it. It also can disinhibit therapists by providing a context for therapeutic behaviors that might seem inappropriate in other settings (T. X. Barber, 1985). For example, the hypnotic context permits the therapist to repeat statements over and over, which enhances their forcefulness and salience. Outside the hypnotic context, this style of communication would seem strange and inappropriate.

INDICATIONS FOR THE USE OF HYPNOSIS

Although hypnosis can be used as an adjunct to almost all psychotherapeutic procedures, its effectiveness has been validated empirically for particular problems. Hypnosis has been shown to be of specific benefit in the treatment of pain, smoking, anxiety disorders, stress-related physical disorders and medical conditions (e.g., hypertension and ulcers), dermatological conditions, asthma, and obesity and eating disorders (Holroyd, 1996; Kirsch, Montgomery, & Sapirstein, 1995; Lynn et al., 2000; Wadden & Anderton, 1982). In the chapters that follow, we discuss how hypnosis can act as a catalyst in the treatment of these disorders and conditions, as well as posttraumatic stress disorder and depression.

Although we do not discuss conversion and dissociative disorders in detail elsewhere in this volume, they do deserve mention. Conversion and dissociative disorders are diagnoses likely to be assigned to patients presenting such symptoms as psychogenic paralyses, involuntary movements, temporary amnesia, hallucinations in various sensory modalities, numbness in various parts of the body, and the temporary belief that one is someone else. Some of these symptoms are also the responses by which levels of hypnotic suggestibility are conventionally measured (e.g., Weitzenhoffer & Hilgard, 1962). Others are seen in the hypnotic demonstrations of stage hypnotists.

The similarity between conventional hypnotic responses and the symptoms of what historically was termed *hysteria* suggests that at least some common mechanisms might underlie these phenomena. This similarity is also indicated by the degree to which the manifestations of hysteria and those of hypnosis go in and out of style. Conversion disorders were far more common in fin de siecle Vienna than they are anywhere in the world today. In a similar manner, the current epidemic of dissociative identity disorder in North America may be due, at least in part, to the influence of movies such as *Sybil* and *The Three Faces of Eve*, and, more recently, *Fight Club* and *Secret Window*.

Dissociative and conversion disorders historically were considered forms of hysteria. Beginning with the third edition of the *Diagnostic and Statistical Manual of Mental Disorders* (DSM–III; American Psychiatric Association, 1980), these conditions were dissociated from each other and the overarching construct of hysteria was eliminated entirely. We think this decision unfortunate because it draws attention away from the psychosocial factors that previously justified grouping conversion and dissociative disorders together and because it dissociates these disorders from their historical context (see Frankel, 1994). It also tends to obscure the link between hysteria and hypnosis. Both may be seen as suggestive phenomena, one pathological and the other curative.

The idea of a link between hysteria and hypnosis is not new. Freud's notion of the unconscious was most directly influenced by Charcot's demonstration of the control of symptoms of hysteria through posthypnotic suggestions. The linkage is further strengthened by current research indicating that conversion and hypnotic responding share common neurological processes (see Moene, Spinhoven, Hoogduin, & Van Dyck, 2003), that patients with conversion disorder have higher suggestibility scores than do patients in a control group (Bliss, 1984), and that hypnotic suggestibility is related to the success of hypnosis-based treatment of conversion disorders (Moene et al., 2003).

In the clinical setting, direct suggestion can be used for symptom management in patients diagnosed with dissociative or conversion disorders. Psychogenically lost functions can be restored, physical pain and emotional distress can be controlled, and the content of frightening dreams can be altered. Hypnosis is not a panacea for these individuals, but it does make their lives more tolerable, it demonstrates the possibility of improvement through therapy, and it enables attention to be devoted to other therapeutic tasks.

CONTRAINDICATIONS TO THE USE OF HYPNOSIS

Because hypnosis is an adjunct to therapy, rather than a form of treatment, it should not be treated as a magic cure for problems that the therapist is unable to address without it. The conventional rule of thumb is as follows: Do not treat any condition with hypnosis that you are not qualified to treat without hypnosis. Nor should a therapist treat a condition, with or without hypnosis, that extends beyond the range of his or her training, expertise, or competence. Attempting to do so is unethical.

Patient characteristics might contraindicate the use of hypnosis. For instance, obsessive–compulsive clients are less hypnotizable than other patient groups and normal control participants (Spinhoven, Van Dyck, Hoogduin, & Schaap, 1991). In addition, patients who are vulnerable to psychotic decompensation (Meares, 1961), those with a paranoid level of resistance to being influenced or controlled (Orne, 1965), unstabilized dissociative or posttraumatic patients, and those with borderline character structure for whom hypnosis may be experienced as a sudden, intrusive, and unwanted intimacy may be poor candidates for hypnosis or require special attention or modification of typical hypnotic procedures to emphasize safety, security, and connectedness. In each case, the pros and cons of hypnosis must be carefully weighed against those of nonhypnotic treatment.

Some patients' histories with parents, authority figures, or helping professionals predispose them to view the hypnotist with mistrust, anger, and fear. Given cultural associations of the hypnotist as having control, power, and authority over the patient, the hypnotic situation may accentuate patients' negative reaction tendencies (Lynn, Kirsch, & Rhue, 1996). Not only may the patient be reluctant to become involved in hypnosis, but hypnosis may be experienced as an emotionally charged, aversive event. This situation is most likely when hypnosis is imbued with connotations of personal dominance and control. However, patients might develop a highly charged positive, idealized, archaic, or even sexualized transference vis-à-vis the therapist (Shor, 1979), which can be equally counterproductive. The therapist must, therefore, be alert to these possibilities and develop a resilient working alliance as a deterrent against such departures from the treatment agenda (Lynn, Kirsch, & Rhue, 1996).

PLACEBOS, EXPECTANCIES, AND RESPONSE SETS: PREPARING THE PATIENT AND ENHANCING TREATMENT EFFECTS

When the effects of a pill depend on its psychological meaning rather than on the specific ingredients that it contains, it is called a placebo. The ability of placebos to produce important therapeutic changes was not established until the 1950s, when placebo-controlled research revealed that many drugs—and even some surgical procedures—were actually placebos (Beecher, 1955). Since then, placebos have been found to produce changes in pain, anxiety, depression, sexual arousal, blood pressure, heart rate, bronchial constriction, skin temperature, contact dermatitis, and angina (Kirsch, 1990). There was even a report of the successful use of placebo medication to treat a malignancy (Klopfer, 1957).

Placebo effects reveal a basic principle of human experience and behavior: When people expect changes in their own responses and reactions, their expectations can produce those changes. Self-fulfilling response expectancies are a cause of psychological problems and an essential part of psychological treatment (see Kirsch & Lynn, 1998). Dysfunctional response expectancies are partial causes of anxiety (Reiss & McNally, 1985), depression (Teasdale, 1985), and sexual dysfunction (Palace, 1995). People can be afraid of their fear and be depressed about their depression. They can suffer insomnia because they worry about not falling asleep and experience an anticipated loss of sexual arousal in the form of a self-fulfilling prophecy.

Because expectations can maintain psychological symptoms, the removal of those symptoms may require that those expectancies be changed.

Placebo effects appear to be particularly strong in the treatment of depression. A quantitative review of the published clinical trial data indicated that inert placebos duplicated the 75% effects of antidepressant medication, regardless of the type of antidepressant used (Kirsch & Sapirstein, 1998). However, a subsequent analysis of the data sent to the U.S. Food and Drug Administration by pharmaceutical companies revealed that the placebo effect was underestimated and the benefits of medication were overestimated (Kirsch, Moore, Scoboria, & Nicholls, 2002). When unpublished data are considered, placebos duplicate 82% of the effects of medication. Indeed, the difference between the effects of placebo and those of antidepressants appears to be clinically insignificant. Therefore, potent means of eliciting the placebo effect clinically should be highly welcome.

There is one legitimate barrier to the manipulation of expectancy by clinicians: The use of placebos typically entails deception. Psychotherapists, in particular, are rightfully concerned about deceiving their patients in any way. Expectancy is only one of the powerful psychological factors on which the outcome of treatment is dependent. Trust is another, and, in the long run, psychotherapists will earn their patients' trust only if they (the therapists) behave in a trustworthy manner. The problem, then, is how to maximize patients' therapeutic outcome expectancies without deception.

Hypnosis is one solution to this dilemma (Kirsch, 1994b). It is seen by many people as a powerful procedure that may help one lose weight, stop smoking, overcome fears, block pain, recover childhood memories, and accomplish a myriad of other goals. Although some of these beliefs are ill-founded (Lynn & Nash, 1994), others are supported by substantial data (e.g., Holroyd, 1996; Kirsch, 1997a; Kirsch, Montgomery, et al., 1995; Lynn, Vanderhoff, Shindler, & Stafford, 2002). At the same time, the data indicate that many of these effects of hypnosis are due to expectancy.

Like placebos, hypnosis produces therapeutic effects by changing patients' expectancies. But, as we mentioned in chapter 1, unlike placebos, hypnosis does not require deception to be effective. Whereas placebos are presented deceptively as pharmacological treatments, hypnosis is presented honestly as a psychological procedure. Furthermore, honestly informing patients about what has been learned through research about the nature of expectancy may reduce resistance and increase responsiveness to hypnotic interventions.

Hypnotic Inductions and Expectancy Modification

Consider the range of procedures that historically have been used as hypnotic inductions: clanging oriental gongs, flashing bright lights, applying pressure to participants' heads, and, more commonly, relaxation. From a review of the diverse methods of induction, it becomes clear that their only common ingredient is the label of hypnosis. When the effect of administering a drug is found to be independent of its specific ingredients (i.e., when an inert preparation produces the same effect), the drug is deemed to be a placebo. In a similar manner, hypnotic inductions must be expectancy manipulations, akin to placebos, because the inductions' effects on suggestibility are independent of any specific component or ingredient.

Not only do expectancies determine when hypnotic responses occur; they also play a large role in determining the nature of those responses. Following a hypnotic induction, patients report increased or decreased involvement, time slowing down or speeding up, logical thought becoming easier or more difficult, the hypnotist's voice sounding closer or farther away, sounds being clearer or more muffled, and so forth (Henry, 1985). Henry's data indicated that the direction of these alterations in awareness depended on the subject's preconceptions about the effects of hypnosis.

Expectations also shape the overt behavior of people in hypnosis. Spontaneous amnesia for the experience of hypnosis, for example, is limited to people who expect to be amnesic (J. Young & Cooper, 1972). In a similar manner, the ability to resist suggestions can be altered greatly by what people are told about that ability (Lynn, Nash, Rhue, Frauman, & Sweeney, 1984; Silva & Kirsch, 1987; Spanos, Cobb, & Gorassini, 1985). Those patients told that hypnotized people can resist suggestions find themselves able to resist, whereas those told that hypnotized people cannot resist suggestions may show an inability to resist. Spontaneous arm catalepsy is yet another response that occurs among people who expect it to occur (Orne, 1959), as was the case with Charcot's patients. These examples underscore the point that therapists can exert a great deal of influence on what patients experience during hypnosis by shaping their expectations about what will transpire.

Individual Differences in Responsiveness

As mentioned in chapter 2, expectancy is one of the few stable correlates of hypnotizability (Kirsch & Council, 1992; Kirsch, Silva, Comey, & Reed, 1995). Most of the correlations between expectancy and suggestibility are moderate, accounting for approximately 10% of the variance in responding. However, substantially higher correlations have been reported in some studies. Very high correlations between hypnotic suggestibility and expectancy are obtained when waking suggestibility is measured or when expectancy is assessed after the provision of a hypnotic induction (but before the administration of test suggestions).

Still, correlation does not establish causality. It is possible that expectancy is an epiphenomenon rather than a cause of responsiveness. More convincing evidence of causality is provided by studies in which participants' responses were shown to vary as a function of experimenter-manipulated expectations regarding their level of suggestibility. Kirsch, Council, and Mobayed (1987) demonstrated that altered expectancies can account for more variance than trait hypnotizability (i.e., premanipulation responsiveness) in subsequent hypnotic suggestibility. Wickless and Kirsch (1989) used a complex, expectancy modification procedure to convince research participants that they were highly responsive to hypnosis. For example, they surreptitiously imparted a red tinge to the room by means of a hidden light bulb while administering a suggestion that the room was becoming more and more red. Participants thus concluded that they were highly responsive to the suggestion. Following the expectancy manipulation, participants were tested for hypnotic suggestibility without any further environmental enhancement. Unlike the normal distribution of response scores obtained among control participants, 73% of those given the experimental treatment scored in the high range of suggestibility and none scored in the low range.

These data provide strong evidence for a causal relation between expectancy and hypnotic suggestibility, but they still leave some variance in responsiveness unexplained. It is possible that expectancy is the sole proximal determinant of hypnotizability and that the residual variance is a result of measurement error. Conversely, the unexplained variance may be due to a talent or personality characteristic, the nature of which is yet to be established.

Enhancing Suggestibility

Although there are individual differences in hypnotic suggestibility, we noted earlier that the increase in suggestibility for most participants is small. A person who responds to 6 of 12 suggestions without an induction (12 is the number of suggestions on the most frequently used scales of hypnotic susceptibility) might respond to 7 after an induction. Furthermore, the correlation between hypnotic and nonhypnotic suggestibility is high enough to indicate that what is being measured is suggestibility rather than hypnotizability (Kirsch & Braffman, 2001).

More substantial effects on responsiveness to suggestion can be brought about by enhancing expectancies. Many of the techniques we present are designed to alter expectancies and modify patients' response sets (Kirsch, Silva, et al., 1995; Lynn & Hallquist, 2004; Lynn & Sherman, 2000; Matthews, Lankton, & Lankton, 1993). In fact, it is of paramount importance to create a context with the patient in which an expectancy for change will occur (Matthews et al., 1993). Before, during, and even after a hypnosis session, it is vitally important that clinicians fortify patients' beliefs and expectancies that they are responsive to hypnosis.

PREPARING THE PATIENT

It is useful to think of hypnotic interventions as composed of three components—preparation, induction, and application—although in practice, the dividing line between these phases may not be distinct. Clinicians often devote considerable effort to the latter two tasks. They attend workshops in which indirect inductions, double inductions, special deepening techniques, and other procedures of this sort are taught. However, research indicates that many of these specialized techniques provide no benefit whatsoever, and some may even decrease the effectiveness of a hypnotic intervention (Lynn, Neufeld, & Matyi, 1987; Matthews, Kirsch, & Mosher, 1985). In general, people who receive traditional authoritative and direct suggestions pass as many suggestions as do people who receive more permissive and indirect suggestions. Although direct or authoritative suggestions may engender feelings of suggestion-related involuntariness more so than would indirect or permissively worded suggestions, these differences are small in magnitude (Lynn et al., 1987). Responding to hypnosis depends more on the abilities, attitudes, and anticipations of the patient than on the skill of the hypnotist. In contrast to special inductions and suggestions, the impact of these three As of suggestibility on hypnotic response has been well documented (Kirsch & Council, 1992).

Instead of devoting energy to learning elaborate inductions and suggestions, we emphasize ample preparation of patients for hypnosis to create positive treatment expectancies. This preparation consists of establishing a strong working alliance, debunking myths and misconceptions, providing an accurate, data-based explanation of hypnosis, and demonstrating that hypnotic experiences can be produced even without a hypnotic induction.

The Therapeutic Alliance

Horvath and Bedi (2002), after a comprehensive review of literature on the therapeutic alliance, concluded that establishing a strong alliance early in therapy is crucial to the ultimate success of therapy. Wampold (2001) went further in stating that the alliance accounts for the largest proportion of systematic variance in psychotherapy outcome. Considerable evidence indicates that rapport is also important in optimizing hypnotic responsiveness (Frauman & Lynn, 1985; Gfeller, Lynn, & Pribble, 1987;

Lynn, Weekes, et al., 1991). It is clearly important for the therapist to forge a strong therapeutic relationship.

One way to do this is to provide a clear rationale for the therapeutic approach that is consistent with the patient's personal goals, objectives, and expectancies. T. X. Barber (1985) noted that patients often enter therapy with expectancies that hypnosis will enhance the effectiveness of psychotherapy and that merely by defining the treatment as hypnotic in nature, it is possible to enhance treatment outcomes (Kirsch, 1997a; Kirsch, Montgomery, et al., 1995). However, not all patients have initially positive expectancies, so it is important to assess their prior experience with hypnosis.

Assessing Prior Experience

At the very outset, it is important to determine whether the patient has had previous experiences with hypnosis. These may have been vicarious or direct. Vicarious experiences derived from watching a hypnosis performance or hearing about hypnotic treatment experienced by a friend can be a source of information or misinformation about hypnosis. The nature of these experiences and the ideas about hypnosis that have been gleaned from them should be investigated thoroughly.

Stage and television performances are particularly poor sources of information, as it is typical in these settings to sacrifice truth for entertainment value. Hypnotized participants often are portrayed as mindless robots who can be made to perform bizarre acts and to believe in outlandish delusions. Age regression may be presented as a literal reliving of the past, even when the regression is extended to past lives. An evaluation of these experiences can be a lead-in for a discussion of the myths and misconceptions of hypnosis.

If the patient has had prior direct experience of hypnosis, there is even more to be learned. When did this occur and for what purpose? What does the patient remember about the induction procedures? Were there any aspects of the induction that were particularly helpful? Were there parts of it that got in the way? How pleasant was the experience? What kind of suggestions were given, and how did the patient respond? Were there any phenomena that the patient would like to reexperience? Answers to these questions can allow the therapist to structure the hypnotic induction and suggestions in a way that is optimal for the patient.

If the patient has not experienced hypnosis before, experiences with procedures such as relaxation training and meditation should be elicited. Because most hypnotic inductions include suggestions for deep relaxation, the experience of hypnosis is likely to be similar to that of relaxation or meditation. Foreknowledge of that similarity can help allay fears of entering an altered state and can foster the interpretation of relaxation as an indication of successful entry into the hypnotic context.

Correcting Myths and Misconceptions

Although some patients have already had direct experiences with hypnosis, others come to therapy without prior experience. Before hypnosis is begun, it is important to clear up misconceptions about it that are likely to have been acquired from the media. As we indicated earlier, many people believe that hypnosis is something that is done to them, rather than something they do. They think that hypnotized people lose control of themselves and can be made to do or say whatever the hypnotist wants. They think that they will feel drastically altered, as if they had taken a powerful drug, and they may fear that they will not be able to come out of this altered state. Some believe that people who have been hypnotized are unable to remember what occurred. Less common misconceptions include the idea that only weak-willed people are capable of being hypnotized or that hypnosis might weaken one's willpower.

The media is not entirely to blame for these misconceptions. Many of them were believed by mesmerists and early hypnotists. But clinical experience informed by the results of controlled research in hypnosis has led to a more accurate understanding of hypnotic phenomena, as we indicated in our discussion of the facts about hypnosis. Many, if not all, of these facts should be provided to patients before hypnosis is attempted.

The idea that hypnosis involves a trance state may be the most pernicious of popular ideas about hypnosis. Decades of research have failed to confirm the hypothesis that responses to suggestion are due to an altered state of consciousness, and as a result, this hypothesis has been abandoned by most researchers in the field (see Kirsch & Lynn, 1995). Many knowledgeable scholars either reject the use of the term *trance* as misleading or use it in a sufficiently broad sense to include such commonplace experiences as being absorbed in an interesting movie, conversation, or daydream. Nevertheless, the idea of trance is the most commonly held view of hypnosis among the general public and is even retained by some clinicians and researchers, as we discuss in depth in the final chapter.

There are several ways in which thinking of hypnosis as a trance can inhibit the experience of hypnotic phenomena. First, many people without prior hypnotic experience are afraid of the idea of going into a trance. They may fear the loss of control that they mistakenly think hypnosis entails. As a result, they intentionally resist the therapist's suggestions. Second, uninformed patients may think that hypnotized people are supposed to take a passive role and merely wait for changes to occur. In hypnosis, as in therapy more generally, therapists depend on the active collaboration of the patient to bring about change. Countering the idea that hypnosis is a trance state allows the patient to interpret relaxed involvement as evidence that the induction was successful, which thereby takes the pressure off of the patient to experience a trance and facilitates response to suggestion. Lynn et al. (2002) found that participants informed that responding to hypnosis involved entering a trance were less suggestible than were participants informed that responding to hypnosis involved their active cooperation.

Priming

Priming refers to the activation or change in accessibility of a concept by an earlier presentation of the same or a closely related concept (see Reason, 1992). By talking to patients prior to hypnosis about various non-hypnotic relaxing experiences they have enjoyed in the past such as listening to soothing music or watching waves on a beach, and by asking patients to have a fantasy about what they would like to experience during the upcoming hypnosis session, therapists can generate useful suggestions and prime subsequent hypnotic responses based on the patient's input. Priming effects can be subtle. Even subliminally presented stimuli can affect interpretations of events (see Greenwald, Draine, & Abrams, 1996; Merikle & Joordens, 1997). Priming effects can also extend to complex social behaviors (Wilson & Capitman, 1982).

In summary, prior to the first attempt at hypnosis, patients' preconceptions about hypnosis should be elicited and misconceptions corrected. They can be told that there is nothing mysterious about hypnosis, that it is a normal state of focused attention rather than a profoundly altered state of consciousness, and that it may not feel much different from meditating or relaxing. Most important, they can be informed that they will remain in complete control of themselves, that they will experience only those things that they wish to experience, and that they will be able to remember everything that occurred within the hypnotic session. These empirically established facts about hypnosis enhance the ability to experience the effects of suggestion.

Facilitative Information

Besides debunking myths and misconceptions, providing patients with facilitative information may make it easier for them to experience suggested effects. Beyond alleviating their fears, this kind of information is designed to elicit the patient's active cooperation. Patients are told that hypnosis is something that they do, rather than something that is done to them, and that hypnotic suggestions are experienced more vividly when people actively imagine their occurrence. Suggested arm heaviness, for example, can be experienced more easily if participants intentionally imagine that their arms are becoming heavier.

For some patients, involvement in suggestion may be facilitated by imagining situations that would make one's arm feel heavy, such as holding a heavy dictionary in the palm of one's hand. However, there is also some evidence that goal-directed fantasies of this sort can detract from the person's ability to focus on generating the suggested experience (Comey & Kirsch, 1999). Patients can be encouraged to experiment with different response strategies to discover what works best for them.

Patients should also be informed that the experience of hypnosis depends on their beliefs and expectations. Having never experienced hypnosis before, they are likely to wonder whether they are really hypnotized or whether they are merely fooling themselves. They may feel divided about the answer to this question, part of them feeling suggested experiences and part of them doubting their experience. They can facilitate the experience of hypnosis by laying aside their doubts and deciding temporarily to go along with the suggested experiences. They will not forget their skepticism, but the doubts can remain in the background until after the hypnotic experience, at which point they can reconsider them if they wish.

Suggestions Without Hypnosis

Telling people that hypnosis is a normal state of focused attention, rather than a drastically altered state of consciousness in which the subject's behavior is controlled by the hypnotist, amounts to providing information that is inconsistent with the views of hypnosis that are often presented in the media. For that reason, it may not be fully accepted by some patients. A useful strategy for reinforcing a more accurate view of hypnosis is to provide patients with hypnoticlike experiences prior to inducing hypnosis.

In an effort to prevent an initial experience of failure, a very easy prehypnotic suggestion should be used. The easiest hypnotic suggestions are ideomotor suggestions, although one of these (arm levitation) is more difficult. Imagining a force moving one's outstretched arms apart or pulling them together is a suggestion to which most people can respond successfully. Suggested arm heaviness is even easier to experience.

The Chevreul Pendulum Illusion

One of the best suggestions to use during prehypnotic preparation is the Chevreul pendulum illusion. This illusion is experienced by holding a pendulum (e.g., a locket on a chain) between the thumb and forefinger of one hand and concentrating on the idea that it will swing in a particular direction (i.e., back and forth, sideways, clockwise, or counterclockwise). The pendulum should not be swung intentionally, but neither should the patient concentrate on holding it steady. Instead, the hand holding the pendulum should be ignored. The patient's concentration should be focused on the bottom of the pendulum and the direction in which he or she wishes it to move. The pendulum typically will begin to move in the suggested direction.

The Chevreul pendulum illusion is very easy, and most people are successful when they attempt to experience it. Nevertheless, it is experienced as uncanny. The pendulum appears to be moving of its own accord, without physical effort. While this is occurring, the therapist can point out that the patient is not in an altered state of consciousness and that the experience is entirely under his or her control. All that the therapist has done is to suggest an experience. It is the patient who is making the suggested experience occur. The patient can stop the pendulum from swinging any time that he or she wishes.

To demonstrate the effect even more convincingly, the therapist can suggest that the patient make the pendulum change directions. The change in direction is experienced as unconnected to any intentional physical movements, yet it is entirely under the patient's control. The locus of control can be demonstrated convincingly by suggesting that the patient concentrate on a particular direction (e.g., side to side) while the therapist suggests movement in a different direction (e.g., back and forth). The patient will observe that the motion of the pendulum is determined by his or her imagination and not by the therapist's words.

The following is an example of a typical preparation of a patient for an initial experience of hypnosis.

Therapist: Before we begin, I'd like to get some idea of your thoughts about hypnosis and what you understand it to be. Have you ever experienced hypnosis before?

Patient: No.

Therapist: Have you ever seen someone be hypnotized, maybe at a stage performance or on television? Or maybe you know someone who has experienced hypnosis.

Patient: Well, I've probably seen it in movies, although I can't think of a particular one right now.

Therapist: Most of us have seen something that's supposed to be hypnosis in movies. I remember taking my son to see the Disney movie, *The Jungle Book*. Have you seen this one?

Patient: Oh yeah! I think I have.

Therapist:	Do you remember the snake in it that used to hypnotize people with its spiral eyes? [*Patient nods.*] I guess that's pretty typical of the image that gets projected about hypnosis in the media. The hypnotist has all the power, and the subject goes into a trance and does anything the hypnotist suggests.
Patient:	Barks like a dog; quacks like a duck.
Therapist:	Exactly!
Patient:	I guess hypnosis isn't really like that, is it?
Therapist:	Not at all! You know, we have a saying that "all hypnosis is really self-hypnosis." In other words, I'm not going to hypnotize you; I'm going to teach you how to hypnotize yourself. In fact, I've never hypnotized anyone. But I have helped many people to experience the effects of suggestion. Hypnosis isn't something that I do to you. It's something that you do for yourself. Many people think of hypnosis as a mysterious altered state of consciousness, in which people go into a trance and lose control over their behavior. Hypnosis really isn't like that at all. Most people describe hypnosis as a normal state of focused attention. When you are hypnotized, you remain awake and in full control of your behavior, and after hypnosis, you can remember everything that happened while you were hypnotized. Have you ever experienced meditation or relaxation training or anything like that?
Patient:	Yeah, I took a yoga class once, and we used to meditate.
Therapist:	What was that like for you?
Patient:	Well, it was very relaxing.
Therapist:	Did you enjoy it?
Patient:	Umhmm.
Therapist:	Well, you may find the experience of hypnosis a lot like that: relaxed, focused, and in control. You were in control when you meditated, weren't you? I mean, if the yoga teacher told you to do something you didn't want to do, would you have done it?
Patient:	Probably not.
Therapist:	Well, that's true in hypnosis as well. I may make various suggestions, but it will be up to you to decide whether you want to experience them. You'll experience only suggestions that you want to experience. If I suggest something that

you don't want to experience, you'll be able to just ignore it. You see, the suggestion doesn't make the experience happen. You do. Let me give you an example of what I mean. [*The therapist holds up a pendulum.*] Now, when I show you this pendulum, it probably makes you think of those old movies we talked about in which the hypnotist says, "Watch the watch! Watch the watch!" Well, I'm not going to use this to hypnotize you. What I want to do with it is show you how you can experience hypnotic suggestions without hypnosis. Let me show you what I mean. I hold the pendulum between my thumb and forefinger, and I concentrate on it moving in a particular direction. Right now I'm imagining it moving back and forth. [*The pendulum begins to move.*] There it goes. Now obviously, my hand must be moving to make the pendulum move, but I don't feel my hand moving. To me it feels as if I'm controlling it with my mind, and my imagination is making it move. Now, I've had a lot of practice with this, so it happens pretty quickly for me. It usually takes longer at first and doesn't move quite as much. But most people can do it, if they try, and it gets easier with practice. Why don't you try it? [*The therapist hands the pendulum to the patient.*] Now, hold the top of the chain between your thumb and forefinger and rest your elbow on the arm of the chair. That's it.

Stabilizing the elbow may facilitate pendulum movement, but because the effect is small, it can be omitted if there is nothing convenient on which to rest the elbow. Next, the therapist stabilizes the bottom of the pendulum and then gently lets go, saying, "Now imagine the pendulum moving back and forth, back and forth." In addition to using words, the therapist can facilitate pendulum motion by moving his or her finger underneath it in the desired direction. Once it begins to move in the requested direction, the therapist continues as follows:

Therapist: That's it, moving more and more, wider and wider. Okay, now let's see if you can make it change directions. How about getting it to move clockwise? [*The therapist's finger begins to move in a clockwise direction under the bob of the pendulum.*] Round and round, wider and wider circles. That's it. Okay! Now who controlled the movement of the pendulum?

Patient: I did, I guess.

Therapist: Right, but let's test it to be sure. I'll suggest it moving in a particular direction, but I'd like you to imagine it moving in a different direction. Okay? Then we'll see which way it moves. What direction would you like to try?

Patient: I don't know. Maybe sideways.

Therapist: Okay! You imagine that and just ignore my suggestion. [*The therapist pauses briefly to allow the patient to begin imagining.*] Back and forth, back and forth, back and forth. [*The pendulum moves from side to side.*] Okay! So who was controlling the movement, me or you?

Patient: [*Chuckles*] I was.

Therapist: Exactly! You ignored my suggestion and gave one of your own, and what happened was consistent with your suggestion, not with mine. That's just what hypnosis is like. In hypnosis, I make a suggestion, and you decide whether you want to experience it. And if you do, you can make it happen by concentrating on it and imagining along with it. Do you have any questions at this point?

Patient: Not really.

Therapist: Okay! Then let's try hypnosis.

Most patients feel quite comfortable with this description and demonstration. They often express amazement when the pendulum starts to move, smiling and exclaiming, "This is weird!" Their fears about giving up control are assuaged. They have learned that taking an active role as a hypnotic subject will make it easier for them to respond to suggestion. More important, they have learned that they must take an active role as patient, rather than wait passively for the therapist to cure them.

Although most people respond easily to Chevreul pendulum suggestions, a few do not. This can indicate that the person may be very unresponsive to the kinds of suggestions used in hypnotic suggestibility scales, but it does not mean that hypnosis is contraindicated. Many people with low levels of suggestibility experience hypnosis to be helpful.

However, it may be useful to attempt to prevent a feeling of failure from developing in the occasional patient who does not respond to the pendulum suggestion. One way to do this is to draw a line on a sheet of paper, hold it under the pendulum, and ask the patient to prevent the pendulum from moving in the direction of the line. At the same time, the patient is to count backward from 1,000 in sevens. Often, the pendulum will begin to move in the indicated direction, and the addition of cognitive load (e.g., counting backward in sevens) can facilitate this by inhibiting the attempt to prevent it (Wegner, 1994).

In the rare cases in which neither form of Chevreul pendulum suggestion has produced the suggested movement, the therapist can continue as follows:

> *Therapist:* Well, it's clear that you have excellent control over your movements, much more so than most people, and I can't make you move involuntarily no matter how hard I try. That's very useful to know. During hypnosis, you can use that control to relax your muscles very deeply, and perhaps you can exert that same control over your imagination, so that you can experience imagined feelings and sensations very vividly.

A Fail-Safe Induction

The Chevreul demonstration capitalizes on what social psychologists (see Dillard, 1991) have dubbed the "foot in the door tactic," which begins by getting compliance with a small request (e.g., moving the pendulum) and then advances to a related, larger request (e.g., responding to more difficult suggestions). Easy initial tasks, such as the Chevreul pendulum, ensure early success, which bolsters the patient's confidence in treatment (Lynn, Kirsch, & Rhue, 1996). Another way to get one's foot in the door is to tie suggestions to naturally or frequently occurring responses or, more broadly, to whatever response the patient made (Erickson, Rossi, & Rossi, 1976). Certain naturally occurring responses, such as lowering of an outstretched arm, provide immediate positive proprioceptive feedback that increases the likelihood of responding. Once patients cooperate with a relatively easy task, it becomes possible to engage them in more difficult tasks.

Consider the following fail-safe suggestions (Lynn, Kirsch, & Rhue, 1996) based on the aforementioned principle. These suggestions can be given before a more formal induction of hypnosis, in the context of relaxation or creative imagination, or they can be incorporated into an induction.

> *Therapist:* You may notice that one of your arms is just a bit lighter than the other, and your other arm is heavier. As we talk, your light arm may become even lighter or your heavy arm may become even heavier. And I wonder just how light your lighter arm will feel, and how heavy the other arm will feel. Will your light arm become so light that it lifts up into the air all by itself, or will your heavy arm become so heavy that it stays rooted to the arm of your chair? And I wonder which arm feels lighter. Is it your right arm or your left arm? And where do you feel the lightness most? In your wrist or in your fingers? In all of your fingers or especially in one of them?

Overt signs of upward movement in one hand or arm provide a signal to focus on suggestions for arm levitation. Otherwise, these suggestions are abandoned and suggestions for arm heaviness and immobility are stressed. In our experience, this method can prevent perceptions of failure, maintain therapeutic rapport, and provide some indication of the patient's level of responsiveness. If the patient is not able to generate responses of either arm lightness or heaviness, it may indicate the presence of recalcitrant negative beliefs and attitudes, which may preclude using hypnosis as a treatment modality.

Prepare the Patient for Gradual Change

The fail-safe suggestions are based on the principle that it is important to ensure that positive feedback will be experienced throughout treatment. Positive feedback can be facilitated by introducing the expectancy early in the course of treatment that improvement will begin with small, gradual changes. As a rule, progress in therapy and involvement in hypnosis, for that matter, are not linear. Therefore, therapists can prepare patients for setbacks by labeling them in the preparation stage as inevitable, temporary, and useful learning opportunities. For example, in preparing the patient, we inform them that they may feel hypnotized more deeply at some times than others, and that they should note what it feels like when they are most deeply hypnotized so that they can recreate the feelings in the future. Or patients can be informed that they can choose whether they will experience a light, a deep, or a medium level of involvement in their experience of hypnosis at any given time and that the only thing that matters is their comfort. In this way, perceptions of failure are minimized when involvement in a particular suggestion or intervention wanes in the later stages of treatment (Lynn, Kirsch, & Rhue, 1996). We describe these later stages of treatment in the chapters that follow.

4

HYPNOTIC INDUCTIONS
AND SUGGESTIONS

This chapter introduces the tricks of the trade of clinical hypnosis. We acquaint you with inductions and suggestions that we have used with considerable success. Many of the procedures we describe, or variants of them, are commonly taught at hypnosis workshops and presented in hypnosis manuals and textbooks (e.g., Lynn, Kirsch, & Rhue, 1996; Rhue, Lynn, & Kirsch, 1993; Yapko, 2003). In the next chapter, we present an array of techniques and strategies designed to promote relaxation, manage negative affect, guide imagery, and catalyze a variety of empirically supported treatments that we review in the remainder of the book. The examples are intended to be used as templates, not to be adopted slavishly with all patients. Inductions are often largely interchangeable. Nevertheless, it is often helpful to tailor suggestions to patients' goals, treatment objectives, and psychodynamics and to have a variety of different strategies and tactics at one's disposal.

Certain patients prefer particular inductions or suggestions. Indeed, Lynn and Kvaal (2004) found in their university studies that some students expressed strong preferences for a traditional relaxation induction, other students preferred a sensory awareness induction that focused on subtle changes in body sensations and imaginative experiences, and still other students preferred an induction composed of suggestions for positive experiences, enjoyment, energy, and inner strength. Although there were definite differences among students in terms of their preferences and satisfaction regarding their participation, there were no differences across the inductions in terms of how the students fared on a test of suggestibility. The first induction we present is a relaxation-based approach that can be easily modified to accommodate a variety of hypnotic procedures (Lynn, Kirsch, & Rhue, 1996).

BASIC INDUCTIONS: RELAXATION-BASED TECHNIQUES

Please make yourself comfortable. Close your eyes and let yourself relax. Take a few slow deep breaths, and notice that as you exhale, you can feel yourself becoming more relaxed. Notice that when you breathe in, your shoulders rise, and that when you exhale . . . fully and completely . . . your shoulders fall. Maybe you hardly notice the easy, gentle, natural way your shoulders move up and down . . . with your breaths . . . and you know, you don't even have to think about it a lot . . . but as you continue to relax in this easy natural way . . . with each breath . . . each time you exhale, let it happen . . . let your shoulders and your entire upper body relax even more . . . that's it . . . more and more . . . more and more relaxed . . . more and more relaxed. Perhaps you notice that as you exhale, you can enjoy a sense of becoming more and more relaxed . . . more and more relaxed . . . as you experience yourself resting more and more easy . . . more and more easy . . . calm . . . relaxed . . . peaceful . . . serene.

And as you go deeper and deeper into a state of comfortable relaxation, you probably are beginning to have a sense of what the experience of hypnosis is like. You probably already have a sense that you are the one relaxing . . . you are the one creating the changes in your state of mind . . . your state of being . . . even though I am the one giving you suggestions. Even as I give you suggestions that help you enter your hypnosis, you are the one who decides whether you want to experience those suggestions. If you don't like a suggestion that I make, you can choose to ignore it and to not have that experience. But if you want to experience a suggestion, you may find it easier to experience than you ever thought possible. So the choice is always yours, and it's safe to enter hypnosis now, as you allow yourself to relax.

Feel yourself becoming more and more relaxed. But no matter how relaxed you become, you will hear my voice, and you will be able to respond to my suggestions. At any time, you can adjust your body to make yourself completely comfortable. And of course, if you need to speak to me, you will be able to do so easily, while you remain so very relaxed . . . very relaxed and at ease.

Right now, you might want to relax even more, and as you relax, you may feel a slight tingly feeling in your fingers . . . or in your toes

. . . and if you do, you will know that it is a feeling of relaxation that some people have as they begin to experience hypnosis. Let your body relax. Just let the tension drain from your body, letting go of all your cares and concerns, and just relaxing . . . more and more . . . feeling more and more at peace . . . more calm . . . more and more deeply relaxed, as you enter into a pleasant, comfortable state of hypnosis . . . becoming so deeply involved in hypnosis that you can have all of the experiences you want to have . . . deep enough to experience whatever you want to experience . . . but only the experiences you want . . . just your own experiences.

And you can focus your attention on your toes . . . your right toe . . . and your left toe. Feel any tension that may be there, and just let it drain from your right toe . . . and from your left toe . . . letting all the tension drain out and letting your toes relax . . . more and more . . . more and more relaxed. And let the relaxation spread from your toes into your feet, and let your feet relax. Let all the tension drain from your feet, and let them become more and more relaxed. And now pay attention to your ankles and to your calves. I wonder if there is any tension in your ankles or your calves, in your right leg or in your left leg. And if there is, you can let it go right now. Just let your legs relax . . . more and more relaxed . . . more and more completely relaxed.

And the relaxation can spread into your thighs . . . your thighs can relax more and more . . . just letting go. And you can let your pelvis relax. Just let it go loose and limp . . . loose and limp . . . relaxing more and more. Relax your stomach. Let your stomach become completely relaxed. Notice how it feels, and if you feel any tension at all, just let it drain from you . . . loose and limp . . . completely relaxed. And let the relaxation spread upward into your chest. Let all the nerves and muscles in your chest relax, completely relaxed . . . loose and limp . . . all the tension draining away. And now let your back relax, and your shoulders. Let yourself feel the relaxation in your back and your shoulders . . . more and more relaxed . . . loose and limp . . . completely relaxed.

Let the relaxation spread through your arms, down into your hands and your fingers. Focus on the feelings in your arms and hands. Notice any tension that may still be there, and let it drain out through your fingers. Focus on your right upper arm . . . right lower arm . . . your right hand . . . and fingers . . . relaxing completely . . . more and more relaxed . . . completely relaxed. And now your left arm . . . relaxing completely, the tension draining out . . . completely relaxed . . . completely relaxed. Now relax the muscles of your neck . . . just let go and relax . . . loose and limp . . . completely relaxed. And relax your jaw muscles. Just let them go limp. All the nerves and muscles in your jaw relaxing completely. And relax all the rest of the muscles in your face . . . your mouth . . . nose . . . eyes . . . eyebrows . . . eyelids . . . forehead . . . all the muscles going loose and limp . . . loose and limp . . . completely relaxed . . . at peace . . . calm and relaxed . . . completely at ease. And now take a minute or two to just thoroughly enjoy your experience of hypnosis.

Some patients fear that if they relax completely they will be vulnerable, and they actually experience an increase in physical tension or anxiety following relaxation procedures (Heide & Borkovec, 1983). The following induction, although relaxation-based, can be used to decrease the likelihood that a paradoxical anxiety reaction will occur during hypnosis (Mellinger & Lynn, 2003):

> Holding on and letting go. During your hypnosis today, I would like you to hold on to only as much tension as you need to feel comfortable and relaxed, safe and secure. You know that you need a certain amount of tension in your body to sustain your everyday functions. You need a certain amount of tension in the muscles of your mouth to talk, but you don't have to talk during hypnosis . . . unless you want to. You need a certain amount of tension in your legs to walk, but you don't have to walk during hypnosis, unless you want to. And you need a certain amount of tension in your eyes to open them and keep them open, if you want to. But you don't have to open your eyes during your hypnosis today, unless you want to. In fact, I would like to invite you to close your eyes right now. Release all of the tension in your eyelids and eyes that you do not need . . . relax your eyes and let them close . . . let them close, knowing you could summon up just as much tension as you would need at any time to open them. Now create just enough tension to open your eyes a little and then release the tension in your eyes and let them relax even more completely . . . more completely, let them close comfortably, and let your body begin to release some of the tension that it does not need. And as you begin to do this, you notice that your body relaxes. Actually, you need to have very little tension in your body for you to breathe, walk, talk, and see, because much of these basic processes occur automatically, with little conscious awareness and relatively little tension required to sustain these activities. So, if you want, your body can become relaxed, very relaxed, perhaps even more relaxed than when you sleep. Today, we will discover just how much tension you need while your body releases and relaxes as much as it possibly can.
> And as your body begins to relax, I would like to draw your attention to your breathing. As you notice your breathing, perhaps you notice a certain amount of tension when you breathe in, and then a relaxation of tension when you breathe out, although your breathing may be very effortless, and you may not even notice the steady rhythm of you breathing in and out . . . in and out. But for now, I would like you to take a very deep breath and hold it for as long as you can. And then you will notice some tension I am sure. And when you can hold that breath no longer, let it out. Release the breath completely. See how good you can feel. Let the tension out and experience how deeply

relaxed you feel when you release the breath completely . . . release the breath completely and hold on to only as much tension as you need to feel relaxed and comfortable, comfortable and at ease. And now take another breath . . . hold it for as long as you can and then release it, just as you did before . . . tensing and releasing . . . releasing and relaxing . . . holding on and letting go. And now feel your breathing becoming easier and easier . . . easier and easier . . . with each breath you release tension you do not need and you become more and more relaxed, peaceful and relaxed.

Actually, you have had a lot of experience in holding on and letting go. When you were a child and learned to walk, you held on to the walls when you needed support. The stronger you became, the more agile and confident you became . . . and as you sensed you could release you did . . . and you were able to let go of the walls. You had to hold on less and less as you became more confident in your abilities. You learned to train your muscles to support the activities your mind wanted you to engage in. And today, you can walk on your own. You can talk on your own. You can stand on your own two feet and make decisions for yourself. And today, you can become more confident in your abilities to experience hypnosis as you experience yourself holding on and letting go . . . releasing and relaxing.

And, with your permission, now we are going to start at the top of your head, and I am going to ask you to tense and release various muscle groups in your body to help you relax and enjoy your experience of hypnosis. Would you like to do this? [If answer is yes, proceed as follows.] Remember, if you need to hold on to tension, hold on to it, but only as much as you need to to sustain the vital workings of your body. When you let go, you allow yourself the privilege of feeling as relaxed and at ease as you would like to be . . . as you can be. Should you ever need any extra tension, it will be there for you to speak, walk, open your eyes, or whatever you need to do.

As you release the muscles in the top part of your body, from your waist up, feel the tension flowing out of your fingers and your body relaxing just the right amount. [Follow general relaxation procedures, as in the previous relaxation induction.] As we move through the muscles in your lower body, you will feel the tension flowing out through your toes. [After all of the muscle groups of the body are relaxed, proceed with other suggestions, as appropriate.]

OTHER INDUCTION TECHNIQUES

The following induction provides suggestions for a literal step-by-step progressive relaxation of the body as the participant is instructed to imagine walking down a staircase.

The Staircase

Now imagine yourself on a magnificent staircase with 10 steps to the bottom. When you reach the bottom I think you will find it of great interest to discover just how relaxed, safe, and secure you will feel. And as you probably have guessed, in a few moments, I will ask you to walk down the staircase . . . and with each count, feel free to move one step down the staircase. Take a nice deep, full, and filling relaxing breath. Good, now take another, and see how calming that can feel. But as calming as simple slow breathing can be, why not discover how with each step down the staircase, your body will relax more and more, more and more. Of course, at this point neither you nor I know just how relaxed you will be, how deep you will go, but even that doesn't matter . . . all that matters is that you are comfortable and at ease . . . comfortable and at ease.

OK, I am going to start counting, guiding you down the staircase, deeper and deeper into a most comfortable state of mind, a most comfortable state of being, calm and at ease, relaxed and secure. In fact, the truth is . . . you don't have to do much of anything, really . . . just listen to my voice. Let my voice go with you.

One . . . one step down the staircase. Let your feet relax as you move down the staircase, feel the calmness spreading. There's lots of time.

Two . . . let your legs relax. Do you feel more relaxed than when you are asleep or would you rather not think at all? Deeper and deeper calm and feeling quite secure.

Three . . . three steps down the staircase . . . can you feel your thighs relax? Can you feel yourself letting go just a little bit more with each breath, can you feel waves of gentle relaxation, or are you not thinking at all, just feeling open and receptive? Do you feel more heavy and warm or an easy floating feeling?

Four . . . can you let the area around your pelvis relax? There is lots of time. Do you feel as relaxed as you feel when you are very tired before you know that you will fall asleep or as relaxed as you feel after you wake up from a deep, sound sleep?

Five . . . five steps down the staircase. Halfway down. Can you feel a sense of calm in your stomach area? Do you want to experience a deeper level of hypnosis, of openness to ideas, receptiveness to images, feeling sure and in control, aware of possibilities for yourself? Or are you so comfortable with your level of hypnosis now that you want to just maintain that feeling in an easy, effortless way? You know you don't have to do anything, unless you want to, like adjust your position to get even more comfortable.

Six . . . down the staircase. Six steps down the staircase. . . . Can you feel the calm, easy feeling spreading to your chest? Can you feel that some parts of your body are catching up with other body parts that are even more relaxed?

Seven . . . down the staircase. Can you feel your arms relax? Nothing to disturb, nothing to bother you. Can you feel time slowing down? Do you think you are ready to go even deeper? Would you like to be even more calm and secure within yourself? And yet it really doesn't matter just how deeply relaxed and at ease you feel, just that you feel comfortable.

Eight . . . eight steps down the staircase. Almost near the bottom . . . soon you will arrive at that place where you feel so comfortable and secure, so much at ease. Can you feel a still, quiet point between inspiration and exhalation of your breath? Can you feel quiet and still inside? I really don't know and it really doesn't matter, because soon you will arrive at your special place, where you are so deeply centered within yourself.

Nine . . . nine steps down the staircase. Are you aware of just how relaxed your face and eyes feel or are you in a dreamy state of mind, perhaps not thinking at all?

Ten . . . ten steps down the staircase. You have arrived! Feeling so good . . . so relaxed . . . so comfortable and at ease.

Eye Closure

The eye-closure induction is a simple variation of the relaxation induction. Instead of being asked to close their eyes, patients are asked to stare at a target. The therapist can provide the target or ask patients to pick a spot on the wall or ceiling ("the target"), preferably somewhat above the normal field of vision so that some eyestrain is provoked.

The patient can be told the following:

As you begin to enter hypnosis, you will feel your eyes becoming tired and heavy, so heavy that they will feel like closing all by themselves. You will notice that the more you focus on the heaviness in your eyelids as you stare at the target, the heavier your eyelids become. This demonstrates one of the principles of suggestion: When you focus on what is suggested, when you carefully attend to what is suggested, you can make it easier for yourself to respond to the suggestion. So why don't you see just how tired your eyes can become, as your body feels more and more relaxed, as you notice yourself beginning to breathe just a bit easier and more comfortably, as your breathing slows down to meet the resting requirements of your body, and how your eyes want to close by themselves, so you can better rest . . . and relax . . . and feel even more comfortable. Wouldn't it be so nice for you to close your eyes . . . and let your whole body relax completely . . . wouldn't it be wonderful to relax completely . . . relax completely.

If the patient's eyes have not closed completely by this point, insert further suggestions for eye heaviness and closure into the typical relaxation instructions, and monitor the patient for such signs as blinking, eyelids beginning to droop, or watery eyes. Note these verbally, as though they provide evidence that the patient is successfully entering hypnosis:

Your eyes are beginning to droop . . . getting heavier and heavier . . . more and more tired . . . they are closing all by themselves as you become more and more deeply hypnotized.

If the patient's eyes have not closed after the preceding suggestions have been given, the therapist can give the patient a directive to "close your eyes now, please, so that you can more fully enjoy the experience of hypnosis and be better able to imagine and get involved with the suggestions that I will give you. Yes, please close your eyes now. That's good."

Arm Levitation

Suggestions for arm levitation can be given to provide the patient with a demonstration of how suggestions can lead to behavioral responses. The patient is told that one arm is becoming lighter and lighter, and that soon it may become so light that it will float up into the air. These suggestions can be combined with relaxation instructions and with the eye-closure procedure previously described. Sample suggestions such as the following can be given to facilitate arm levitation:

I'd like you to experience how thinking of an action can lead to a most interesting hypnotic response. All you have to do is think and imagine along with what I am suggesting and do your very best to have the experiences I suggest to you . . . to go with what I suggest and lift your arm in response to the suggestion I will give you for it to be light . . . to float up . . . gently up . . . and let your body experience a comfortable sense of relaxation in the process. Now I know that if my arm had a helium balloon attached to it, it would feel so very light, just like it wanted to lift up off the resting surface. That would be very interesting to see. And wouldn't it feel good to imagine that it was a very lovely day, with a gentle wind blowing, and that there was a bright-colored helium balloon attached to your wrist? To the wrist of one of your hands? Perhaps when I mentioned a beautiful day, you could begin to picture it . . . the clouds that take shape in the sky . . . the sun's comforting warmth on your skin . . . the green grass . . . the sounds of life . . . the lovely scents as you take a deep, relaxing breath. That's right. A deep, relaxing breath. And if you look down at that hand of yours, and that wrist . . . in your mind's

eye ... perhaps you can see that balloon tied to your wrist with that
oh ... so ... long ... piece of string. I'm not sure exactly what color
the balloon is. It's your balloon. But I'm wondering whether you would
be willing to share the color of the balloon with me. If you are, please
tell me the color. [If yes, proceed as follows.] Ah, that's so nice ...
a [red] balloon. Can you feel the balloon that is ever so light, beginning
to tug at your wrist ... can you feel how it is beginning to lift your
wrist up off the resting surface, as the wind blows it ... watch the
balloon ... is it dancing in the sky? Feel this balloon lift that hand
up ... up ... beginning to lift more and more ... off the resting
surface ... feel how light your hand is becoming ... how it just wants
to lift up ... lift ... lift up ... let it happen ... go with it ... if
you need to, help the hand follow the balloon in the sky ... let it
lift up toward the balloon ... almost like you want to shake hands
with the balloon ... funny, huh? ... let it go up and up and up ...
lighter ... lifting higher and higher ... very good.

Self-Hypnosis

T. X. Barber (1985) contended that most hypnosuggestive procedures
can be truthfully defined as self-hypnosis (see also Orne & McConkey, 1981;
Sanders, 1991). We agree. Ultimately, patients are responsible for generating
suggestion-relevant imagery, experiences, and behaviors. By teaching patients to orchestrate their experience of hypnosis, it is possible for them to
practice implementing hypnotic techniques in many real-life situations and
to take credit for the success they achieve. Other advantages of defining
procedures as self-hypnosis include bypassing resistances and fears associated
with being under the control of another, fear of being unaware or unconscious, fear of revealing secrets, and fear of not coming out of a trance.
Practicing self-hypnosis, the patient can become the active agent during
the therapy hour and beyond, and the therapist can settle into the congenial
role of a coach, facilitator, or advisor, rather than an authoritarian figure.
Self-hypnosis is most frequently taught by first introducing the patient to
traditional (heterohypnotic) techniques and then encouraging the patient
to assume increasingly greater responsibility for devising suggestions appropriate to achieving treatment goals (Hammond, 1992; Lynn, Kirsch, &
Rhue, 1996). This can be done as follows:

> Remember how you learned to ride a bike? If you were like me, at
> first you might have wondered whether you could do it ... whether
> you could experience the pleasure of riding a bike. Coasting along,
> feeling the gentle wind. And after awhile, you learned that you could
> do it. And you were able to just get up on the seat and ride, and feel
> the wind in your hair and the pleasure of moving along ... at your
> own pace ... going in a direction of your choice. And didn't it become

easier and easier, so that after awhile, you didn't even have to think about staying in control, but you knew that you were in control of where you went and how you got there? And, you know, it's the same thing with hypnosis. You do it; you go in a direction of your own choosing. You decide whether to respond or not, to cooperate or not, to imagine or not, to try to make the suggestion seem real. And it gets easier and easier, just like riding a bike. After we practice with me giving you suggestions at first, you realize that all hypnosis is self-hypnosis. You make it happen, you create the experiences for yourself. I can't do it for you. And you, too, can devise helpful suggestions tailored just for you. Made just for you, by you. I can help if you like, but you can do it too. After all, you know yourself even better than I know you. But for now, just relax, settle in, and I'll give you some suggestions that you can make seem real . . . real to you, in your own mind, in your own way, as we discussed when I introduced the idea of hypnosis to you. And after that, after you experience hypnosis for yourself, you can begin to generate suggestions of your own, suggestions that can and will help you to achieve your goals, just for you, your suggestions. Not mine, but yours. And we can work together too, to devise suggestions, and these suggestions can be ours.

Within this framework, we encourage patients to write down clear, specific (e.g., how they would like to think, feel, and act in a given situation and in general) suggestions and develop scripts consistent with their goals that can be incorporated into self-hypnosis sessions and their everyday lives. The suggestions and scripts can be recorded on 10- to 20-minute tapes that can be played before the patient enters self-hypnosis on a regular or as-needed basis. After a period of experimenting and discovering what suggestions work best, shorter, more focused and customized tapes can be made, recorded in the patient's or the therapist's voice, as the patient prefers. In either case, patients should be encouraged to integrate helpful suggestions into their internal dialogue or self-talk on a routine basis.

Deepening Techniques

There are times when the therapist would like a patient to feel more deeply hypnotized, such as, when the patient appears to be having some difficulty in achieving a desired therapeutic effect. In these instances, a brief deepening procedure can act as a catalyst, enabling the patient to experience phenomena that could not be accomplished earlier.

Deepening techniques and the components of hypnotic inductions are interchangeable, the only difference between them being the time at which they are used. For example, a simple counting procedure like the following can be used to deepen the subjective experience of hypnosis:

And with each count you can drift more and more deeply into your hypnosis . . . you can go deeper and deeper . . . and as you go even deeper, it will help you move closer and closer to realizing your goals . . . to experience whatever you want to experience. One . . . deeper and deeper into your hypnosis . . . even deeper . . . more and more relaxed . . . two . . . more and more comfortable . . . three . . . four . . . deeper and deeper . . . wouldn't it feel good to let yourself relax even more? Would you like to experience hypnosis even more completely? Feel even more calm and at ease? five . . . halfway there . . . six . . . can you feel even more safe . . . secure . . . seven . . . even deeper than before . . . so deep that you can experience whatever you wish to experience . . . think of all that you can discover about the experience of hypnosis . . . or maybe you don't even have to think to go deeper and deeper . . . it just happens quite naturally . . . eight . . . nine . . . ten . . . very deep now . . . very deep . . . completely engrossed . . . completely engrossed.

Any metaphor that implies progressive deepening of response is appropriate. For example, the staircase induction previously described can be easily modified so that the participant is instructed to go "twice as deep" with each step down the staircase. As patients "go down" the staircase at their own pace, they can verbalize what step they are on as they descend the staircase, not moving to the next step until they are twice as deep as the step before. Or patients can select a favorite step to alight on, where they feel most comfortable and secure.

You can instead invite patients to imagine themselves on a beach watching the waves and to feel themselves go deeper and deeper as each wave they watch rolls in, or to imagine themselves sitting by a pond or lake and throwing small pebbles into the water. Each pebble makes small concentric circular waves that create a sense of peace and relaxation. When the waves merge completely with the water, you can invite the patient to throw another pebble into the water and to go deeper and deeper as each pebble is thrown and each wave moves outward and merges with the water. After awhile, suggest that the client is perhaps too relaxed to even toss another pebble in the water, although he or she could if he or she really wanted to do so. Indeed, he or she might prefer to just thoroughly enjoy being in this wonderful place of comfort and security.

Simple instructions for becoming more deeply hypnotized will generally suffice:

And now I would like you to become even more deeply hypnotized . . . more deeply than before. With each breath you take, you can become more and more deeply entranced . . . so deep that you will be able to do whatever you need to do in hypnosis today . . . whatever you want . . . deeper and deeper . . . deep enough to experience anything you wish to experience.

Posthypnotic Suggestions

Preparing for Subsequent Sessions

Before the initial hypnosis session ends, it is useful to prepare the patient for subsequent sessions, so that the time required for inducing hypnosis can be shortened. This can be accomplished in two ways. First, patients can be told that hypnosis becomes easier to experience with practice, so that each time they experience hypnosis, they will find it easier and easier to become hypnotized and they will enter hypnosis more and more quickly.

Suggestions along the following lines can be given:

> Like many things, your response to hypnosis will improve with practice. Each time you practice relaxation, it's easier to relax. Each time you experience hypnosis, your ability to do so will improve, and you will be able to have a more complete experience of hypnosis . . . experience even greater relaxation, and go deeper and deeper into your hypnosis. Wouldn't that be nice? And you can enter hypnosis more and more quickly . . . more and more quickly and easily.

Second, a posthypnotic suggestion can be given, establishing a cue or signal for quickly becoming involved with the experience of hypnosis. For example:

> From now on, it is going to be very easy for you to become hypnotized when you want to. In fact, we are going to establish a cue that will allow you to become hypnotized instantly. We can use any word or phrase you like. I wonder if there is a particular word or phrase that can symbolize this experience for you . . . or whether you prefer that I suggest the phrase. [The patient or therapist selects a phrase.] Okay! From now on, the words hypnosis now will be a signal to enter hypnosis. But the interesting thing is that it will work only when I say those words and when you want to become hypnotized. When you want to enter hypnosis and I say the words hypnosis now, you will immediately become deeply engrossed in the hypnotic experience. But it won't happen if someone else says those words. If you hear those words in normal conversation, they will have no effect at all. And it won't work if you do not wish to experience hypnosis. But if I say "hypnosis now," and if you are ready to be hypnotized, you will be able to enter hypnosis immediately or at your own comfortable speed.

In subsequent sessions, once the patient is comfortable and indicates readiness to begin hypnosis, the therapist says "hypnosis now," either alone or embedded in a phrase, such as "You can enter hypnosis now," stressing the cue words so that the signal intent is not missed.

Posthypnotic Suggestion: Developing an Anchor

Anchoring techniques are easy ways of transporting what is learned in session to everyday life. Physical cues for relaxation or the activation of a particular suggestion are relatively unobtrusive and easy to implement, as follows:

> Is there any tension in your body, even a little bit, that you would like to release now? If you have even a bit of residual tension in your body that you would like to release so that you can relax even more completely, make a fist now. That's it. Make a fist. That's good. A strong fist. Scan your body now, from your head to your toes. Be aware of any tension that remains that you would like to let go of . . . release . . . because you don't need it, now, do you? And now you can do something you will find interesting. See whether you can gather all of that tension into your hand and make your fist even stronger with this tension you have gathered. Take your tension and convert it into a feeling of strength. A strong and powerful fist. A fist of strength. This strength that you can feel will remind you that strength is within . . . strength is within. And as you release the fist, you let go. . . . You learn more about holding on and letting go. And as you learn, you perhaps notice something very interesting. . . . You notice that you can release any and all tension that is within your body that you do not need. And that you can be strong without being tense at all. Say to yourself strength is within . . . and if you wish . . . relax more and more. Feel your entire body becoming more and more comfortable as you become more in tune with the strength that is within your body, strength you can access any time you wish . . . and as you are even more aware of this strength, you can relax and feel so comfortable . . . if you wish . . . to just the degree that feels comfortable.
>
> And now I would like to suggest to you that you can have this feeling of strength combined with relaxation any time you wish. You can establish a cue or what I call an anchor to remind you in any situation that you can remain strong, even while you relax. All you have to do instead of making a fist is to simply bring your thumb and forefinger together in a way that nobody will notice . . . nobody but you, that is. . . . In fact, you notice that when you bring your thumb and index together, as you can do now, that you can remember what it was like to be relaxed, and feeling strong. You can feel relaxed and strong after your hypnosis. And you can do this quickly, and easily. And you can do this better and better with practice. You make your anchor, and you feel yourself calming down . . . calming down. You can be wide awake, alert, and you can calm yourself . . . soothe yourself . . . ease into a

comfortable, relaxed state . . . even when you are fully awake, alert, and going about your everyday life after our hypnosis today. [*Now terminate the hypnosis procedure.*]

Develop Multiple Cues

The anchoring cue can be tied to a suggestion for a feeling, thought, or action to occur in the future. Hammond (1992) recommended the following format: "When I feel _____, I will _____. He observes that many different cues can be attached to posthypnotic suggestions that include visual cues (e.g., "When I see a person smoking, I will remind myself that smoking is bad for my health"), sounds ("Whenever I hear _____ on the radio, I will list five reasons to not smoke"), thoughts ("When I think I need to smoke, I will have an image of myself as a nonsmoker"), and physical sensations and emotions ("When I feel an urge to smoke, I will tell myself that the urge will pass"). Each of these suggestions can be anchored with a sense of strength and resolve to resist any urge to smoke.

Terminating Hypnosis

Ending a hypnosis session is even easier than inducing it. One can terminate hypnosis by simply telling the patient, "Wake up now" or "You can come out of hypnosis as soon as you are ready." Often a brief counting procedure, spoken in an increasingly energetic tone, is used, such as the following:

> I am going to count backward from five, and with each count you are going to become more and more alert and energized. At the count of one, you can open your eyes. At zero, you will be fully alert and wide awake, feeling better than you did before we began. Five . . . four . . . three . . . feel the energy flowing into you . . . two . . . one . . . open your eyes . . . zero . . . wide awake.

Be sure that your patient is completely alert before he or she leaves the office.

In the next chapter we present hypnotic techniques and strategies that, along with the basic inductions and suggestions we described, are the backbone of the use of hypnosis as an adjunctive treatment.

5

TECHNIQUES FOR CATALYZING EMPIRICALLY SUPPORTED TREATMENTS

In this chapter we describe methods that clinicians should have at their disposal to craft individually tailored interventions based on empirically supported principles and procedures. In subsequent chapters, we address many of the techniques that follow, or variants of them, in the treatment of smoking, eating disorders, depression, anxiety, posttraumatic stress disorder, and pain and medical conditions.

PROMOTING FEELINGS OF SAFETY AND SECURITY: THE SAFE PLACE

Suggestions for participants to experience a place of safety and security have been reported in the treatment of many disorders and conditions including eating disorders, pain, sexual abuse, and dissociative disorders (see Lynn, Kirsch, & Rhue, 1996; Rhue, Lynn, & Kirsch, 1993). Suggestions along the following lines can be embedded in virtually any hypnotic induction:

And now you can experience yourself in a place of comfort and security, safety, and peace. A special place. Perhaps you are alone, enjoying the sights and sounds in this place . . . captivated by all the possibilities . . . all that you can experience in this place. . . . Perhaps you are with someone else . . . perhaps you have experienced this place in your past, or perhaps you create it in your imagination. . . . I don't know. You know, it really doesn't matter. All that matters is your comfort . . . your comfort and ease. Experience this special place. Go to it now, in your mind, your imagination . . . go if you are not already there . . . approach this place, if you haven't already . . . experience it . . . experience the peace . . . the serenity . . . you are entitled to be in this special place . . . to enjoy it . . . to be there . . . you deserve it . . . go there now . . . enjoy your opportunity to feel so secure in this special place . . . move toward it . . . or perhaps let it draw you ever so gently . . . like a magnetic force. Wouldn't it be restful and relaxing to feel so comforted, so good . . . so good . . . breathe easy . . . feel comfortable . . . calm . . . free, easy . . . breathe in . . . and out . . . in . . . and out. As you breathe in and out, let yourself feel even more safe and secure . . . let it happen . . . wouldn't it be nice? Comfortable and soothed . . . relaxed and serene . . . safe and secure . . . at ease . . . good enough . . . good enough . . . no one to please here . . . secure . . . at ease . . . peaceful . . . isn't it nice?

And wouldn't it feel right to feel your senses come alive in this place . . . seeing and touching and tasting and hearing and feeling? You can be you in this place . . . nothing to bother, nothing to disturb . . . deeper and deeper, deeper and deeper levels of comfort . . . deeper and deeper security, deeper and deeper into your hypnosis . . . deeper and deeper as you learn even more about feeling safe and secure. Safe and secure, at rest . . . at ease.

The following suggestions can be used to generalize treatment effects beyond the immediate hypnosis session:

Would you like to take some learnings and insights from this special place with you? Would you like to take them wherever you go? Wherever you are? Make them a part of yourself? If you would like to do this, please feel free . . . please feel free . . . free and easy . . . easy and free. Wouldn't it be wonderful? Would you like to give yourself permission to feel more secure as you move throughout your life? As you walk your path through your life . . . wherever you go? Would you like to learn more and more about how to do this . . . what you need . . . how to take care of yourself? Perhaps you are so relaxed and at ease that you just want to enjoy this special place and know that you can take with you whatever you have learned and experienced. And now go deeper and deeper . . . deeper and deeper . . .

BUILDING SECURE BOUNDARIES AND
DECISION-MAKING CAPACITY: THE BUBBLE

When one of our patients imagined arriving at the bottom of the stairs, during the staircase induction, she would imagine that she entered a healing and protective vitamin E capsule. We recognize that some participants might find it a bit of a sticky situation to be in a vitamin E capsule, but the following suggestions, adapted from D. P. Brown (1992), accomplish the same purpose of helping the participant to experience a sense of being in control and of regulating personal and interpersonal boundaries.

Would you like to have a sense of being safe, secure, and in control? [*If answer is yes, proceed as follows.*] Good. I would like to invite you to imagine you are in a bubble where you feel protected and in control. Would you like to do this? [*If the answer is yes, proceed as follows.*] Good. Maybe this bubble is colored with a fine iridescence, or maybe it is translucent. Maybe the bubble fits tightly yet comfortably around you, or maybe it is large and there is plenty of room. Perhaps you feel yourself floating gently and easily in this bubble, floating freely and easily . . . light and free . . . so light and free . . . completely comfortable because it is safe in your bubble . . . you are safe in your bubble. In your space. It is your space. You control what goes on in this space . . . what goes on inside your bubble . . . your bubble of safety. Feel comfortable . . . in control. Wouldn't it be wonderful to let yourself enjoy this feeling? Is it surprising that the bubble can move up? The bubble can move down. It can move to the side, left or right. You can make the left decision or the right decision. You control this bubble. You can even control how thick the bubble is . . . thick or thin . . . thin or thick . . . you decide.

You can let people in . . . you can keep people out. . . . It is your decision. Your decision . . . you decide. You can get close to people in the bubble, or you can keep your distance. . . . It is your decision. You can share your feelings with others in the bubble, or you can keep your feelings to yourself. . . . It is your decision. You can say yes in this bubble, or you can say no. . . . It is your decision. You are free to decide. You have the right to decide . . . yes or no, no or yes. . . . You can decide now, or you can decide later. . . . There's no hurry. Lots of time . . . lots of time. Feel your sense of security deepen.

And with this deepening sense of control, I wonder whether you would enjoy giving yourself permission to relax even more? Would you like to go even deeper into your hypnosis . . . would you like to enjoy a sense of floating . . . or are you at peace now, with no need to move at all? Maybe you don't have to go anywhere or do anything to feel more safe and in control . . . safe and in control. Now I will be quiet for a minute or so to let you explore the bubble and how safe you can feel within its protective surfaces.

Yes, more and more you can have this sense of control. . . . Isn't it nice to feel this? Yes, and you become more aware of your power to decide, as you realize there is a comfortable and flexible boundary around you that you . . . and only you . . . control. You can learn more about expanding the boundary of your bubble . . . or contracting it . . . any time you like. And I think you will find it interesting to discover that after hypnosis you can do this . . . you can do this . . . after hypnosis you can continue to explore your boundaries . . . your boundaries with people . . . your ability to make capable decisions for yourself and those you care about. . . . Wouldn't it be nice to discover how after your hypnosis today you can acquire more learnings? Wouldn't it be interesting to discover how comfort flows from your awareness of new possibilities? I am sure you can feel more comfortable and secure in your everyday life as you control who you let in and who you keep out of your space, and you control in what ways you choose to relate to others in everyday life, filled with confidence in your power to make decisions that enhance your sense of security and safety.

ACCESSING A HIGHER SELF: FACILITATING PROBLEM SOLVING AND FRUSTRATION TOLERANCE

Suggestions of a higher self or a wise inner advisor can be given in conjunction with imagery of a special place or as independent suggestions in their own right. The following suggestions are designed to facilitate problem solving and frustration tolerance. These suggestions can be readily combined with imaginative rehearsal of problem-solving activities, which we describe in the section that follows:

You can make a strong connection with the wisdom you have acquired in a lifetime of learning in this special place, begin to get a sense of what I hope we can agree to call your higher self or your inner adviser . . . take some time to feel connected with this aspect of yourself . . . this higher self of wisdom and sound judgment . . . this higher self that holds the power to make good decisions . . . evaluate situations. Soon you will discover that you can get closer . . . closer . . . closer, as you move toward discovery of this higher self. . . . Soon you will discover that it can become stronger and stronger . . . within your reach . . . within your grasp.

I will count from one to five. And with each count, you will take a step toward your higher self of wisdom, strength, and decision-making ability. With each count . . . with each step that you take . . . you can take a deep, slow, easy breath, as you discover how you can move even closer to your higher self. That's right. A slow, easy breath. And I think you will agree that it is much easier to get in touch with your ability to think clearly . . . logically . . . to maintain a calm focus . . . to solve problems . . . to find solutions . . . when you are calm and at ease.

One. That's right . . . take your first step. Notice that you are starting to focus more on your higher self. . . . Be aware of a sense of inner peace and calmness spreading . . . calmness accompanying this inner peace. Enjoy this sense of calmness . . . serenity. Your mind is becoming clearer . . . sharper as you become more and more relaxed and at ease. Your ability to think and reason is becoming even more focused. Two. And with your second step, perhaps you can notice how relaxed you feel. Do you feel more relaxed than when you are asleep? Would you be willing to release any tension you do not need as you go deeper and deeper? . . . deeper and deeper as you move to discover that higher aspect of your being? Is your breathing as relaxed and steady as you would like it to be? Would you like to go even deeper? Moving closer . . . moving closer. And three . . . take a third step. Learning . . . more and more . . . more and more . . . with each breath. Plenty of time. Your higher self is like a magnet, gently drawing you toward it. Would you like to learn even more about your higher self, discover, sense even more aspects of it? Yes? Then approach the space close to your higher self . . . get in touch with your ability to think through problems . . . consider alternatives . . . deal with frustration. And four . . . take that fourth step. Yes. You are almost there. Almost touching that higher part of yourself, almost one with it. Just breathe . . . that's right. In and out . . . in . . . and out. You don't really have to do anything, nothing to bother, nothing to disturb as you turn inside to discover peace and serenity, along with the ability to focus your mind. And five . . . with that fifth step you are in touch with your higher self . . . the wisdom you have accumulated over the course of a lifetime . . . you are in touch with your ability to stay calm and focused . . . your ability to think clearly and remain calm . . . remain calm . . . stay balanced . . . stay focused . . . even when you experience stress . . . let yourself be informed by your feelings . . . yet don't think with your feelings. Isn't it helpful when you stay focused on your goals? Yes, you *can* stay focused on being the person you respect . . . the person you want to be . . . when you think about what you want to achieve . . . when you contact . . . access this higher self . . . when you think before you act. When you develop strategies . . . ways of being and acting . . . think of the possibilities before you act. . . . Yes, you discover that this higher self is within you . . . that strength and wisdom and power are all within you.

Anecdotes and Metaphors

Earlier, we noted that priming is a way of increasing the accessibility of a concept to build therapeutic response sets. Anecdotes, stories, and metaphors allow therapists to seed therapeutic change in patients in a nondirective manner and to activate concepts and ideas consistent with therapeutic goals. For example, Erickson (Rosen, 1982) told the detailed story of precisely how children learn to stand up and walk as a way of building a learning response set and suggesting to patients that they would accomplish difficult tasks in therapy by completing many small tasks. P. Brown (1993) observed that metaphors can implicitly structure experience and determine responses to events, often without explicit conscious awareness.

Imaginative Rehearsal

Asking people to think about, imagine, rehearse, and problem solve possible situations or to explain hypothetical outcomes is another effective means of priming and altering the accessibility of facts in memory. Hypnosis can be used to increase the salience of particular outcome expectations and to bring to mind concepts and ideas consistent with positive outcomes and inconsistent with negative outcomes (see Sherman & Lynn, 1990). When subsequent judgments or decisions are made, these ideas will then be most accessible and will serve as a basis for action (Sherman, Skov, Hervitz, & Stock, 1981).

For example, in the cognitive–behavioral therapies we present later in this volume, we describe how imagining negative outcomes of smoking and overeating and positive outcomes of not doing so can make it easier to resist those urges. Often imaginative rehearsal is used to help patients prepare for situations they will confront in the future. We present examples of how patients can be instructed to (a) anticipate and prepare for stressful events; (b) engage in imaginative rehearsal by visualizing themselves on a television screen, for example, implementing successful coping strategies; and (c) generate a positive internal dialogue (e.g., "good job," "well done") for successfully implementing the strategies.

Another tactic, recommended by solution-focused therapists (Fish, 1996; de Shazer, 1985), is to direct the patient's attention to exceptions to the problem (e.g., "Tell me when you do not feel anxious"), thereby priming adaptive thoughts and behaviors. Posing questions to patients such as "How would your life change if you did X?" or "What would you have to change in your life in order for you to relinquish your fear of public speaking?" also is likely to increase the accessibility of adaptive activities (Kirsch & Lynn, 1998).

Age Progression

Imaginative rehearsal and finding exceptions to the problem can be done in the context of age progression in which patients are asked to imagine a future time in which they have resolved their problems and take note of the steps taken to improve their lives. Gevertz (1996) recommended a technique in which patients are asked to imagine standing between two mirrors, with the mirror in front representing how they wish to be and the mirror behind them representing how they are now. In our experience, most patients, when given a choice, step through the mirror in front of them and, as suggested, become the image, describing how they change to accomplish their goals as they enter the mirror on successive trials, with each trial representing increasingly distant times in the future. Patients can also be asked to progress in time by (a) riding an elevator to floors or tuning channels on a mental TV set, in which they watch events unfold, with numbers corresponding to years of their lives; (b) walking up a staircase with each step representing a year ahead in the future, and each step down representing a year in the past; (c) looking into an imaginary crystal ball in which they can see their future self; (d) observing scenes on a stage of the future; and (e) moving forward a year with each count of the hypnotist. In fact, many patients need little more than a suggestion to "move into the future" to age progress.

Age Regression

Many of the same techniques can be used to promote the experience of age regression to an earlier time in life (see Hammond, 1990, for a useful compendium of age-regression techniques). For example, the therapist can ask the patient to walk down a staircase, with each step representing a year in the past, or ask the patient to observe scenes on a stage of the past. Patients can also be given simple suggestions to "go backward" in time (Yapko, 1993). Alden (1995) described an interesting variation of the bubble technique in which suggestions are given to "float back to an event and review it from the safety of the bubble" (p. 67). Whatever technique is used, patients are typically asked to mentally re-create events or feelings that occurred at successively earlier periods in life or to focus on a particular event at a specific age, with suggestions to fully relive the event. To help patients manage anxiety during age regression to childhood events, for example, the therapist can "come along" with patients to give them advice; patients can give adult advice to their child self, as events unfold in memory; and patients can use relaxation anchoring procedures that can be transported to the past. When past stressful events are targeted, it is often advantageous to precede such exploration with suggestions to experience happy or joyful times in life.

Experiences during age regression can be compelling to both therapist and patient, yet they do not necessarily mirror historical events. A televised documentary (Bikel, 1995) showed a group therapy session in which a woman was age regressed through childhood, to the womb, and eventually to being trapped in her mother's fallopian tube. The woman provided a convincing demonstration of the emotional and physical discomfort that one would experience if one were indeed stuck in such an uncomfortable position. Although the woman may have believed in the veracity of her experience, research indicates that her regression experiences were not memory based. Instead, age-regressed participants behave according to situational cues and their knowledge, beliefs, and assumptions about age-relevant behaviors. According to Nash (1987), age-regressed adults do not show the expected patterns on many indices of development, including brain activity (as detected by electroencephalograms) and visual illusions. No matter how compelling, age-regressed experiences do not represent literal reinstatements of childhood experiences, behaviors, and feelings.

Nevertheless, when age regression is not used to recover accurate memories of past events, it can be a useful technique. For example, in our experience, inviting a patient to revisit a well-remembered past event with the goal of examining how she coped, in order to cope more effectively in response to future events, can be productive.

In the chapters that follow, we also provide examples of how age regression can be used in the context of exposure-based cognitive–behavioral treatments to help patients habituate to anxiety-provoking stimuli and learn new, adaptive ways of responding to stressful life events. However, age-regression procedures warrant great caution. For example, certain individuals may not be able to access happy times in life, and age-regression suggestions can touch on sensitive issues and unsettling memories such as when patients have been abused or traumatized in some way. A careful assessment of family history and dynamics and traumatic events should be undertaken before age-regression suggestions are administered. It is imperative that therapists evaluate the probable effects of hypnotic procedures prior to implementing them.

Managing Negative Affect and Anger: The Closed Fist

Some patients, especially those in crisis, require assistance in attenuating negative affect and concomitant physical tension. Patients can observe themselves on TV, using dials or a remote control to control feelings, or imagine themselves in a command and control center in the hypothalamus in the brain (see Hammond, 1992) in which they can regulate specific feelings with computers. Such imagery can assist patients in damping strong emotions, especially when combined with suggestions for the benefits of finding constructive solutions to anger-eliciting problems or situations. In the closed-fist technique that follows, making a fist that many people associate with anger can come to represent a means of containing and controlling anger or other negative emotions. This technique is a variation of the anchoring technique presented earlier that involves making a fist.

Scan your body and identify any places where you feel your anger [or anxiety, etc.]. Find this place and get in touch with your anger, with the knowledge that you will be able to discharge it and let go of it so safely, not hurting yourself or anyone else, letting it go in such a way that you are free of it, at least for now. At least for now, you will learn to let it pass, let go of it, in this way. Start with your feet. Do you feel anger there? If so, let it move up, up into your body and settle right on your hand that you will place in your lap now, good, place your right hand in your lap, palm up, that's it, palm up. Let the anger settle there, and let the angry feelings in all of the lower part of your body move up, up, right up to the surface of your open hand. And now, with your body scan, you can identify anger in the upper part of your body, yes, starting with your head, let the anger move down into that right hand, that right hand sitting on your lap, and settle there, moving down and away from your face, let the anger drain down, drain out, drain out completely, into that hand, and yes, any anger, any anger in the upper part of your body, let it move down, drain down, right into your right hand . . . yes, and let all your anger go there, no need to keep it in any other place in your body. . . . Let's limit it, keep it limited, no need to make any other part of your body tense, and yes, can you feel it happening, let all the anger in your entire body settle in that right hand . . . and now . . . can you feel your hand closing around the anger, making it smaller, compacting it? Let it happen, let your hand close, closing tighter, tighter around the anger, yes, that's it, make a tight fist, close your hand, make a fist of strength, strength that can contain, it's OK, it's safe, you are in control because you are stronger, wiser, smarter than your anger, you can contain it, yes, you are much stronger and bigger a person and stronger than your anger, it is so much smaller now, so much more contained, compacted, you can control and contain it, getting even smaller, all of the tension in your body focusing in your hand, your strong hand, yes, but it's so much effort to make such a tight fist, isn't it . . . it takes so much out of you to be angry, to hold onto it, and you want to release it in a healthy, safe way, a way that doesn't hurt anyone, much less you . . . let the anger go, release the tension that goes with it. . . . Wouldn't it be nice to be free of it, mind clear, body relaxed? So let it go, you don't need it, let it go, be rid of it, let it go, let your entire body relax, and when you are ready, open your fist, open your fist and feel the anger dissipate, let it go, away from you, you can be distant from it . . . let it go into thin air, not hurting anyone, not hurting you, you are safe, everyone around you is safe, and you are rid of the anger, let it pass, let it drain from you, drain, yes, dissipate, let your entire body relax, breathe it out as well and relax . . . relax completely . . . that's it, let it go, let it go, at least for now . . . at least for now. . . . If there's a lesson to learn from your anger, we can talk about it, perhaps a choice to make, I don't know, but you can learn and grow and make choices with your body and your mind relaxed, not angry . . . your mind and body working together . . . yes, good, I can see your entire body is relaxing now, you deserve it, let it go, whatever tension is left that you don't need, let it go, let your hand and body relax, your hand feels quite normal now, and you are in charge, stronger than your anger.

The Anger Rock

Krakauer (2001) advocated use of a technique modified from an intervention suggested by Watkins (1980) called the *anger rock* in which the patient smashes an imaginary rock into smithereens, while retaining the awareness that it is just a rock, and not a person, and that the anger can be expressed in such a way that it hurts no one. The size of the rock can vary with the intensity of the felt anger, and a small fragment of the smashed rock can be sanded down to a smooth pebble that can represent a symbol of transformation. Favorite or special place imagery can be incorporated, such that after the rock is smashed, the patient can experience absolute peace and comfort in a special place and learn new, constructive ways of problem solving and coping with the situation that stimulated the angry feelings.

CLINICAL HYPNOSIS WITH CHILDREN

Many of the techniques we have reviewed can be applied with children who are developmentally prepared to attend to suggestions; be involved in a bedtime story, fairy tale, or book; or be engaged and participate in a story on audio- or videotape (Kohen & Olness, 1993). According to Rhue, Lynn, and Pintar (1996), the following suggests a capacity for imaginative involvements and involvement in hypnotic procedures: the belief that dolls and stuffed animals are alive; imaginary friends, animals, and objects; and pretending, and in some sense believing, to be someone else (e.g., a fairy tale character). In contrast, cognitive deficits, poor reality contact, a poor attention span, and an impoverished fantasy life are contraindications for hypnotic methods, or diminish their effectiveness. The child's developmental level, not so much the child's chronological age, determines the appropriateness of using hypnotic procedures. Age is generally regarded as secondary to the child's ability to concentrate, focus attention, imagine, and understand what is suggested.

Formal inductions are rarely useful with children younger than 7 or 8 years old. Naturalistic, spontaneous interventions often produce desirable outcomes in young children. In our experience, children often respond well when the procedures are embedded in games of "play pretend," "let's do an experiment," or "let's have a daydream" and storytelling, as described in a number of resources for working with children (Kohen & Olness, 1993; Olness & Gardner, 1988; Rhue & Lynn, 1993). Consider the following example of an "experiment," done with the parent and child, taken from Kohen and Olness (1993):

> Let's do an experiment. . . . Everyone close your eyes and just pretend you're not here . . . pretend maybe you're at home . . . or maybe somewhere else . . . where you are very happy and comfortable and be there for a few moments. Good. See who's there with you, hear what's going on, enjoy it . . . and you can either tell about it after or you don't have to because it's your imagining and your inside mind and your self-hypnotizing and you're the boss of it. And you have probably noticed already, in just these few moments, that you also changed a little. Your breathing became slower, you were sitting real still and it's like your body and brain were talking with each other. Your body knew that your brain was imagining and it got relaxed . . . Isn't that interesting? . . . Nice going! (p. 363)

This example also reveals that it is important to speak to the children in language appropriate to their developmental level. After this brief experiment, Kohen and Olness (1993) noted that seeds can be planted to facilitate future imaginative interventions such as, "And next time you come, you and I will meet in private and do some more imagining and learn how to use this to help those tummyaches that used to bother you!" (p. 363).

Rhue and Lynn (1993) described how storytelling can be used with children whereby they can interact with imaginary characters who are in situations analogous to theirs, give them advice, and, in the case of sexually abused children, for example, help them not to blame themselves and teach them what adults should and should not do. In storytelling, the therapist often tells the child a story, but the child can also construct a story with the assistance of the therapist, who provides suggestions and helps shape the imaginative narrative as it unfolds.

Virtually all inductions for children involve imagery. Children often respond well to stories with images of a favorite or safe place and protective images to alleviate anxiety (e.g., a 10-foot-high velveteen rabbit, Gandalf, magic shields). With preschool children, especially, relaxation is less important than fortifying involvement in what is suggested. Deepening procedures involve the intensification of imagery through multisensory suggestions (e.g., "See who and what's there, smell the smells, hear the sounds"; Kohen & Olness, 1993, p. 365). Moreover, it is essential to establish a positive rapport with the child and to tailor the procedures to the child's unique profile of interests, imaginative proclivities, and attentional capacities.

Hypnosis has seen a wide range of application with children including the treatment of learning problems, acute pain, general medical problems, and nausea and emesis from chemotherapy. The lion's share of the 15 studies of hypnosis with children that Milling and Costantino (2000) reviewed focused on the relief of chemotherapy distress and acute pain. The authors noted that research on hypnosis with children is in a relatively early stage of development. However, one study by Edwards and van der Spuy (1985) of clinical hypnosis for nocturnally enuretic children was particularly well controlled and compelling. Other promising studies reviewed include research on imagination-focused hypnosis for nausea and vomiting related to chemotherapy (Zeltzer, Dolgin, LeBaron, & LeBaron, 1991), pain from bone marrow aspirations and lumbar punctures (Zeltzer & LeBaron, 1982), and pain reduction in suggestible children undergoing venipuncture and bone marrow aspirations (Lambert, 1999; Smith, Rosen, Trueworthy, & Lowman, 1979).

THE IMPORTANCE OF COLLABORATION

Whether used with children or adults, hypnosis is, at its best, a collaborative enterprise, a partnership. Involve your patients at all levels, including assisting you in devising meaningful and personalized suggestions. For example, one of us recently treated a woman with sleep terrors whose husband had a difficult time calming her during frenzied, agitated sleep terror episodes. She decided that the phrase *beautiful flower* would have a calming influence on her, and she repeated this to herself before she fell asleep and asked her husband to whisper it to her during a sleep terror episode. It worked very well in calming her and allowing her to return to a comfortable sleep.

Invite your patients to preview the suggestions and tactics you plan to use in each session. Most patients appreciate clear, specific suggestions that are consistent with their stated goals. Solicit and value your patient's feedback. For example, you might ask about your pace ("Should I slow down, or speed up a bit?"), tone of voice ("Am I speaking a bit too loud, or too soft, or just right?"), wording of suggestions (e.g., "During self-hypnosis exercises, should I use first person ('I am') or second person ('You are')?"), and your patient's preferences for visual or auditory imagery, and more authoritative versus permissive suggestions. In collaborating with your patient, you will at once deepen the therapeutic relationship, demonstrate your respect for your "partner," and increase your patient's sense of agency and ownership of the therapeutic endeavor.

6

SMOKING CESSATION

Smoking is paradigmatic of a self-destructive habit. Each year, 1 million Americans join the ranks of new smokers ("Cancer doctors," 2003). This statistic is alarming given that smoking (a) is responsible for one third of all cancer deaths and increases the risk of lung, breast, larynx, oral cavity, esophagus, pancreas, cervix, and urinary bladder cancer (Haxby, 1995); (b) doubles a person's chance of dying from either coronary heart disease or stroke (McBride, 1992); and (c) is the primary cause of chronic obstructive pulmonary disease among men and women (U.S. Department of Health and Human Services [USDHHS], 1990).

If current trends continue, 1 billion people will die this century from tobacco-related illnesses compared with 100 million in the past century (Reuters, 2003). Although as many as 80% of current smokers wish to stop smoking (U.S. Department of Health, Education, and Welfare, 1990), only about 5% of the approximately one third of U.S. smokers who annually attempt to stop on their own succeed (American Psychiatric Association, 1994). Can hypnosis help the vast at-risk population of smokers to achieve abstinence? The answer is yes. In fact, hypnosis has a long history as a habit-control technique that dates to efforts to control the use of tobacco in the mid-19th century.

In this chapter, we summarize a sizable literature indicating that hypnosis can play a useful role in smoking cessation. We then describe a two-session cognitive–behavioral program to achieve smoking cessation as an example of the way that hypnosis can be used to master long-standing habitual patterns of self-destructive behaviors.

An early, single-session version of the smoking cessation program was developed in the 1980s by Lynn and Neufeld in conjunction with the American Lung Association of Ohio (Neufeld & Lynn, 1988). The program included many elements of the American Lung Association's Freedom from Smoking program, as well as techniques and strategies culled from the hypnosis and cognitive–behavioral treatment literature on effective smoking cessation programs. The current program that we present herein is a refinement of both the original single session program and the earlier two-session program described by Lynn, Neufeld, Rhue, and Matorin (1993; see also Green, 1996, 2000).

HYPNOSIS AND SMOKING CESSATION: THE EVIDENCE

Johnston and Donoghue's (1971) first major review of the hypnosis and smoking cessation literature reported extravagant success rates as high as 94% (Von Dedenroth, 1964). Unfortunately, no experimental evidence was reported to substantiate his claims. Several years later, Hunt and Bespalec (1974) compared six methods of modifying smoking behavior: aversive conditioning; drug therapy; education and group support; hypnosis; behavior modification; and miscellaneous, including self-control, role-playing, and combination treatments. They concluded that hypnosis "perhaps gives us our best results" (p. 435), with reported success rates varying between 15% and 88%. Because success rates were similar across studies, they suggested that the choice of treatment was secondary to engaging smokers in treatment.

Holroyd's (1980) review of 17 mostly clinical reports concluded that more sessions are better than fewer sessions, that individualized treatments are superior to standardized suggestions, and that adjunctive treatments such as telephone contact and counseling increase the likelihood of successful outcome. Holroyd concluded that when these conditions were fulfilled, more than half of those treated remained abstinent at 6 months. However, the best controlled investigations (Barkley, Hastings, & Jackson, 1977; MacHovec & Man, 1978; Pedersen, Scrimgeour, & Lefcoe, 1975) yielded outcomes of 0% to 50%, the lower range of the studies reviewed by Holroyd.

Viswesvaran and Schmidt (1992) more recently performed a meta-analysis on 633 studies of smoking cessation and examined 48 studies in the hypnosis category that encompassed a total sample of 6,020 participants. Hypnosis fared better than virtually any other comparison treatment (e.g., nicotine chewing gum, smoke aversion, 5-day plans), achieving a success rate of 36%.

Law and Tang (1995) analyzed 188 randomized controlled trials of smoking cessation studies in their systematic review of the literature and further restricted their review to trials in which the duration was 6 months or more. Although the 10 randomized trials of hypnosis indicated an estimate of efficacy of 23%, the authors argued that the effect is unproved in that none of the trials measured biochemical markers (e.g., thiocyanate) of smoking to confirm verbal reports.

In the most comprehensive review to date, Green and Lynn (2000) examined 59 smoking cessation studies and concluded that, as judged against Chambless and Hollon's (1998) criteria for evaluating the empirical support of diverse psychotherapies, hypnosis was a "possibly efficacious" treatment. That is, hypnotic interventions appeared to be more effective than no treatment or waiting-list control conditions. However, in many studies it is difficult to disentangle the specific effects of hypnosis from the behavioral and educational interventions it is combined with. In addition, hypnosis is not necessarily superior to alternative treatments (e.g., rapid smoking), and the evidence concerning whether hypnosis is superior to a placebo is mixed (Green & Lynn, 2000). It is therefore premature to claim that hypnosis per se is responsible for the treatment gains observed or that hypnosis is superior to a number of other treatments. These caveats notwithstanding, hypnosis procedures are brief and economical and represent a viable entry-level treatment for smoking.

A PROGRAM FOR SMOKING CESSATION

Given that cognitive–behavioral techniques are effective in the treatment of smoking cessation in their own right and that many individuals are motivated to participate in smoking cessation programs that incorporate hypnosis, we believe that hypnosis can be a useful addition to a more comprehensive treatment for smoking cessation. Indeed, behavioral and cognitive–behavioral procedures are the lynchpin of numerous treatments that are reported in successful smoking cessation studies (e.g., T. B. Jeffrey, Jeffrey, Grueling, & Gentry, 1985; L. K. Jeffrey & Jeffrey, 1988; MacHovec & Man, 1978; Schubert, 1983). The cognitive–behavioral treatment program we describe can be implemented in both group (range = 5–50 participants) and individual treatment contexts. The program retains many of the features of the initial single-session program that were originally described in Lynn, Neufeld, et al. (1993).

Treatment Components

Hypnosis as Self-Hypnosis

Training in self-hypnosis is an integral part of many successful smoking cessation treatments (e.g., Barabasz, Baer, Sheehan, & Barabasz, 1986; Basker, 1985; D. Spiegel, Frischholz, Fleiss, & Spiegel, 1993). The program informs participants that their active participation and involvement is required. Indeed, as noted in chapter 4, it is legitimate to present hypnosis as self-hypnosis (T. X. Barber, 1985).

Cognitive and Behavioral Skills

Self-hypnosis is described as one of a number of important skills that participants can master to achieve abstinence. Techniques such as minimizing negative self-talk while emphasizing the benefits of nonsmoking and the ability to become a nonsmoker, stimulus control, self-administered reward, and cue-controlled relaxation (i.e., anchoring) are used to promote self-control and teach important skills.

Education

Education is a basic component of many smoking cessation programs (Green & Lynn, 2000). We describe smoking as a learned behavior pattern that can be replaced with adaptive behaviors. Along with elucidating the deleterious physical effects of smoking, we encourage participants to generate positive personal (e.g., health) and interpersonal reasons to be a nonsmoker.

Enhancing Motivation and Self-Efficacy

Motivation enhancement is a crucial aspect of successful smoking cessation programs (see Perry, Gelfand, & Marcovitch, 1979; Perry & Mullen, 1975). Neufeld and Lynn's (1988) research on a preliminary version of the program indicated that of the participants abstinent at 6-month follow-up, all indicated that they were either *strongly* motivated to stop smoking or *somewhat strongly* motivated to stop. That is, all scored at least 3 on a 5-point scale that indexed participants' motivation to stop smoking. The program includes many positive suggestions regarding increased control, mastery, and feeling healthy and alive to counterbalance withdrawal-related discomfort. Nicotine replacement (e.g., nicotine patches, gum, inhaler, nasal spray, lozenges) as well as medications (e.g., bupropion, nortriptyline) is recommended to bolster confidence and engender positive treatment expectancies.

Being a Nonsmoker

Research indicates that the degree to which people see themselves as a nonsmoker is a strong predictor of long-term abstinence (Tobin, Reynolds,

Holroyd, & Creer, 1986). Participants are asked to see themselves as non-smokers; to say to themselves, "I am a nonsmoker"; to experience on a deep level the positive personal and interpersonal benefits of abstinence; and to provide substitute rewards for avoiding tobacco.

Relapse Prevention and Gain Maintenance

Participants identify high-risk or trigger situations associated with increased probability or risk of smoking. Identification of trigger situations linked to places, situations, and times characterized by especially powerful smoking cues is facilitated by self-monitoring of smoking behaviors during the week between smoking sessions. At the same time, participants generate coping responses that constitute an alternative to smoking for each of the trigger situations identified.

The degree to which smokers perceive themselves as effective copers in high-risk smoking situations is a significant predictor of long-term abstinence (e.g., Colletti, Supnick, & Payne, 1985). Hence, participants are asked not only to identify high-risk situations but also to visualize themselves using personally meaningful, desirable, and effective coping strategies that replace smoking behaviors in the situations so identified. Maintenance of treatment gains is encouraged by instructing participants to avoid high-risk situations, teaching participants strategies to cope with smoking urges, and identifying and instituting self-rewards for nonsmoking.

Minimizing Weight Gain

Weight gain that follows smoking cessation increases relapse risk (see Perkins, Epstein, & Pastor, 1990). The program therefore uses a minimal intervention based on recommendations by Black, Coe, Friesen, and Wurzmann (1984). We instruct participants to eat a well-balanced diet from the four basic food groups, to increase nonstrenuous physical activity, and to lose weight slowly and gradually (no more than 2 pounds per week), along with other suggestions presented in a handout described below. More aggressive approaches to weight maintenance and loss are also discussed in the context of individual treatment with smokers.

Contracting and Social Support

In the initial session, participants sign a contract that affirms their intention to stop smoking on the stop date of the second session, a week later. The signing of this contract is witnessed by another group member, and participants are instructed to give copies of the contract to a spouse, living partner, or best friend and their employer. To promote social support, a buddy system is instituted wherein participants are invited to pair up with one another to call each other if they wish to rely on another person for social support outside their family.

Program Description

We recently revamped our program on the basis of the feedback of 11 participants who achieved abstinence for at least 6 months. Within 2 weeks of treatment, these individuals read the original script and identified passages that were not useful or counterproductive in that they evoked thoughts or anxiety that interfered with their involvement or diminished their sense that they could achieve abstinence. For example, 7 of the individuals who provided feedback noted that they had difficulty "ignoring urges." The revised program thus has a greater emphasis on accepting urges, "riding the urge out, like surfing a wave" (see Marlatt, 2002, p. 47) and "letting them go," and using active coping strategies to contend with urges, rather than simply ignoring them. Over the years, we have learned that nicotine fading is not easy for many participants. We therefore present nicotine fading as an option, rather than as a prerequisite to successful completion of the program. Finally, we made many changes in wording on the basis of the feedback we received. For example, we removed all references to *quitting* because of the connotations it has with being a *quitter*.

Description of Session 1

The first session can be completed in about 2 hours; the second session typically requires an hour to an hour and a half to complete. In the first session, the trainer introduces him- or herself to the participants, describes the origins and history of the program, and presents an overview of the workshop. Participants then introduce themselves and discuss their reasons for attending the program.

The trainer then proceeds along the following lines:

> I am confident that this program will be an educational experience for you. Education, of course, involves learning. Let's get a fix on how you "learned" to smoke, because smoking is not a natural act. How many of you felt awkward when you first began to smoke? Did you feel sick or nauseated? It often takes weeks or even months of practice and perseverance to condition your body to learn to accept the noxious agents contained in tobacco smoke. Many of you probably smoked to fill a specific need (e.g., be "in" with your friends, remain alert and awake). What were your reasons for smoking? [*Discussion follows.*]
>
> Many of you probably smoked at first only in very limited situations. However, as time passed, the strength of your habit grew and you probably extended your smoking to many other situations (e.g., on the

telephone, at work, after you eat). Each time you lifted a cigarette to your lips, you strengthened your habit.

Just think of how many times you have lifted a cigarette to your lips. Why don't we calculate the number of times you have lifted a cigarette to your mouth? If you smoke a pack a day: 20 cigarettes per pack; average number of inhalations per cigarette is 10; number of inhalations per day is 200; 365 days per year × number of years smoked × 200 = total number of times you have lifted a cigarette to your mouth. Now that's a habit! The goal of this program is to teach you how to break your habit, or to unlearn your habitual behavior.

We have many ways we will teach you to give you the edge—the advantage you will need to break this habit. You should know that more than 40 million Americans have successfully stopped smoking. So it certainly is possible. We will help you turn that possibility into a personal reality.

We will teach you the skills you need to learn to break habitual patterns, deal with any discomfort you might experience, and maintain the gains you achieve here. We want you to have skills and techniques you can choose from. Your task will be to find the ones that work best for you. We will not only point out some of the costs of smoking but make you more aware of the benefits of being a nonsmoker, and how achieving this status can fill you with a sense of pride as you learn you are protecting and preserving your health, becoming more competitive in sports, becoming more kissable, and keeping your living environment free of smoke odors.

And of course, hypnosis will be one part of the program, one way to give you the edge. If you follow this program, really work it, we are confident you can stop smoking. We cannot do it for you, but we can make it a lot easier for you to become smoke free for life.

We have learned that motivation is one of the most important factors in being a nonsmoker. The best hypnotist in the world will not help if you are not motivated to stop smoking. I would now like to pass out a 3×5 index card. As you will see, it has a 1–5 scale on it of how motivated you are to stop: 1 = *not at all motivated*; 3 = *somewhat*; 5 = *extremely motivated*. I would like you to complete this scale at the end of our first session. If you are not strongly motivated (at least 3), then you should consider not coming back for the second session, and we will give you a full refund. Our research indicates that successful participants score between 3 and 5 on this scale.

But if you do want to stop smoking forever, if you are ready to complete the program, then I will ask you to sign a contract and have it witnessed by another group member. The contract will also be signed by your spouse, living partner, or best friend, and also by your employer if you are employed. We want you to enlist their support. We want you to announce your intention to stop smoking. We want them to understand the efforts you are making. We want them to know you are doing your best, and we want them to help *you* any way they can. How can they help you? Why don't we brainstorm as a group to get some ideas you can share with the people in your life. [*Discussion follows.*]

At this point, I would like to discuss your previous attempts to stop smoking. If you had been able to stop smoking successfully, you would not be here today. You have heard the phrase *know thine enemy*. To conquer the smoking habit, you need to let go of blaming yourself and cut out the sorts of statements you make to yourself such as "I'm weak" or "I have no willpower." If you smoke 15 or more cigarettes a day, you may be physically addicted to nicotine, and it is possible that withdrawal symptoms will occur when you do not receive your dose of nicotine. We will teach you ways to deal with these withdrawal symptoms if you should experience them. You can also avail yourself of nicotine lozenges, nicotine patches, and even medicines to help you stop smoking. Consult your doctor at your earliest convenience for any aid he or she can give you. But there is one thing to remember: Even some heavy smokers do not experience withdrawal symptoms, and withdrawal symptoms may not be very intense in even heavy smokers. In fact, 20% to 45% of abstainers report absolutely no withdrawal symptoms. Our goal is to prepare you for whatever you will face when you stop smoking. This program is designed to help even heavy smokers put an end to their habit. This program will help you to be a nonsmoker for life.

By gradually cutting down on the number and nicotine content of cigarettes you smoke, any withdrawal you might experience will be reduced in intensity. But what is important to remember is that withdrawal reactions are temporary, and you can learn to combat smoking urges. Urges are also temporary; they come and, it is important to note, they go. Consider this: After a month, two thirds of those who stop smoking do not report strong urges. In fact, several months after ending their habit, most ex-smokers feel less anxiety and depression than they did while they were smoking.

Let's focus more on withdrawal reactions now. Withdrawal is actually a sign that your body is coping with your decision to be a nonsmoker. It is a short-term reaction that you can deal with. Some of the reactions are a direct result of the body's healing itself. Let's consider some of the uncomfortable feelings some of you have had and what you can do about each reaction. [*Discussion follows.*]

If you have a cough, this can be a healthy sign, a sign that your lungs are clearing out. Not being able to concentrate is a short-term reaction; it represents your body's adjusting to decreases in nicotine in your body. Feelings of depression may arise because of your mistaken belief that you are losing a friend; actually, you are vanquishing a deadly enemy by stopping smoking. Feelings of anxiety may arise because of the association that you have made between smoking and situations in which you feel anxiety. But in the long run, you will be a calmer, less anxious person, perhaps on a more even keel than before you started smoking. To combat any feelings of lack of energy, you can get the boost you need from eating right and getting exercise. And there's the old cure for problems sleeping—drink milk before you go to bed. It contains a natural sleep-promoting substance—tryptophan—that will also help to calm your nerves. We have no surefire cure for irritability, but one reason why we ask you to have other people in your life sign the contract is so they can better understand what you are going through. At any rate, feelings of irritability will pass in a week or two.

What is important to keep in mind is that any discomfort you may experience is short-term, but many of the long-term effects of cigarette smoking are not. [At this point the program leader reviews the short- and long-term health consequences of smoking.] But the good news is that the body begins to repair itself almost as soon as you stop smoking. After a year of being a nonsmoker, your risk factors for cancer and heart disease return to about what they were before you began smoking. Is this powerful motivation for you to stop? I hope so.

Some people get discouraged and begin smoking again when they gain a few pounds after stopping. We have some recommendations for you that are simple but effective. First, be sure that you eat a well-balanced diet from the four basic food groups; increase physical activity such as walking, jogging, swimming, and playing sports; and lose weight slowly, but do not lose more than 2 pounds a week. Focus on your sensations of fullness when you eat. Enjoy what you eat. Enjoy it very much. But when you feel full, stop eating. To show that you have restraint, leave some food on your plate on a regular basis or every so often. And keep snacking to a minimum. If you feel you must snack, plan what you snack on. Plan on snacks that are low in calories and limit what you eat. I think you will find this simple plan will work for you. I will pass out a handout at the end of our session with additional suggestions for eating in moderation. Remember you *can* do it. You *can* change your life.

Think for a moment about what it would mean to you to be a nonsmoker. I will pass out some index cards, and I would like you to list at least five reasons for never smoking again. List your reasons in order of importance on this stop-smoking card. Now visualize two roads. The first road is a high road where you imagine your future if you stop successfully. Think of all the rewards of stopping the habit: the social rewards, the monetary rewards, and the health rewards. Take your time. Think of all you have to gain by being a nonsmoker. Now imagine a low road where you see your future if you are not truly motivated to end the habit. The choice is yours. Which road will you take? How many think or fear that you may not be able to stop? [show of hands] Keep your hands up. Now, if I told you that you would receive a million dollars if you could stop for a year, do you think you could do it? [show of hands] But a question I would like you to ask yourself is whether your health is worth a million dollars. Close your eyes now and tell yourself all the reasons you have to be a nonsmoker, and see yourself walking down the road of health and well-being as a nonsmoker. Add any additional reasons to stop smoking on your index card.

What I would like you to do this week is to review your reasons to stop, and to do this on a frequent basis. Carry your stop-smoking card on your person. During this week, I would also like you to identify trigger situations. Trigger situations are places, situations, and times that trigger the urge to smoke. An urge is an internal smoking cue or a prompt for you to smoke. Smokers tend to have urges linked with specific experiences. When a specific situation is linked with the feeling or urge to smoke, it is a trigger situation. What triggers your desire to smoke? [*Encourage discussion.*]

Now let's talk about how you can cope with urges. Let's brainstorm. How can you cope with smoking urges? [*Encourage discussion. If no coping methods are mentioned, the trainer lists a number of coping methods that center on (a) doing something else, (b) letting it pass, and (c) distraction techniques. Participants are encouraged to devise their own coping responses that might include exercising, taking a shower or bath, playing a sport, stretching, drawing, doing deep breathing, using imagery, bicycling, chewing sugarless gum, observing the urge and letting it go, drinking water, breathing the urge out, and using self-talk and self-hypnotic techniques.*] Now on the reverse side of your stop-smoking card, write your alternative coping responses in the trigger situations you identified.

One technique that many participants in our workshop have found useful is what we call the *urge zapper*. First, say to yourself, "I am aware of an urge to smoke." Second, say to yourself, "No! I do not have to smoke" or another key phrase that will help you. Three, read your reasons for being a nonsmoker listed on your stop-smoking card. Four, take a deep breath, breathe out all the tension in your body that you do not need, and feel yourself let the urge to smoke go. Let it go. It will pass, it will fade, to be replaced by something more comfortable. Ride it out, like you might surf a wave. Take another few breaths. Go on with your life. Urges will come, urges will go, until you are free of them forever. And finally, engage in one of the alternate coping responses on the back of your stop-smoking card.

During this first week, and thereafter, it is important that you avoid high-risk or trigger situations, whenever possible. Think about situations that you can avoid. Think about how you can reduce stress in your life this week. There may be some situations you cannot avoid, so I would like you to anticipate a situation that might come up this week, imagine it now, and see yourself coping effectively in this situation.

We recommend that after this week you never put a cigarette to your lips again. However, some people do slip. This does not mean that you are a total failure and that you should end your efforts to stop smoking. A slip can be a learning experience, a sign of the strength of the smoking habit. A sign that you have a choice. But remember this:

A lapse does not mean relapse! A relapse is a full return to the original pattern of behavior. Keep in mind, though, that you are playing with fire if you think you can control your smoking by smoking a few here or there. It is my belief that you will begin to feel better as you convince your body that you are serious about giving up the habit. Make that resolve firm! Firm it up! Do it now!

To help you to maintain the important gains you have achieved, you need to reward yourself. Make a list of things you enjoy and that are easy to obtain. A few can be expensive, but not all rewards have to be material. Make this list of rewards now on the paper provided. One thing you might wish to do is to put money ordinarily spent on cigarettes in a highly visible container and then spend it for a pleasurable activity when it accumulates.

Self-hypnosis is an important part of this program. It is a skill that you can learn. It can help you to be a nonsmoker by promoting relaxation, by strengthening your motivation to stop smoking, by helping to change your self-image from a smoker to a nonsmoker, and by providing you with a vehicle for administering useful self-suggestions that have the power to change your life. [*Trainer answers questions about self-hypnosis and fosters positive attitudes about hypnosis by demystifying hypnosis and correcting misconceptions, such as that hypnosis involves a trance, contact with reality is lost, and responses occur compulsively. Hypnosis is framed as involving the willingness to experience and imagine what is suggested and being open to useful suggestions.*]

The trainer then administers the self-hypnosis induction, which consists of the following elements and are described in the earlier chapters on inductions (see chap. 4) and advanced techniques (see chap. 5): (a) suggestions for calmness and releasing excessive tension; (b) deepening and relaxation suggestions of walking 20 steps to a place of safety and security; (c) developing a key phrase to catalyze motivation and desire to stop smoking; (d) developing a physical anchor (touching first and second fingers together) to access inner strength and anchoring reasons for being a nonsmoker; and (e) imaginally rehearsing resisting smoking urges in a trigger situation and using relaxation and anchoring techniques. After the induction, the trainer provides participants with a self-hypnosis tape that recapitulates the suggestions and recommends practice on a twice-daily basis.

Participants are given a number of instructions for homework on a daily basis that include the following assignments:

1. Record the number of cigarettes smoked.
2. Practice self-hypnosis.
3. Buy cigarettes by the pack, not the carton.
4. Start a "butt jar" and place cigarette butts in the jar.
5. Use urge management techniques.

6. Review reasons for being a nonsmoker.
7. Write a list of triggers and alternate behaviors.

Some participants benefit from nicotine fading, which is presented as an option. Participants who wish to try nicotine fading are instructed to reduce the number of cigarettes they smoke by about 10% a day and switch to a brand with lower tar and nicotine. Participants are told that they should not be discouraged if they are unable to reduce their nicotine intake substantially before the stop-smoking day of the second session. All participants, regardless of whether they attempt nicotine fading, are instructed to bring an empty pack of cigarettes to the second session.

Before the first session comes to a close, the trainer passes out the motivation scale and the contracts for participants to complete. At the end of the group, participants are invited to pair up with another person to telephone for support, if they wish to rely on another person for social support outside the family.

Description of Session 2

Welcome to our second session! By coming here you again affirm your wish to become a nonsmoker. We will start our work today with a stop-smoking ceremony. What we will do is walk, one by one, to the front of the room, crumple up your last pack of cigarettes, and throw it in the wastebasket that you see here. If you would like, feel free to make a statement, a positive affirmative statement about your feelings about being a nonsmoker as you throw out your last pack. If you are willing, say this in front of the group, along with a personal statement such as "I am a nonsmoker" or "I can stop smoking forever," and we will all show our support by clapping as you toss your last cigarette away.

Before we do this, though, let's briefly review our reasons for ending the smoking habit. Let's share a bit and talk about what we became aware of during the week. Let's talk about how our lives can change for the better when we stop smoking. I know that throwing your cigarettes away may seem to some of you like you are losing your best friend. But as we talked about last week, cigarettes are not really your friend but a deadly enemy. Reviewing our reasons for being a nonsmoker will only firm your resolve. Let's take a few minutes to review our reasons. [*Stop-smoking ritual takes place.*]

I would like us to start with your experiencing hypnosis again. You have had some practice doing this. I will give you suggestions for deepening this experience you are already familiar with. Here goes. Just close your eyes now and begin to relax, with nothing to worry, nothing to disturb . . . and moving into the familiar ground, the territory of your private relaxation . . . you can close your eyes, yes, you can close your eyes . . . so easily . . . so gently . . . eyes closing, closing, closing. Please close your eyes now to help you relax even more. I wonder if you can let yourself relax even more, calm and at ease, relaxed and secure, your mind and body working together, your conscious and your unconscious mind working together for your best good . . . partners . . . partners to protect your health, your well-being, your life . . . your breath. With each breath, let go of more and more tension, let go of whatever tension you don't need. You don't need it . . . you don't want it . . . you don't have to have it. Let any tension you don't need move out of your body, flow away from you. You don't need it; you can let go of it to feel even more comfortable. Even if your attention wanders, it's all right, but keep coming back to my voice, as I give you helpful suggestions . . . suggestions you can use.

Calm . . . peace . . . at ease . . . serene . . . nothing to bother, nothing to disturb . . . calm . . . relaxed and secure . . . centered . . . feel the strength that is within you, as you let any remaining tension that you don't need, don't want . . . drain out of you . . . leave you with each breath . . . feel even stronger as you feel the tension you don't need . . . and who needs a lot of tension? . . . flow out of your fingertips, out of your toes . . . with you feeling calmer and calmer . . . more and more open to suggestions . . . more and more tuned into your best interests . . . wouldn't it feel good to move even deeper into a wonderful state of mind, of being. . . . Imagine a favorite scene, a scene of a special place, your spot, your place, where you feel just right, so centered, so secure. Don't fall over the edge of sleep, remain awake, yet so deeply relaxed, just on the edge, with me communicating with the deepest levels of your understanding . . . all the while knowing you can tap the strength that you need from inside yourself . . . strength you will discover . . . strength that is within . . . wisdom that is there for you . . . courage that is a part of you . . . strength and courage to be what you can be . . . to do what you need to do . . . to be a nonsmoker as you were for so many years before you first smoked. Just like you let go of the tension you don't need, you can let go of any urges to smoke . . . just let them go . . . if they come back . . . let them go . . . they will pass . . . but you don't even have to think about that now . . . as you are aware of a deepening sense . . . a sense of the strength that is within . . . within you . . . discover it . . . it's there. . . . Now move toward this place in your mind . . . in your imagination . . . in your being . . . this place where you are centered and secure . . . where you can return any time you wish . . . any time you want . . . moving and moving and moving . . . flowing and flowing and flowing. . . . Change your position any time you want to go even deeper, go even deeper into your desire to preserve your health to be a nonsmoker . . . your need to free yourself from this habit . . . nothing to bother now . . . nothing to disturb . . . you can do this . . . you can be smoke-free . . . you can do this . . . yes . . . learning to do this . . . more and more . . . more and more . . . on so many levels . . . your mind more calm and clear . . . different muscle groups relaxing . . . wouldn't it be nice to relax even more? I wonder which muscles are more relaxed . . . your neck or your eyelids . . . it doesn't matter for now . . . does it . . . it really doesn't matter . . . as you approach this place . . . or are you there now . . . I don't really know . . . and is your breathing becoming slower . . . as you relax . . . as you let go . . . or are you feeling heavy or light, floating or heavy . . . or perhaps a relaxed, heavy floating feeling all in one . . . can you feel comfort and security wrapping around you like a blanket that is so comfortable? Or is your conscious mind wandering while your unconscious mind tunes into the deepest meanings, your deepest desires to be a nonsmoker . . . or are you ready to relax even more?

Go deeper now if you like . . . so comfortable and at ease . . . strength is within . . . move toward that place or maybe you are there . . . taking the steps you need . . . learning . . . to get where you are going . . . to where you want to go . . . notice words and images coming easily and naturally to you . . . healing words and images . . . cleansing words and images . . . freeing words and images . . . perhaps a key phrase is coming to you . . . something you can say any time you want . . . any time you wish . . . a phrase that touches the deepest core of your being . . . a phrase that cushions you . . . supports you . . . maybe it's an image . . . I don't know. . . . You can say this phrase or visualize your image any time you want . . . say it to yourself now . . . use it to anchor your resolve to be a nonsmoker forever.

As you do this . . . think of all the many reasons you have to stop smoking forever. Can you see a writing board? . . . Is it black or is it green . . . I don't know . . . write . . . and hear your words while reading your reasons . . . write why you will stop smoking . . . listen to your voice saying to yourself . . . talking to yourself . . . about why you will stop smoking . . . think of all the benefits . . . all you have to gain . . . health . . . money saved . . . so many benefits . . . think of even more reasons . . . let them move you deeper and deeper . . . swell your confidence . . . help you as you move toward your goal . . . your life can mean so much to you . . . so much you have to look forward to.

Perhaps your hands feel more relaxed than your feet . . . your breathing so easy . . . perhaps, if you like, you can feel your head moving ever so slightly . . . just a nod to signify a *yes* to your intention to stop smoking, just a little nod, feel your head nod, move up and down ever so slightly, a slight nod to signify *yes*, *yes* . . . *yes* to your intention to stop smoking, your unconscious mind communicating with your conscious mind your desire to be free of smoking . . . *yes* . . . *yes* . . . *yes* . . . *yes*, or if you did not feel your head move, just say *yes*, *yes* to yourself, *yes* to your intention to stop smoking. Whether you moved your head or not, let your head and body settle into a comfortable resting position and begin to create a sense of yourself, perhaps an image of yourself as a nonsmoker . . . perhaps you see yourself with others . . . or perhaps you are alone . . . feeling a sense that you can say *yes*, *yes* to your health . . . say *yes* to yourself . . . *yes* . . . take a few minutes to see yourself as a nonsmoker . . . create this image . . . see it, feel it becoming more and more real to you . . . feel a sense of the strength that is within . . . can you feel it . . . or is it becoming so much a part of you that you do not notice it? So comfortable now . . . your need to smoke . . . any urges to smoke once a part of you are fading . . . they are dissolving . . . detaching from you . . . breaking up . . . like clouds in the wind . . . like clouds on a day that the sun begins to shine through . . . the light . . . the diffuse light . . . the breeze . . . the wind . . . the gentle calm . . . it all helps you to believe you can be a nonsmoker for life . . . see yourself doing something else in situations in which you smoked in the past . . . now in your past. . . . You can resist smoking . . . any urges that come up . . . you can watch them fade . . . fade . . . like clouds in the wind . . . use your key phrase now . . . you know your strength is within . . . see yourself as a nonsmoker . . . it is coming clearer to you . . . the light is illuminating you, your reasons to stop smoking . . . your will . . . your resolve . . . the power is within you . . . you know that smoking is a poison . . . you respect yourself . . . you will protect your body . . . you need your body . . . it needs you . . . your strength . . . your willpower. . . . Watch the urge fade should it arise after our session today . . . let it come and feel it go . . .

Think about what you can do besides smoking . . . so many things . . . your conscious working with your unconscious mind . . . help you to decide what to do . . . you know that you are capable of taking care . . . taking good care . . . of others . . . of yourself . . . get in touch with your kindness . . . your caring . . . direct this toward yourself . . . learn the art of flowing with an urge . . . riding it out . . . observe it . . . breathe it out . . . it leaves your body with each breath . . . let the tension go . . . let the urge go . . . it will pass . . . ride it like a wave . . . it passes . . . go on with your life . . . don't smoke . . . go on with your life . . . don't smoke . . . breathe any urge out . . . observe it, and let it go . . . it will be replaced by something else . . . trust that it will pass . . . remember your commitment to respect your body . . . take care of yourself . . . trust that the urge will pass . . . you are your body's keeper . . . you can do so many things besides smoking . . . any urge passes . . . ride it like a wave . . . a wave that flows into the water and exists no more as it once was . . . let it flow away . . . fade away . . . you ride it out . . . you choose not to smoke . . . you get to know the person you can be as a nonsmoker . . . you do it . . . do it today . . . it is important . . . you do it.

See yourself in social situations . . . notice others supporting you . . . noticing you are not smoking anymore . . . feel their respect for you . . . you are in control . . . avoid situations in which you would be likely to smoke . . . you care about yourself . . . you take care of yourself . . . you know what you have to do . . . say *yes* to this. Reward yourself for not smoking . . . you are saving money . . . you are preserving your health . . . you are letting urges pass . . . exercise . . . eat in moderation . . .

take care of yourself . . . feel pride . . . reward yourself . . . you deserve it . . . how can you do this? Show yourself you can be good to yourself . . . yes . . . see yourself as the person you want to be . . . move toward strength . . . be that person . . . be that person. . . .

Wouldn't it be nice to feel your senses awakening? As a nonsmoker, your senses will come alive . . . touch . . . smell . . . as a nonsmoker . . . you begin to taste . . . really taste . . . you smell fresh . . . free of the stench of cigarettes . . . free of their clinging odor . . . fresh . . . beginning to regain your senses . . . becoming aware . . . like a newborn baby . . . before your senses were dulled . . . your body is healing . . . healing . . . able to taste your foods . . . as you chew them slowly . . . with enjoyment . . . eat in moderation . . . not too much . . . exercise . . . if you wish . . . you are a nonsmoker today . . . from this moment on . . . say this to yourself . . . "I am a nonsmoker from this moment on." . . . yes . . . say yes to it . . . yes . . .

Go deep into your comfort . . . deep . . . deeper and deeper . . . learning, firming your resolve . . . at ease . . . nothing to bother, nothing to disturb . . . as you go deeper and deeper and deeper, you become more aware of what you are and what you can be . . . how you can use what you have learned . . . how you will help yourself to be a nonsmoker for life . . . a new you . . . see yourself not smoking in situations in the past in which you were tempted to smoke, see yourself substituting healthy behaviors for smoking . . . choosing health and well-being . . . your senses alive . . . proud, in control . . . you do it . . . use your key phrase . . . your anchor . . . find ways to reinforce your sense of accomplishment . . . control what you do and what you do not do . . . you are no longer a slave to smoking . . . yes . . . more in charge of your life . . . say this firmly to yourself . . . I am more in charge . . . I am more in control . . . my strength is within . . . discover the strength that is within . . . I am a nonsmoker . . . realize what you can do . . . yes . . . capable of so much . . . perhaps now you can absorb this fact—every day of your life you are a nonsmoker . . . you do not smoke when you sleep . . . perhaps for 8 hours a day you do not smoke . . . perhaps more . . . perhaps less . . . you do not feel deprived yet you are not smoking when you sleep . . . your conscious and unconscious mind working together . . . your body relaxed . . . your body healing . . . now when you do not smoke during the day . . . you will heal your body even more . . . you can relax too . . . with what you have learned . . . with what you have learned.

Wouldn't it be so good to feel good . . . really good . . . peace . . . peace and serenity . . . comfort and ease . . . relaxed . . . even more secure in yourself . . . a sense of feeling worthwhile. . . . Now, as you experience these feelings, please bring your thumb and forefinger together . . . make your anchor . . . just lightly touch . . . make your anchor and feel so good and relax . . . more and more . . . more and more . . . even more confident . . . even better . . . gentle relaxation . . . gentle waves of relaxation . . . flow with a sense of ease . . . secure . . . deep . . . deep . . . relaxed . . . so good . . . so calm . . . at ease . . . yes . . . feel this in your entire body . . . relax even deeper, if you like . . . it is you who creates the feelings . . . so deep . . . you create the feeling . . . your strength . . . your security . . . is within . . . create these feelings . . . make the feelings move and flow together with your need to be a nonsmoker . . . relaxing . . . coping effectively . . . that anchor . . . a symbol of your conscious and unconscious mind working together . . . your mind and body working together . . . to help you control your thoughts and feelings in ways that are productive . . . good for you . . . for your health . . . for your self-respect. The more you practice . . . the more you develop your skills, the better you feel. . . . Practice early in the morning . . . practice during the day . . . as you do the things you do in your life . . . as you live and learn . . . more and more and more . . . more and more . . . you can program your own mind . . . to be a nonsmoker . . . tune yourself . . . tune your feelings . . . like you would tune a precision instrument . . . use your anchor . . . say your key phrase . . . review your reasons for not smoking. . . . If you experience any urges . . . use your lifetime of learnings to focus on your health and well-being as you let the urge fade away . . . it will fade away . . . it will move past you, it will drift away from you, it will dissipate, like clouds in the wind . . . like a wave of water fades into the ocean. . . . Use your anchor . . . perhaps take a deep breath and hold it in for four counts, and then as you slowly exhale, say your key phrase . . . be sure to anchor those feelings . . . you are a *nonsmoker*.

Go deep . . . even deeper . . . deeper still . . . anchored . . . grounded in your being . . . centered in yourself . . . visualize yourself in a situation in which you might in the past have been tempted to smoke . . . now anchor your resolve to be a nonsmoker . . . this sense of yourself as a nonsmoker . . . feel so good . . . lock your resolve to be a nonsmoker with good feelings . . . and the knowledge that thoughts of smoking will fade away . . . they will be gone . . . feel good, whole and together . . . your body . . . your unconscious . . . working together with your conscious . . . all of your senses working together to help you do what you need to do . . . to be a nonsmoker for life. [*Give participants suggestions to practice self-hypnosis and to use what they have learned in real-life situations, and terminate the hypnosis.*]

Research on the Program

Research on the program indicates that it achieves continuous abstinence rates ranging between 24% and 39%, across trainers, at 6-month follow-up ($N = 236$). Even though trainers used the same training manual, somewhat different outcome rates were achieved by different trainers. It is significant that at follow-up, more than one third (36%) of the participants who did not achieve continuous abstinence reported reducing the number of cigarettes smoked per day. Finally, 42% of the people who did not stop smoking were interested in either participating in follow-up treatment or acquiring additional information about other smoking-cessation treatments.

CLINICAL CONSIDERATIONS

The program can be adapted and tailored in individual work with patients to meet their unique treatment needs. However, many patients, regardless of their level of hypnotic suggestibility, can benefit from the suggestions and strategies included in the generic program. For the most part, even low suggestible individuals can easily experience suggestions that require no more than the ability to relax, focus attention, and imagine resisting smoking in different situations, for example. These observations are consistent with many studies that have failed to find a relationship between suggestibility and treatment gains in smoking cessation programs (see Green & Lynn, 2000).

Motivation to stop smoking consistently emerges as a predictor of abstinence (Green & Lynn, 2000). Every effort should thus be made to identify the unique circumstances and thoughts (e.g., negative self-talk) that perpetuate smoking behaviors. One way to do this is to videotape participants as they say "I am a nonsmoker" and ask them whether they believe the statement. Patients can be repeatedly taped and questioned until they are satisfied that their affirmation that they are a nonsmoker is credible. Often 3 to 5 tapings are needed, but it may take as many as 10 trials before the patient expresses a modicum of satisfaction. After each taping, participants can carefully examine and challenge thoughts that precluded their stating, with conviction, "I am a nonsmoker." Often this technique reveals specific thoughts that stifle motivation to stop smoking; following are some examples, along with possible rebuttals in parentheses:

- "I can't stop now; it will disrupt my life." ("Perhaps, but a short-term disruption is worth the long-term benefits of being a nonsmoker. Cancer, or a serious smoking-related disease, is much more disruptive and can be fatal.")
- "Cigarettes are my best friend." ("Consider the evidence; cigarettes are a health hazard, your dire enemy.")
- "I'll be miserable if I stop smoking." ("Maybe, maybe not. But even if stopping is difficult at first, I can help you cope with discomfort, and in the long run, you will be much happier.")
- "I'll balloon in weight." ("Weight gain can be minimized or prevented by following a straightforward plan for weight management. Even if you gain a few pounds, the health risks of

continuing to smoke are far greater than the risks associated with gaining a small amount of weight.")

- "I've tried before and failed." ("True, but with each attempt to stop you increase your odds of success. If you work hard at it this time, it is likely you will be able to stop.").

Another approach to identifying treatment-interfering cognitions involves a two-chair technique in which patients take a seat in a chair opposite their own and are instructed to "speak with the voice of your addiction and say something along the lines of 'You need me; what would you do without me? You can depend on me.'" In this context, the patient is told to elaborate all of the positive things they get from smoking, with the goal of uncovering secondary gains associated with smoking as well as doubts and ambivalent feelings about being a nonsmoker. Patients then take a seat in their own chair and counter their positive statements about smoking and ambivalence about being a nonsmoker with reasons it is vitally important that they achieve abstinence. In the dialogue that unfolds, as the patient alternates from chair to chair, the therapist has the opportunity to challenge maladaptive thoughts and reinforce reasons for ending the smoking habit.

Age-progression techniques can assist patients in envisioning a future in which they are free of the urge to smoke and confident in their ability to be a nonsmoker for life. Participants can then be asked how they achieved this smoke-free status. Often, specific impediments and negative thoughts that preclude this possible future from coming to fruition can be identified and addressed with this protocol.

WEIGHT LOSS

One common roadblock to being a nonsmoker is the fear of weight gain. This fear is based in reality: More than three fourths of people who try to stop smoking will gain weight (USDHHS, 1990), with weight gain averaging 6 pounds for men and 9 pounds for women (Williamson, Gleaves, & Lawson, 1991). We provide participants with a handout with the following recommendations for participants concerned about stabilizing their weight in the long term: (a) eat a well-balanced diet; (b) monitor and limit caloric intake and portions; (c) avoid or limit snacking (i.e., restricting the time and place of eating); (d) exercise three times a week or more; (e) use fullness cues to moderate eating; (f) practice restraint by leaving food on the plate at some if not all meals; (g) use cue-controlled relaxation in situations that trigger excessive food consumption; (h) eat slowly and take time-outs from eating during meals; (i) when there is a dawning sense of bingeing, rinse out the mouth to diminish sensory cues (see also Levitt, 1993); and (j) increase physical activity. If obesity is already a problem, additional tips and strategies for losing weight can be found in chapter 7.

Multiple treatment attempts and a range of interventions are often required to achieve more than temporary abstinence from smoking (Ziedonis & Williams, 2003). Hypnosis, combined with cognitive–behavioral methods and pharmacological treatments to ease withdrawal symptoms, can be a viable approach to a pervasive and often intractable problem. Our program is time efficient, cost effective, and rated positively even by participants who do not achieve complete abstinence. It can be individually tailored and presented to participants as hypnosis, relaxation, or a strictly cognitive–behavioral intervention, with references to hypnosis deleted.

7

EATING DISORDERS AND OBESITY

Since the late 1970s, interest in hypnotic techniques for eating disorders has burgeoned as it became apparent that hypnosis could supplement a variety of therapeutic procedures. In this chapter, we describe how hypnosis can be used as an adjunct to a well-established and empirically supported cognitive–behavioral therapy (CBT) for eating disorders (Fairburn, 1985) and obese patients (Fairburn, Marcus, & Wilson, 1993). Because interpersonal problems often contribute to disordered eating, the treatment we present incorporates interpersonal interventions into a multifaceted CBT treatment.

Our discussion centers on the treatment of bulimia and obese binge eaters for the following reasons: (a) Bulimia and obesity are much more common than anorexia; (b) treatment effectiveness has been well documented for women with bulimia and obese women but not rigorously evaluated for women with anorexia; and (c) women with bulimia are more responsive to hypnotic suggestions than both women with anorexia and normative samples of college students (Covino, Jimerson, Wolfe, Franko, & Frankel, 1994; Griffiths & Channon-Little, 1993; Pettinati, Horne, & Staats, 1985; Pettinati, Kogan, Margolis, Shrier, & Wade, 1989). In fact, Gross (1983) found that only 10% of 500 patients with anorexia were amenable to hypnotic treatment; the remainder expressed an underlying fear of losing control over their ability to lose weight. Before we discuss

---

This chapter was coauthored with Maryellen Crowley and Anna Campion.

specific hypnotic procedures, we present information pertinent to the prevalence of eating disorders in the population as well as empirically supported techniques for treating bulimia and anorexia and, later in our discussion, overeating and obesity.

PREVALENCE OF EATING DISORDERS

Although the number of men endorsing bulimic symptoms has risen in the past decade, bulimia nervosa (BN) is still a woman's disorder. Indeed, 95% of people who receive an eating disorder diagnosis are women (Hoek, 1991). Bulimia is the most common major eating disorder, with a prevalence of about 1% to 3% of the population (L. W. Craighead, 2002). The essential symptoms of bulimia are (a) recurrent episodes of binge eating, at least twice a week for 3 months; (b) compensatory measures to prevent weight gain such as purging, excessive exercise, and misuse of laxatives, diuretics, and enemas; and (c) self-evaluation that is unduly influenced by weight and body shape (American Psychiatric Association, 1994). The symptoms of bulimia fluctuate in frequency and severity for a large percentage of people, but for a small subgroup, the symptoms persist despite many treatment attempts (Fairburn & Beglin, 1990).

Obesity is a serious health problem that increases the risk of coronary heart disease, stroke, cancer, osteoarthritis, hypertension, Type II diabetes, gallbladder disease, sleep apnea, and respiratory problems. According to federal guidelines released in 1998, individuals with a body mass index (BMI; a description of body weight in relation to height) of 25 or more are overweight and those with a BMI of 30 and above are obese. Approximately 55% to 65% of the American population is obese or overweight, and the number is growing.

Anorexia nervosa (AN) is less common than bulimia and obesity, with rates of AN ranging from 0.5% to 1% (L. W. Craighead, 2002). AN is diagnosed when there is a refusal to maintain body weight at or above a minimally normal weight for age and height (e.g., body weight less than 85% of that expected), along with an intense fear of gaining weight or becoming fat. Fear of fatness is accompanied by a disturbance in the way in which body weight or shape is experienced. Concerns about body shape can become paramount so that women with anorexia stubbornly deny the seriousness of their low body weight and strongly resist pressures from family and others to gain weight. Some researchers estimate the mortality rate for AN at 10%, one of the highest mortality rates for all psychiatric conditions, with a 5% mortality rate over each decade of follow-up (P. F. Sullivan, 1995). Amenorrhea (i.e., the absence of at least three consecutive menstrual cycles) also must be present to warrant a diagnosis of AN, which may be either the food restricting or the bingeing–purging type.

In contrast with the relatively low rates of bulimia and anorexia, the rates of subclinical eating disorders, or eating disorder not otherwise specified, is alarmingly high. The fact that an additional 8% to 16% of young women fall short of a diagnosis of bulimia by only one symptom or display significantly disordered eating patterns (L. W. Craighead, 2002; Spitzer et al., 1992) implies that many women are predisposed to develop eating disorders. Bulimic symptoms often do not occur in isolation: At least half of patients with bulimia are eligible for a second diagnosis, most frequently depression, anxiety, or substance abuse, and half of patients with bulimia have a personality disorder (Lewinsohn, Striegel-Moore, & Seeley, 2000; Wonderlich & Mitchell, 1997).

RESEARCH ON TREATMENT

Psychotherapy can restore normal eating and improve the lives of many women with eating disorders. A meta-analysis (Thompson-Brenner, Glass, & Westen, 2003) of psychotherapy trials for BN published between 1980 and 2000 revealed that approximately 40% of patients who complete treatment recover completely. The most effective treatments for eating disorders are CBT and interpersonal therapy (IPT). CBT is semistructured and problem focused (Wilson & Fairburn, 1993). Primary treatment goals include (a) modifying dysfunctional attitudes toward body shape, weight, and dieting; (b) replacing dangerous dieting behaviors with healthier eating patterns; and (c) developing coping skills to combat urges to binge and purge. CBT is typically conducted over 20 weekly sessions, after which a limited number of bimonthly posttreatment sessions can be added to evaluate progress (Wilson & Fairburn, 1993).

CBT is widely regarded as the treatment of choice for BN. Note that CBT research participants typically do not have comorbid diagnoses. In fact, some research shows that certain patients, including those with borderline features (e.g., Coker, Vize, Wade, & Cooper, 1993), do not derive much benefit from CBT. Hence, researchers have investigated IPT as a viable treatment option. This treatment was originally developed for depression (Klerman, Weissman, Rounsaville, & Chevron, 1984) and focuses on the identification and modification of current interpersonal problems based on adaptive coping with interpersonal stress and conflict (Fairburn, 1997). IPT is based on the observation that most eating disorders emerge toward the end of adolescence when interpersonal issues are most prominent. Binge eating serves as a maladaptive coping mechanism for dealing with negative emotions associated with problematic relationships with family and friends (Fairburn & Wilson, 1993). The treatment course of IPT is typically 19 sessions over an 18-week period, with eight initial semiweekly sessions, followed by eight weekly sessions and three final sessions separated by two-week intervals (Fairburn & Wilson, 1993).

Empirical Support

The empirical support for both treatments is impressive. Fairburn (1985) developed a detailed manual for the treatment of binge eating and BN, with adaptations for individuals with other eating disorders (Fairburn, 1985; Fairburn, Marcus, & Wilson, 1993). His manualized protocol has played an indispensable role in fostering the widespread use and evaluation of CBT for bulimia. CBT is successful in eliminating bingeing and purging in approximately half of patients with bulimia (Wilson & Fairburn, 2002). CBT is superior to antidepressant drug treatment, supportive psychotherapy, focal psychotherapy, purely behavioral therapy, and exposure therapy (Wilfley et al., 1993; Wilson & Fairburn, 2002).

IPT rivals the long-term effectiveness of CBT in head-to-head comparisons. The controlled outcome studies of IPT reported to date are based on Klerman et al.'s (1984) depression treatment manual, adapted for eating disorders. In one study (Fairburn, Jones, Peveler, Hope, & O'Connor, 1993), binge eating was reduced by 95% and maintained over a 12-month follow-up period for both CBT and IPT treatment groups. There also was a 90.9% reduction in purging at 12-month follow-up across the two groups, as well as a reduction in degree of dietary restraint for both groups. Six-year follow-up revealed that half of the treated participants no longer binged (Fairburn et al., 1995). Wilfley et al. (1993) found that both group IPT and CBT were equally effective in significantly reducing binge-eating behavior for up to 1 year following treatment. In the most recent study (Agras, Walsh, Fairburn, Wilson, & Kraemer, 2000), after treatment, CBT was found to be superior to IPT. However, at longer follow-ups, ranging from 4 to 12 months, the treatments were comparable in terms of remission from binge eating and purging, as assessed over the preceding 4 weeks.

CBT treatment effects likely emerge more rapidly because of the focus on eating habits and dysfunctional thoughts, which may translate more directly into better psychosocial functioning (Fairburn, Jones, et al., 1993). Nevertheless, the fact that CBT and IPT yield reasonably equivalent long-term outcomes underlines the importance of considering interpersonal factors in the treatment of bulimia (Wilfley et al., 1993; Wilson & Pike, 2001).

Anorexia

Much less research has been conducted on effective treatment methods for AN than for bulimia because of the chronic course of the disorder, treatment resistance associated with reluctance to adopt more normal eating patterns, and, in certain cases, the need for inpatient or hospital treatment necessary to restore healthy weight levels (Gross, 1983). Nevertheless, the core mechanisms of anorexia are very similar to those operating in bulimia, and it is "therefore reasonable to expect that CBT, suitably adapted, would be a useful treatment for anorexia" (Wilson & Fairburn, 2002, p. 576). Conversely, methods that have shown promise with patients with anorexia are likely to benefit individuals with bulimia. The treatment of anorexia can be prolonged and typically runs 12 months, with a recommended 6- to 12-month follow-up (Wilson & Fairburn, 2002). A multifaceted approach to treatment is often adopted that combines elements of IPT, insight-oriented approaches, and family therapy, along with CBT.

HYPNOSIS IN THE TREATMENT OF EATING DISORDERS

Crasilneck and Hall (1975) were among the first to report the successful use of hypnotic techniques with patients with anorexia. They noted marked improvement in more than half of the 70 cases of anorexia they treated with suggestions for enjoyment of eating and increased hunger. Kroger and Fezler (1976), Kroger (1977), and H. Spiegel and Spiegel (1978) reported that hypnosis could be used as an adjunct to behavior modification programs to increase treatment compliance.

Since the early 1980s, clinical case reports have touted the ability of hypnosis to increase patients' self-control and solidify cognitive restructuring. Although rigorously controlled studies are lacking, research and clinical case reports suggest that hypnosis can be useful in treating both bulimia and anorexia (M. Barabasz, 2000; Griffiths, 1989; Gross, 1983; Hornyak, 1996; Lynn, Rhue, Kvaal, & Mare, 1993; Nash & Baker, 1993; Torem, 1992; Vanderlinden & Vandereycken, 1988; Yapko, 1986; D. Young, 1995). For example, Nash and Baker (1993) described a multimodal treatment for AN that succeeded in treating 76% of 36 women at 12-month follow-up. The protocol combined hypnotherapy with individual therapy, group therapy, and psychotropic medication. Hypnosis was used to reduce tension, enhance mastery and independence, foster feelings of self-control, and support realistic body awareness. The authors reported that only 53% of a group of 31 women who were treated identically but without the use of hypnosis achieved the same level of symptom remission and weight stabilization.

Thakur (1980) reported substantial improvement in 10 of 18 individuals with anorexia treated with hypnotherapy, after a 6-month to 5-year follow-up. The most detailed description of hypnotic methods was provided by Gross (1983) in reference to a sample of 50 patients with anorexia. Gross used hypnosis to correct distorted body image, increase awareness of internal cues, build self-esteem, and engender a sense of control over eating. Gross contended that hypnosis is appropriate with AN only when a nonauthoritarian approach is taken that avoids the use of direct suggestions for weight gain.

As previously alluded to, a variety of behavioral and cognitive–behavioral methods were used in early clinical studies. Vanderlinden and Vandereycken (1988) more recently systematically integrated hypnosis into a multidimensional bulimia treatment that included cognitive–behavioral as well as interpersonal elements. For example, patients were asked to imagine themselves sitting at the table while they eat and enjoy a meal. Suggestions were then given for eating slowly, enjoying the taste of the food, and relaxing afterward. Vanderlinden and Verdereycken (1988) also described a variety of other cognitive–behavioral and hypnotic suggestions for planned reduction of binges, adaptive coping and relapse prevention, cognitive restructuring and reframing, and age regression to a time prior to the onset of BN and age progression to a time when the patient is no longer vexed by bulimic symptoms. Jacka (1997) has suggested that hypnosis can be used to catalyze a variety of cognitive–behavioral interventions including eating only at set, regular times; letting hunger become a trigger for eating by reducing the amount eaten at meals (not to be used with AN); avoiding fast foods and lengthening food preparation; eliminating unnecessary temptations; sticking to the shopping list; ensuring that a meal is eaten slowly, prolonged to at least 20 minutes; and identifying and disputing irrational eating-related thoughts (e.g., "If I eat chocolate, I'm finished"). And most germane to the approach we present, Griffiths presented several case studies (1984, 1997) illustrating how hypnosis can be incorporated into a CBT program like Fairburn's (1985), and she published a brief treatment manual for her approach (Griffiths, 1995), which she termed *hypnobehavioral treatment*.

Introducing Hypnosis

Given deep concerns about control held by women with bulimia, the administration of hypnotic suggestions should be presented in the context of self-hypnosis in which wholehearted cooperation is essential (see Lynn, Neufeld, & Mare, 1993; Nash & Baker, 1993). Generally, we postpone hypnosis until after a positive therapeutic alliance has been established, and hypnosis is viewed as congruent with overarching goals and objectives. We strive to convey the idea that hypnosis can enhance control over eating as well as the ability to tolerate, accept, and contend with difficult feelings.

If patients balk at the prospect of learning self-hypnosis, especially after we do our best to disabuse them of common misconceptions about hypnosis, we do not persist in trying to sell hypnosis. Instead, we note that a variety of techniques that are not strictly speaking hypnosis but nevertheless involve imagery and suggestion can be used to achieve control over eating. Indeed, all of the hypnotic techniques we recommend can be implemented without defining them as hypnosis. If hypnosis is attempted with patients with borderline features or major dissociative tendencies, the procedures should be modified to emphasize safety, security, and self-soothing on an ongoing basis.

Assessment

Apart from determining whether hypnosis is appropriate, the assessment of patients with eating disorders entails garnering the following information: (a) the patient's current mental status and diagnosis; (b) motivation for treatment; (c) the personal, interpersonal, and familial context in which the eating disorder is enmeshed and maintained; (d) developmental milestones and major life events, (e) problems with self-esteem, depression, anxiety, and personality disorders, as well as other potentially comorbid conditions (Wonderlich & Mitchell, 1997); (f) body image distortion and fear of fatness, dieting history, and bingeing–purging patterns; (g) excessive exercise, diuretic and syrup of ipecac (a dangerous poison used to vomit) use, and diet pills and laxative abuse; (h) suicide potential; and (i) screening for physical and sexual abuse.

The selection of specific tactics, including the extent to which interpersonal themes and interventions are incorporated into treatment, depends on a behavioral or functional analysis (i.e., antecedents, accompaniments, consequences) of disordered eating. To canvass the nature and quality of the patient's interpersonal functioning, the therapist should scrutinize the patient's entire social network and support structure. Because sociotropy—the need for approval from others and "people pleasing"—is related to eating disorder symptoms (M. A. Friedman & Wishman, 1998), it merits evaluation, as does perfectionism, which has emerged as a long-term predictor of dysfunctional eating behaviors (Joiner, Heatherton, Rudd, & Schmidt, 1997). We strongly recommend formalizing ongoing assessment by administering well-validated instruments such as the Eating Attitudes Test (Garner & Garfinkel, 1979), the Eating Disorders Inventory—2 (Garner, 1991), the Eating Disorders Examination (Cooper & Fairburn, 1987), and the Beck Depression Inventory (see Beck, Steer, & Garbin, 1988).

Incessant dieting can lead to a potpourri of serious and potentially life-threatening medical complications including endocrinological disturbances (e.g., amenorrhea), cardiovascular complications (e.g., hypertension, bradycardia, and arrythmias), and gastrointestinal, hematological, and immunological difficulties (see Garske, 1991; Sheinin, 1988). Therefore, a thorough assessment of health status that includes consultation with medical practitioners, when appropriate, should be undertaken. Typically, hospitalization is recommended when weight loss reaches 20% to 30% below ideal body weight because when starvation becomes severe, cognitive disturbances prevent patients from benefiting from outpatient treatment (Andersen, 1995). Day treatment or partial hospitalization has become more popular in recent times. Andersen's (1995) review of 25 controlled trials indicated that in only a small percentage of cases is inpatient or day hospital treatment necessary. However, inpatient treatment is mandatory for individuals in medical or physical danger, as well as for patients who exhibit a poor response to outpatient treatment or severe psychological problems.

Cognitive–Behavioral Therapy and Hypnosis

Fairburn's cognitive–behavioral approach is divided into three stages, which we describe in the following section, along with hypnotic techniques that can potentially augment treatment effects. Because learned techniques build on each other, the ordering of stages is more critical to the success of treatment than is the precise timing of their introduction (Fairburn, Marcus, & Wilson, 1993).

Stage 1: Sessions 1 Through 10

The primary goals of Stage 1 are to introduce CBT and its basic tenets and to begin to supplant disordered eating behaviors with healthier, more balanced eating patterns. Key goals of this stage are (a) educating the patient about the adverse cyclical effects of dieting, bingeing, purging, and compensatory measures; (b) offering more adaptive alternatives for weight regulation; and (c) teaching the patient how to self-monitor eating behaviors (Wilson & Fairburn, 1993). The therapist and patient also agree on a healthy weight range based on BMI, and cautions are proffered about the ineffectiveness of compensatory methods.

Introducing hypnosis into treatment typically adds one to three sessions to the 20-week program. After a working rapport has been established and the patient has experienced self-hypnosis, suggestions along the following lines can be administered not only to introduce self-monitoring but to help the patient better understand the vicious circle of dieting, bingeing–purging, and laxative abuse (Polivy & Herman, 1985).

Let's try to understand this vicious circle by your entering self-hypnosis and doing the following: Sit back, relax, close your eyes, and imagine you are watching a special television. You can watch and experience yourself on this television. With each channel you go back a number with your remote control (starting with the patient's current age), you move a year back in time, and with the fine-tuning control on your remote, you can tune into the exact time when you first experienced a binge and a purge. At any point, you can stop the action, or slow it down with the stop and the speed controls. You will be able to describe what is happening in a calm, detached manner, as an objective observer, a complete reporter.

Now, slowly, slowly, tune . . . go back, one year at a time . . . slowly . . . to the year, and when you get there let me know . . . just say, "I'm there" . . . good. Now fine-tune to the time just before the binge. Tell me exactly what is happening . . . what you are thinking and feeling . . . what is going on. . . . What prompts this first experience? . . . Good. Now watch the binge unfold. What foods are you eating? How much? What are the exact circumstances? What are you thinking . . . feeling? Good. And now the purging episode . . . What are you thinking and feeling? . . . What are you doing? Now the binge is over. What are you feeling? What are you thinking? What do you do next, or feel like doing?

By repeating the exercise with the most recent binge as well as a number of intermediate episodes the target of age regression, the therapist can track the progression of the disorder and determine whether thoughts, feelings, and behaviors have changed or rigidified since the inception of the binge–purge cycle, the exact nature of which is revealed to the patient by way of Socratic questioning (Beck, 1976). The goal of the questioning is to elucidate the nature of the vicious circle of dieting and bingeing–purging and to convey the following points. First, purging is rewarded and likely to recur because it relieves anxious feelings after excessive eating and averts weight gain. Purging sets up subsequent bouts of overeating because vomiting allows the patient to compensate for or "undo" the binge and to rationalize subsequent overeating (e.g., "I can always get rid of the ice cream"). In addition, it is easier to purge with a fuller stomach, which abets overeating. Second, guilt, shame, diminished self-esteem, and other negative emotions, which attend binges, are mitigated by the resolve to adhere to a rigid diet. However, dieting increases preoccupations about weight and physical appearance, while food deprivation engenders the temptation to binge eat. Third, the imposition of strict dieting rules leads to the notion that all control over eating is lost in the event of even small lapses or deviations from "the rules." And fourth, as eating spirals out of control, self-esteem continues to plummet, which in turn increases concerns about dieting and the likelihood of a binge, thus completing the self-destructive circle.

The exercises also constitute an introduction to self-monitoring and afford an opportunity for the therapist and patient to gain an initial and crucial understanding of the situational antecedents and interrelated thoughts, feelings, and behaviors surrounding binge eating and purging. Patients are asked to maintain written diaries of their eating behavior and weight. Forms are typically provided for this purpose. Eating behavior entries may include date, time, situational context, type and amount of food eaten, and motivation for eating (e.g., hunger, pleasure, emotional comfort).

Posthypnotic suggestions, as follows, can be given to self-monitor between sessions and record eating and any tendencies to binge, noting in particular situational triggers, and accompanying thoughts and feelings:

> During the coming week you will be able to harness all of your observational powers, your creative intelligence, your insight, and your motivation to learn more about your eating behaviors and the vicious circle we talked about. You will be able to tune into yourself and your surroundings, to be alert and aware as you go through your day, eat your food, and record your observations on the sheets I will provide. ... You will note what you eat, how much, what you feel and think, and, if you overeat or binge, you will have a keen, clear sense of what you are doing, feeling, and thinking just before and when you overeat, as well as thereafter. This will start you on the road to gaining more awareness, to tuning in instead of checking out. You can start nurturing yourself by treating your body with respect, giving yourself a choice, taking charge of your life, what you put into yourself, when, and how much. In this way, you will be able to identify high-risk situations, such as a party, work, dinner at a friend's house, or shopping at a mall, in which you are most likely to binge or be tempted to binge. I'd also like you to weigh yourself. Not every day. Once a week. In the morning. Perhaps Wednesday, perhaps Thursday. Maybe you will select another day. It really doesn't matter. You choose. Surprise me. Know that what you are doing is important. This will allow you to look for meaningful changes in weight, rather than multiple weigh-ins, which reflect too much variability. We will learn together, we will work together in this way, a team, learning and using the knowledge we glean to help you to achieve your goals.

Stage 1 paves the groundwork for the tasks that follow. In three or four sessions, it is possible for the patient to identify high-risk situations and thoughts such as "I'm a pig and totally out of control," "I blew it; just look at how fat I am," "So much for my diet; I might as well get into the chips and chocolate," and "I've got to eat even less; I'm turning into a blimp" that might occur after as well as before a binge. The goal is to achieve a dawning recognition of the connection among thoughts, feelings, dieting, and bingeing behaviors, which will be fleshed out in the next stage.

Many patients with eating disorders equate change in therapy with threat as well as opportunity. After all, successful treatment demands that they relinquish behaviors that relieve anxiety, at least in the short run. Many patients are so demoralized by the time they embark on therapy that they question whether therapy will make much of a difference. Early in therapy, it is important to empathize with the patient's fears and doubts and to acknowledge the value placed on bingeing as a means of coping with the demands of everyday life. However, the following positive suggestions regarding the benefits of risk and change provide a necessary counterpoint to consideration of the difficulties of relinquishing bingeing and dieting:

> Go deep, deeper and deeper into your self-hypnosis. . . . Realize, recognize that bingeing is a quick fix that fixes nothing. . . . The anxiety relief you experience is only for the very short run, and then it is replaced with concerns about dieting and physical appearance, and the inevitable bad feelings about yourself. . . . Now I'd like you to look into what I will call the mirror of the future. See yourself in this mirror, a healthy weight, at a time when your life does not center on food and eating, when you realize that you are more than what you eat, and how much you eat, and you have a sense of yourself as a whole person, nurturing and caring for your whole self, in control of your life, not overeating, not purging . . . not dieting but eating in moderation . . . sensibly. . . . Take your time . . . think of the many reasons you have for learning to better tolerate discomfort, to find better ways of coping, comfortable and at ease . . . without resorting to quick fixes. . . . See yourself as being more accepting of who you are, what you are, the person you are, better able to let go of needless self-criticism, able to express your needs to others, no longer embarrassed by your eating behaviors. . . . Wouldn't that be nice, more in control, feeling good about yourself, nothing to bother, nothing to disturb, your weight in the healthy target range; what you see in the mirror of the future can and will become your present. You have the strength that is within, the strength within to make what you see your future reality. At any time you want, recapture this sense of yourself, close your eyes, even for a moment, and gaze into the mirror of the future, and fortify your resolve.

In the next four or five sessions, considerable attention is devoted to record review, reinforcing the model, and education, including a discussion of the idea of a set-point weight that the body tries to protect. Hypnotic suggestions to enhance imaginative rehearsal can be very useful at this point to normalize eating patterns. The following suggestions also are geared toward expanding the patient's interpersonal horizons and moving away from eating and its vicissitudes as the focal point of life.

> Now let's review our eating plan, with you attending very, very carefully to my words, absorbing everything, taking in just as much as you need to, doing it for yourself, translating suggestions into actions you carry out today, tomorrow, and the next day, and on and on . . . into the future, aware . . . living fully in the best way possible. You have a strong sense of yourself . . . able to follow through with what we have agreed on. Develop images of carrying out each task, doing what you

need to do . . . acting in your own behalf . . . meeting with success . . . your strength and will . . . shining through . . . you can do it . . . moving toward more normal eating patterns . . . moving in the right direction . . . moving with deliberation, planning your steps, small and easy, planning your meals, putting thought into what you take into yourself, not just swallowing anything, but thinking, deliberating, each day . . . each day . . . exciting in its own way, new . . . full of surprises, but what you eat is no mystery, and there's a comfort in that, a surety in that, knowing what and when to eat . . . at least for now . . . eating three planned meals, and three snacks that you plan to eat each day . . . yes . . . we'll start with the first meal of the day, breakfast, break your fast, but stick to your plan. We'll talk about what you will do, what you will eat after this exercise, but already you have some ideas. . . . You are in the early stages of planning, now see yourself eating food, food you plan to eat, food that is good for you, healthy, see yourself eating slowly, slowly, chewing your food slowly, tasting it and enjoying it, feeling the food in your body, aware of the nutrients providing your body with what it needs . . . to be healthy . . . feeling good about it, sticking to your plan, staying with it, you can do it, prepare or eat only as much food as you have planned, that's how you start, small steps, and you can keep it all in you, all the food you planned to eat . . . as in the interpersonal arena of your life, you begin to have more access to your feelings, hiding less behind your eating problems . . . coming out of yourself . . . expressing yourself . . . feeling comfortable . . . assertive . . . you have needs . . . caring about yourself, caring about others, avoiding the foods you binged on in the past, new habits forming, growing, see yourself saying *no* to your favorite junk food—ice cream—see yourself avoiding it, and see yourself avoiding the places you used to binge, see yourself removing the ice cream from your study at the desk where you would overeat in the past, see yourself saying, "I won't binge." Say to yourself, "No, I can do something else, and I will." . . . Dispose of the junk food, say *no* to the old ways, start fresh, as you eat fresh fruits and vegetables we talked about, healthy meals. . . . If you feel tempted to overeat you can interrupt the urge, let it pass . . . ride the urge out . . . surf it like a wave . . . do one or more of the things we talked about, take a walk which makes you strong, engage in active coping . . . read a book, work on a school assignment, call a friend . . . realize this . . . you have many options to choose from, especially if you slow down to see them. . . . See yourself feeling tempted but resisting temptation . . . say *yes* to saying *no*, feel the good feeling of nurturing and protecting your body, feel your strength, feel your resolve firming, your strength growing . . . and now take another look into the mirror of the future, see yourself no longer trapped in the vicious circle we have talked about, see yourself smiling . . . feeling healthy, fit and strong, a sense of accomplishment.

Even at this relatively early point in treatment, patients can enter self-hypnosis and practice progressive relaxation and impulse management techniques to cope with high-risk situations and incipient urges to overeat. We recommend frequent body scans to isolate tension spots and practice in tension reduction, by "releasing all the tension you don't need," as described in chapter 4. However, a caveat is in order. With individuals who report increased negative body obsessions with progressive muscle relaxation, it is necessary to use other techniques, including (a) anchoring methods in which the thumb and forefinger are brought together as a cue to experience a sense of calm and resolve (see chap. 4); (b) the use of key phrases such as "strength is within" or "healthy eating is self-nurturing" to combat the urge to binge; (c) observing the urge to binge until it dissipates; (d) visualization techniques such as at the first signs of overeating, interrupting the habitual behavior and observing the self on a TV not avoiding the problem but calling a friend and disposing of the food; (e) when snacking excessively or overeating, getting a sense that one can stop at any time and become aware that one is consuming excessive amounts of food; feel one's entire body slowed to the point that it takes great effort to continue dysfunctional eating; (f) focusing on the costs of the binge–purge cycle and the rewards of breaking it; and (g) binge postponement, which is analogous to worry postponement (described in chap. 9), in which patients cope with the urge to binge by deferring overeating for increasing lengths of time (Cooper, Todd, & Wells, 2000). Patients can be encouraged to say something to themselves along the lines of "I won't say I can't binge, but I must do X errands first." Maneuvers of this sort can reduce the urge to binge.

Stage 2: Eight Sessions

Successful completion of Stage 2 involves achieving certain goals set forth in Stage 1, particularly reducing the frequency of binge eating and purging. Once the pattern of binge eating is interrupted and less consistent, cognitive restructuring and problem solving can begin. A behavioral analysis is conducted by the patient and therapist together to identify situational precursors (high-risk situations) as well as irrational or dysfunctional thoughts and mood swings reliably associated with binge eating, as determined by a review of self-monitoring records and an increased focus in therapy on problematic thoughts and their relation to subsequent eating behaviors. By this time, the patient may be well aware that depression, interpersonal stressors (e.g., tension at work, relationship difficulties), and certain thoughts reliably precede a binge.

Cognitive restructuring begins with an explanation of the link between thoughts and feelings and actions, as well as a description of the key features of unbidden, automatic thoughts, which frequently recur in everyday life, as described in detail in chapter 8. Common dysfunctional thoughts in BN (Garner & Bemis, 1982) often fall into the categories of dichotomous reasoning (e.g., "I ate a chocolate; I'm a total failure"), overgeneralization (e.g., "I ate a chocolate. It just shows I can't resist eating anything sweet"), magnification (e.g., "I ate a chocolate. It proves I have little self-control"), and emotional reasoning ("I feel fat, so I must be fat"). Many patients freely report these thoughts and are at least vaguely cognizant of their irrational or distorted nature.

However, identifying dysfunctional attitudes, which give rise to the automatic thoughts, is often more difficult because the patient is unaware of them and they must be inferred from patterns of behavior. These attitudes are commonly entangled with global issues of perfectionism ("I must be perfect in everything I do"), self-worth ("I'm worthless and not lovable"), self-control ("I'm totally out of control"), and guilt ("I'm a bad person and don't deserve to feel good about myself"; Fairburn, Marcus, & Wilson, 1993).

Cognitive restructuring techniques can be readily applied to challenge the dysfunctional beliefs of patients with bulimia. These techniques, described in greater detail in later chapters, include objectively assessing the evidence for a particular thought or prediction (e.g., Has the situation turned out that way before? What's the person's recent track record? If it were another person would the inference be the same?), reestimating the probability of a negative outcome (e.g., "Is there a 100% likelihood that you will binge if you eat a single chocolate?"), and directly challenging specific ideas ("Is it true that you must never binge again, to be loved?"). Another cognitive restructuring technique is to evaluate the pros and cons of holding a particular belief. For example, the therapist might ask if anything is to be gained when the patient tells herself that she is totally out of control when she eats a cookie and that she must be in control all of the time. Acceptance of how one feels at a given time and a consideration of healthy alternative, self-nurturing actions and positive coping statements can be much more helpful than all-or-nothing thinking (i.e., seeing the world in starkly black-and-white terms) and negative self-labeling. Although one patient we treated initially verbalized that these sorts of self-critical statements minimized the likelihood of bingeing, a careful review of her records indicated that such thoughts predictably generated negative emotions and preceded bingeing.

Interventions along the following lines can broaden the patient's definition of self-worth beyond issues of shape and weight and help her to develop a more positive self-evaluation independent of her dysfunctional eating behaviors.

Now move deeper and deeper into your self-hypnosis. That's good. I'd like you to tell me about a person you admire. See this person in your mind's eye. Click the snapshot when you are ready. It might be a person you know in everyday life, or it might be a person you have never met. It doesn't matter. What is important is that you get a sense of this person. You know what they are like at the deepest levels of their being. What are they like? What do you respect about this individual? What do you like about this person? Imagine you are doing something with this person. How do you feel in the person's presence? When you feel you have a clear picture and a sense of this person, please share your impressions with me.

Often patients make no mention of the admired individual's weight or physical appearance. Rather, their respect stems from personal qualities including consideration, caring, kindness, empathy, intelligence, sense of humor, work ethic, artistic or athletic abilities, and the self-acceptance and comfort the patient feels in the person's presence. The glaring disparity between the patient's valuation of others and her self-evaluation affords the therapist the opportunity to vigorously challenge the patient's single-minded concentration on superficial criteria of self-evaluation that center on appearance.

After patients engage in this exercise and effectively challenge distorted beliefs, they can again be given suggestions to gaze at themselves in the mirror of the future, or if this image is too emotionally loaded, a television of the future, changed by their new self-perceptions and more adaptive thoughts. Can they envision themselves as happier? Can they tune into their positive qualities? Can they begin to believe "I am more than my weight" and "I am more than my physical body"? Can they have greater respect for the person they see in the mirror (or television screen)? Do they feel more in control? If the answers are not in the affirmative, a careful assessment of why this is the case can suggest avenues for subsequent cognitive restructuring. If patients prove resistant to cognitive interventions, more emphasis should be placed on behavioral and interpersonal approaches (Fairburn & Wilson, 1993).

Apart from cognitive restructuring, an important goal of Stage 2 involves reinforcing the idea that the root of the problem is in extreme dietary rules and underscoring the importance of eliminating dieting. As in the following example, hypnosis can be used to create a hierarchy of forbidden foods—that is, junk foods that can be gradually introduced in the diet in healthy amounts, starting with the food that evokes the least anxiety or concern.

Go deep into your self-hypnosis. . . . Imagine a large table that is set with the foods that you like, foods you have binged on in the past and are most tempting. The table is beautifully set, the foods presented in an inviting way. Perhaps you can see the scrumptious vanilla silk ice cream, or another flavor you like even more . . . and there are the potato chips you love to munch on, and the chocolates are piled high. What other foods do you see? You can sit or stand at this table if you like, in front of the foods. They look so good, and doesn't the faint aroma of the chocolate smell good, and the popcorn, and you can almost hear the crunchy sound of the potato chips. But because these foods have been associated with binges and that out-of-control feeling, you avoid these forbidden delights. The problem is that now you cannot enjoy even small, normal portions of these foods. Wouldn't it be nice to change that? To have a better relationship with these foods? And with yourself? Let's take the food that is of the least concern to you. What is it? Popcorn? Good. There is no good or bad food. Let food be food.

Now remember that you have already shown yourself that you can plan healthy meals each day and snack and tune in to moderation. Let's do this in your imagination with the popcorn. OK, now reach into that bowl. It smells so good. How much would satisfy your taste for popcorn but leave you feeling in control? Two handfuls? OK. Now taste it. It's OK. You know that you won't eat more than two handfuls. Relax. Relax deeply. Tell yourself that you can eat the first few bites and enjoy them, savor them, and relax. Think to yourself something along the lines of "I can eat without bingeing." You can eat a predetermined amount. Go for it. Enjoy the taste, feel the texture of the food. Let it linger on your tongue. Really taste a small amount. Eat it slowly. Make the most of it. Eat a handful. Feel it filling you up. You don't need much more. Chew slowly. As you feel yourself getting fuller and fuller, you slow down more and more . . . more and more. You will stop after the second handful, maybe even a little before. Let your fullness be your guide. If you eat the second handful, if you'd like some more, tell yourself you have had enough, time to stop . . . time to stop. . . . If you would like, drink some water, swirl it around your mouth . . . clear the taste. Walk, read, do something active, if you like. And now tell yourself that you are taking care of your needs, not depriving yourself but not engaging in overeating. Good. Now let's try a food that is next likely to trigger a binge after popcorn and approach the food just as you did with the popcorn. Ah, it's the chips . . .

Posthypnotic suggestions can be very useful in reinforcing these sorts of suggestions in everyday life. The patient then proceeds through the remaining items in the hierarchy of forbidden foods in an analogous manner. The going may be slow if patients doubt their ability to resist a full-blown binge in the face of strong temptation. To progress through the hierarchy, the therapist may find it sometimes necessary to more fully develop impulse management techniques (e.g., cue-controlled relaxation) or to implement a problem-solving approach to interpersonal stressors that engage a temptation to binge. Steps for training in problem-solving skills are outlined by Fairburn, Marcus, and Wilson (1993).

One of the greatest challenges is to identify what feelings fuel the binge and from what situations the feelings stem. Often the initial assessment and ongoing examination of self-monitoring records reveal that interpersonal stressors and conflicts are the prime culprits. Problem solving that guides the person in contending with difficulties and conflicts with friends, bosses, coworkers, and lovers, for example, often suffices to calm emotional tides of feelings of inadequacy, failure, loneliness, rejection, or abandonment that trigger bingeing.

Self-hypnosis can be used to visualize problematic or conflictual interpersonal situations with significant people, noting feelings, avoidance tendencies, catastrophic thoughts, and anticipations that arise. The goal of the intervention is to shift the patient's focus toward empathic attention to the needs of others, while tolerating and working through interpersonal conflict and avoidance patterns to facilitate openness, spontaneity, and vulnerability in relationships. During hypnosis, clarifying needs and wants in relationships can be combined with problem-solving approaches that use imaginal rehearsal to (a) brainstorm solutions to interpersonal problems, (b) evaluate possible solutions, and (c) delineate steps to solve the problem that anticipate potential obstacles. After nonhypnotic brainstorming, two distinct solutions to a problem often emerge as possible contenders for implementation. One tactic we have used involves the patient generating imagery of one problem and its potential resolution played out on one side of a split-screen TV, while another resolution to the same problem is played out on the other side. Commentary and feelings can be spelled out in subtitles as the action unfolds. Observing the scenes from this perspective engenders a more objective consideration of possible solutions, the pros and cons of which can be evaluated after one or both of the scenes are observed. Coping responses that seem most viable can then be enacted in real life and actual outcomes evaluated to calibrate interpersonal responses to mitigate the likelihood of future conflict and binge behavior.

Stage 3

The goal of Stage 3 is to ensure that treatment gains endure. The majority of patients with bulimia remain somewhat symptomatic at this point and may express concern about terminating therapy (Fairburn, Marcus, & Wilson, 1993). The patient can be comforted with information that there is often progressive improvement following treatment, if he or she continues to practice the techniques learned. Nevertheless, unrealistic goals, such as never again bingeing or purging, can set the stage for a relapse, much as unrealistic dieting rules predispose bingeing. The patient should thus be prepared for and able to take in stride occasional setbacks that occur during stressful or emotional periods. Written plans of action that detail coping strategies for contending with fears of failure and discouragement that arise at such times can be very useful (Fairburn, Marcus, & Wilson, 1993).

A distorted body image can be as disturbing as dysfunctional or irrational thoughts about diet and eating. Fairburn, Marcus, and Wilson (1993) underscored the importance of attending to the patient's distorted body image over the course of treatment. However, body image is often the last hurdle to overcome in treatment, insofar as behavioral change often precedes meaningful changes in body image. Nash and Baker (1993) recommended asking patients first to project their body images on screens or to draw them on blackboards, and then to explore the roots of their distorted self-perceptions in "malevolent interactions with family members" by way of age regression (p. 390). They then recommended that the patient use imagery-based techniques to confront body-image distortions and suggest constructive changes in body image. This task can be accomplished by inviting the patient to erase and redraw the distorted aspects of the body image drawn on the imaginary blackboard. Suggestions for calm, ease, and relaxation can be administered if the procedure elicits anxiety. Although Nash and Baker (1993) discussed this technique in the context of treating AN, we have found it to be useful in treating patients with bulimia as well.

The patient should be reminded to use the self-hypnotic and cognitive–behavioral skills learned in therapy to avoid a lapse. In addition to post-hypnotic suggestions and the urge management techniques we have elucidated, H. Spiegel and Spiegel (1978) suggested giving the bulimic patient the following suggestions: "(1) overeating and undereating are insults to body integrity, in effect they become a poison to the body; (2) you need your body to live; (3) to the extent that you want to live, you owe your body this respect and protection" (p. 227). We also recommend that patients periodically practice imaginal rehearsal in which they visualize themselves in high-risk situations and see themselves resisting temptations to binge, eating slowly and in control, for example, and feeling a sense of pride and well-being afterward. Finally, self-hypnosis tapes that contain individualized suggestions, including key phrases generated by the patients and that highlight salient features of the treatment, are also likely to reinforce and help maintain treatment gains.

Hypnosis with CBT (HCBT) has been compared with CBT without hypnosis in six studies (see Levitt, 1993) in obese binge eaters. Averaged across these studies, mean weight loss with hypnosis added to treatment was approximately double that of CBT alone. This effect increased over time, so that the difference between HCBT and CBT was greater the longer the follow-up period. This is particularly important given that most weight loss programs produce initial weight loss, but the weight tends to be regained over time. In the longest of the studies comparing HCBT with CBT, participants in the hypnosis group maintained their weight loss over a 2-year period (Bolocofsky, Spinler, & Coulthard-Morris, 1985).

A TREATMENT PROGRAM FOR OBESITY

As in the treatment of BN, HCBT combines approaches associated with CBT and those associated with the addition of hypnosis. Research indicates that obese individuals can benefit from Fairburn and his colleagues' (Fairburn, Marcus, & Wilson, 1993; Telch, Agras, Rossiter, Wilfley, & Kenardy, 1990; Wilfley et al., 1993) CBT approach when it is modified to treat the unique characteristics of obese bingers. For example, whereas persons with bulimia typically seek treatment to control chronic binge eating, obese patients' primary goal is to lose weight; binge eating is a subordinate problem. In addition, obese bingers may not have a sense of how large they really are, rarely purge or obsess about weight control, and tend not to diet excessively, unlike patients with bulimia (Fairburn, Marcus, & Wilson, 1993).

Stage 1

Stage 1 focuses on educating the obese patient about the relation between weight loss and binge eating. Obese individuals must learn what constitutes normal food intake during a given period and become more involved in an exercise regime and in nutritional counseling to increase awareness of low-fat eating habits and proper body weight regulation. However, the patient must also be informed about the complex genetic factors that affect body weight and limit patient control over weight to some degree (Fairburn, Marcus, & Wilson, 1993). The focus of treatment is consistently on lifestyle changes over the long term.

Therapists must convey empathy for the negative personal, social, and physical consequences of obesity (Fairburn, Marcus, & Wilson, 1993). Because many obese patients have made repeated attempts to lose weight to no avail and are resigned to being compulsive eaters with an addiction, they may resist engaging in self-monitoring. Hypnotic suggestions geared to instill a sense of hope and the ability to eat in moderation, along with imagery of successful experiences and taking pride in making a concerted effort to lose weight, are often useful.

Stage 2

The main goal of Stage 2 is to modify dysfunctional thoughts, attitudes, and beliefs using cognitive restructuring techniques. Because obese individuals often think of themselves as addicted to food, it is essential to distinguish binge eating and true addictions (e.g., alcohol and drug abuse) as follows: (a) unlike food, drugs and alcohol have toxic or addictive properties and related withdrawal symptoms; (b) unlike drugs and alcohol, total food abstinence is neither feasible nor desirable, so patients must strive to maintain self-control and healthy eating patterns (Fairburn, Marcus, & Wilson, 1993); and (c) genetic and metabolic factors may constrain weight control efforts in obesity.

Cognitive restructuring techniques can be used to challenge patients to recognize that although binge eating is a behavioral problem that can be subject to control, obesity is only partially controllable. As in the treatment of BN, body shape and weight concerns should be addressed with hypnosis and cognitive restructuring techniques, guided exposure should be initiated, and the therapist should focus on broadening the patient's definition of self-worth beyond issues of shape and weight and developing a more positive sense of self. Obese patients need to learn that aside from their actual weight, low self-esteem and negative feelings only exacerbate feelings of fatness and ugliness (Fairburn, Marcus, & Wilson, 1993).

The three prongs of treatment of BN are recapitulated in the treatment of obese patients. First, patients engage in self-monitoring in which they maintain eating diaries. Second, patients learn stimulus control in which they are instructed to limit the situations in which they will eat and to reduce the presence of cues that can stimulate overeating. Examples of stimulus control rules for obese patients include the following:

- Eat only in specific locations (e.g., at the kitchen or dining room table).
- Do not engage in any other activities (e.g., watching television) while eating.
- Serve food in small quantities.
- Leave the table as soon as the food is finished.
- When shopping, use a shopping list and buy only foods that are on the list.
- Make snack foods difficult to get to.

And third, obese patients are instructed in eating behavior modification. We give our obese patients a sheet with the following instructions aimed at slowing down the eating process so that less food is consumed within a given amount of time:

- Take small bites.
- Chew slowly.
- Savor the food, so that maximum pleasure is derived from it.
- Swallow the food in your mouth before taking another bite.

- Pause between bites.
- Put down your eating utensil between bites.

These behaviors can be practiced in extreme forms during a treatment session. In doing this, it can be helpful for the patient to come in relatively hungry and to bring in a healthy, low-calorie food (e.g., an apple). The patient can be asked to rate hunger before and after the exercise. Typically, a relatively small food intake over a prolonged period (e.g., half an apple in 20 minutes) leads to a very noticeable abatement of hunger. This is experienced as surprising and builds confidence in the value of practicing slow eating.

Eating behavior modification can also be facilitated by imagery rehearsal in which patients first imagine being in a high-risk situation. Next, the response that the person wishes to make is imagined. Finally, the positive consequences of making the desired response are imagined. These may include losing weight, fitting into different clothes, feeling pride in one's accomplishments, and so on.

Stage 3

The difficulty in treating obesity is not bringing about weight loss, but keeping it off. Once again, the focus is on lifestyle change and how to maintain it, not on the numbers on a scale. This objective may be facilitated by relapse prevention procedures. Stage 3 of CBT for obese individuals parallels Stage 3 for patients with bulimia; however, it usually continues for an additional month or more. This extension is necessary because additional time is needed to establish healthy eating patterns. Relapse prevention is discussed in great detail, along with the danger of emotional eating or allowing food to be the main source of reinforcement or self-gratification in life. Patients are encouraged to continue a balanced lifestyle after treatment, guided by moderation. Hypnotic techniques such as self-hypnosis can be used here to improve generalization of techniques learned in therapy to the patient's own environment to prevent relapse. And as in the treatment of BN, relapse prevention includes identifying high-risk situations (e.g., parties, restaurants) and developing cognitive and behavioral strategies for coping with those situations (e.g., planning what will be ordered in a restaurant, practicing assertive responses to invitations to eat more at a social dinner).

CBT is a promising first-level treatment for eating disorders and obesity. We strongly recommend a multifaceted treatment that targets interpersonal issues when assessment reveals they play a significant role in the development and maintenance of dysfunctional eating patterns. Although controlled research has not established whether hypnosis adds to the effectiveness of well-established treatments, the anecdotal literature as well as our personal experience suggests that it may well enhance treatment outcomes. Research is clearly needed to determine whether treatment failures benefit from hypnotic interventions. Because at least one study (Mitchell et al., 2002) indicates that neither interpersonal therapy nor drug treatment contributes much to the successful treatment of individuals with bulimia initially treated with CBT, research examining the effects of hypnosis on treatment nonresponders is a priority.

8

DEPRESSION

Everyone feels depressed from time to time, but some people experience depressive episodes that last for weeks, months, or years. Depression is the most commonly diagnosed psychiatric disorder, with prevalence rates hovering in the neighborhood of 25% (American Psychiatric Association, 1994; Kessler et al., 1994). Approximately 1 in 5 women and 1 in 10 men experience a major depressive disorder within the course of their lives. Most depressed people recover (with or without treatment), but relapse is a common problem and many people experience recurring depressive episodes throughout their lives. Some people remain chronically depressed and do not recover at all.

Depression has physical as well as psychological consequences. Almost two thirds of people who commit suicide are clinically depressed, and the impact of depression on physical health rivals that of diabetes, arthritis, and hypertension. There are also high social costs of depression. It is one of the leading causes of disability, leading to reductions in family income and increased financial burdens on society.

Before the development of antidepressant medications in the 1950s, cocaine, opium, and electroconvulsive therapy were used as treatments for depression. Two classes of antidepressants—MAO inhibitors and tricyclics—were discovered in the 1950s. Although both seemed to be effective, side effects were a serious problem, leading many depressed patients to discontinue them. Developed in the 1980s and 1990s, selective serotonin reuptake inhibitors (SSRIs) have fewer side effects than do the older antidepressants and for that reason they quickly became the treatment of choice for depression.

Data indicating that SSRIs may increase the risk of suicide among depressed patients (e.g., Healy, 2003; Healy & Whitaker, 2003) have led to growing concerns about their widespread use. This, coupled with the evidence we reviewed in chapter 3 that antidepressants are not much more effective than placebos (Kirsch, Moore, Scoboria, & Nicholls, 2002), makes the identification of safe and effective alternative treatments important. Psychotherapy, especially brief, structured therapy aimed specifically at depression, has proven to be very effective in the treatment of a wide range of depressed clientele, both with and without the addition of antidepressant medications. The effect of therapy alone is similar to that of antidepressants in the short run and greater than antidepressants in the long run, as the relapse rate following psychotherapy appears to be lower than that following medication (Hollon, Shelton, & Loosen, 1991). Although the addition of hypnosis to psychotherapy for depression has not been evaluated directly, there is indirect evidence that it should be effective. In particular, the placebo response seems to be particularly strong in the treatment of depression (Kirsch & Sapirstein, 1998), and conditions that are responsive to placebo treatment generally seem to be responsive to hypnotic treatment as well.

The apparent success of antidepressants in general and of SSRIs in particular has led to biochemical theories of depression. If changes in neurotransmission could cure depression, it was argued, then depression could be due to a malfunctioning brain. This conclusion sometimes leads people to question the suggestions that depression be treated without medication. If depression is a biochemical disorder, should it not be treated biochemically? However, what most people are unaware of is that there is no direct evidence for these theories. They are based entirely on the effectiveness of antidepressant medication. If the therapeutic benefits of antidepressants are not due to their chemical action, as meta-analyses indicate (Kirsch et al., 2002; Kirsch & Sapirstein, 1998), these biochemical theories of depression are cast into doubt.

TREATMENT OF DEPRESSION

Cognitive–behavioral therapy (CBT) and interpersonal therapy (IPT), introduced in our discussion of eating disorders, have the strongest empirical backing as treatments of depression (Craighead, 2000). The most thoroughly assessed CBT for depression is Beck's cognitive therapy (Beck, Rush, Shaw, & Emery, 1979). The focus of CBT is on identifying and modifying (a) irrational (e.g., inflexible, distorted, exaggerated), highly negative beliefs about the self, the past, and the future; (b) rumination about problems and failure experiences; and (c) the idea that painful life circumstances are stable—"unchanging and even unchangeable" (Yapko, 1993, p. 344). IPT addresses conflicts and problems in interpersonal relationships, rather than distorted cognitions, and targets the areas of interpersonal disputes, unresolved grief, role transitions, and interpersonal deficits (e.g., lack of empathy, social skills; Klerman et al., 1984).

In light of both cognitive and interpersonal models, depression appears to be associated with rigid, negative response sets regarding the self, interpersonal relationships, and the world that inflame and perpetuate depression: Pessimism and ineffectual coping and problem solving engender negative outcomes and self-evaluation that, in turn, abet dysphoria. Because depression is, to some extent at least, self-generated, it can be reversed by changing the way people think, the way they make decisions, and the way they interact with others that invites rejection.

CBT for depression is typically conducted over 20 sessions or fewer. The treatment depends heavily on the patient accepting the rationale that there is an intimate connection between negative thought patterns and schemas (i.e., beliefs underlying negative thoughts), depression, and negative life experiences. The cornerstone of treatment is a functional analysis of the specific thoughts, beliefs, and expectancies that contribute to depression. Self-monitoring, with the goal of identifying and ultimately challenging depression-related automatic thoughts and distorted ideas and expectations (e.g., personalization, mind reading, overgeneralization, black-or-white thinking), is thus fundamental to the assessment and treatment of symptoms (Beck, 1976). IPT, which is conducted over the same time interval, uses self-monitoring in interpersonal situations to identify specific problem areas and skill deficits relevant to treatment. We recommend that therapists assess and target both cognitive distortions and interpersonal problems and deficits that a comprehensive behavioral or functional analysis identifies as antecedents to depression.

It is also imperative to assess the frequency and severity of symptoms, including suicidal ideation, alcohol and drug use, prescribed medication use and depression as a possible side effect, medical history to evaluate presence of a co-occurring illness, family history of depression, and past treatment for depression. We strongly recommend administering well-established psychological tests to index depression and chart the course of treatment (Beck Depression Inventory; see Beck, Steer, & Garbin, 1988).

Automatic Thoughts as Self-Suggestions

Automatic thoughts are central to a cognitive–behavioral understanding of depression and anxiety (Beck, 1976; J. S. Beck, 1995). These are the thoughts that constantly enter one's mind during the day. Most automatic thoughts come and go without being focused on, and they are therefore quickly forgotten. According to Beck (1976), emotional disorders depend on the content of these automatic thoughts. Among depressed individuals, automatic thoughts focus on themes of loss, whereas in anxiety disorders, the focus is on the perception of threat. In particular, depressed patients tend to have automatic thoughts that belong to what Beck has described as the cognitive triad. These are persistent negative thoughts about the self, the world, and the future. Changing these thoughts and the cognitive distortions that give rise to them is a key feature of cognitive therapy.

In a hypnotic context, automatic thoughts can be viewed as spontaneous self-suggestions. The task of therapy is to discover the dysfunctional self-suggestions that patients have been giving themselves, challenge them, and replace them with more adaptive self-suggestions. With many patients, dysfunctional self-suggestions can be uncovered by having them imagine situations in which they felt sad and depressed and try to recall or imagine the thoughts that had entered their mind.

The therapist should keep in mind, however, that recall is a reconstructive process. Whether people are hypnotized or not, memory does not function like a video recorder in which one literally replays what has happened. Instead, whenever one attempts to recall something, fragmentary memory traces are combined with cognitive schemas, beliefs, dispositions, and coincident thoughts and feelings (see Mazzoni & Kirsch, 2002). This process, however, does not hamper the use of hypnotic imagery in uncovering the automatic thoughts that are linked to depressed moods. Among depressed patients, negative appraisals of situations are habitual. So it really does not matter much whether the focus is on an actual event that occurred or on an imagined prototypical event. What is likely to be uncovered is the kind of automatic thoughts that these events elicit.

The first step in using hypnosis to uncover, challenge, and change negative automatic thoughts is establishing the connection between thoughts and feelings, as shown in the following example of a therapist working with a depressed student:

Therapist: People often think that it is the events in their lives that lead them to feel sad, but in fact, it is not really the event itself that is causing the emotion. Instead, it is the way we interpret events that determines the kind of feeling we will have. Imagine that one of the students in your class has received a B on an exam. How will she feel?

Patient: Well, it depends.

Therapist: On what?

Patient: I don't know. On how she thought she'd do, I guess.

Therapist: Right! So if she thought she'd get an A, she might think, "I really did lousy on that exam," and she might feel pretty bad. But if she expected a C, she'd think, "Hey, I did pretty good," and as a consequence, she'd probably feel good as well. So it's not the grade that made her feel bad, it's the way she thought about the grade.

The way we think about events functions like spontaneous suggestions that we give ourselves, just like the suggestions that we use in hypnosis. Depending on the nature of those suggestions, we might feel sad, mad, glad, or afraid in response to them. So when people feel bad, it can help to figure out what suggestion they gave themselves that led to that bad feeling. For example, when was the last time you can recall yourself suddenly becoming aware of feeling down?

Patient: That's easy. It was this morning on my way to school.

Therapist: And what were you thinking that was associated with that feeling?

Patient: [*Pauses*] Gee, I don't really know. I can't remember what I was thinking about. I was just driving to school, and I started feeling bad. It seems to happen all the time. I drive to school, and if I'm not already feeling lousy, I start.

Therapist: Yes, thoughts are like that. We are thinking all the time, giving ourselves suggestions that influence our moods, but we don't make note of our thoughts, and two minutes later, we might have forgotten what they were. Let's see if we can uncover the kind of thoughts you tend to have in circumstances like driving to school in the morning. It's morning. You are driving to school. See what's around you. Where you are. But this time, be aware of your thoughts and say them out loud as they come to mind. The thoughts connected to feeling lousy can come to mind easily, all by themselves.

Patient: I'm thinking about my history class. It's the first class in the morning. I'm so far behind. I'll never catch up. I can't do the work. I'm just no good.

In this example, the patient has come up with spontaneous negative self-suggestions involving the future ("I'll never catch up") and the self ("I can't do the work" and "I'm just no good"). These can be challenged through Socratic questioning, either within or outside of hypnosis. Our experience suggests that this part of the process of cognitive restructuring can be best managed outside of hypnosis. Hypnosis can then be used again to reinforce the alternative positive self-suggestions that emerge from this process.

As an aid to identifying habitual negative self-suggestions, patients can be taught to monitor their thoughts during the day, taking special note of the thoughts that occur just prior to changes in mood and writing them down as soon as possible. These notes can then be brought into the therapeutic session and evaluated. Both positive and negative moods can be used as cues to self-monitor cognition. Self-monitoring cognitions associated with negative mood states are likely to reveal the negative self-suggestions that elicit them. Self-monitoring cognitions associated with positive mood states can be equally important. Besides revealing positive self-suggestions that can be reinforced during hypnosis, they provide the patient with examples of the link between cognition and emotion. These positive examples reinforce the notion that mood states can be changed for the better, thereby combating hopelessness and fostering positive expectations.

Assessing and Changing Cognitive Distortions

Cognitive therapists have identified a number of cognitive distortions that give rise to negative automatic thoughts. Identifying and challenging these rigid and irrational ways of thinking can diminish the frequency of negative automatic thoughts and increase the frequency of positive alternatives. They also provide patients with a means of identifying and challenging negative self-suggestions on their own. The following are among the most common cognitive distortions.

Overgeneralization

Overgeneralization is a tendency to overgeneralize from relatively scant data. A key to its identification is the use of words such as *always, never, everyone,* and *no one.* A patient complaining that "no one likes me" might be asked "Who specifically doesn't like you?" followed by "Who else?" Invariably, the list will include fewer people than *everyone.*

Mind Reading

A patient who claims that someone does not like him or her may be engaging in a cognitive distortion known as mind reading. This can be ascertained by asking, "How do you know that X doesn't like you?" If the patient answers that this was concluded from a direct statement by X, he or she is probably not mind reading. Often, however, the behavioral evidence is much less conclusive. An answer that suggests mind reading might be "Sometimes when I pass him in the hall at work and say 'Hi,' he doesn't even answer me. He just ignores me, as if I didn't even exist." Through

Socratic questioning, patients who mind read can be encouraged to consider alternative explanations of the behavior of the person whose mind they are reading. "Can you think of any other reason why X might not have responded?" "Have you ever been so absorbed in something you were thinking about that you failed to be fully aware that somebody was even talking to you?" Projected self-appraisal is a common type of mind reading. Here the person assumes that his or her own negative self-impression is also held by others (e.g., "I sound really boring to myself, so they must think I'm boring").

Besides contributing to depression and other emotional disorders, mind reading is a frequent source of problems for distressed couples. There are two ways in which mind reading can create trouble. One is when a member of the couple may assume that he or she knows what the other is thinking or feeling and acts on that assumption as if it were fact. The second way in which mind reading can be a problem is when people expect their partners to know what they are feeling without having to tell them. In fact, no matter how well people know each other or how long they have been together, they will often incorrectly guess what their partners are thinking or feeling. So it is almost always better to ask and tell than to guess and keep silent.

Fortune Telling

Fortune telling is the anticipation of a negative outcome with the feeling that it is already fact. As in the treatment of anxiety disorders, the key here is to challenge two aspects of the predicted outcome: its probability and its reinforcement value. How likely is it that the anticipated outcome will occur, and what is the empirical basis on which the patient is making that judgment? How terrible would it be if that outcome did occur, and what makes it seem so terrible?

Disqualification

Some patients manage to dismiss positive outcomes in their life by disqualifying them. Having done well at a particular task, for example, the patient may decide that the task was easy. Learning that a particular person likes the patient might lead to devaluation of that person. The key to disqualification is the conclusion that a particular instance that counters a negative belief doesn't count.

Magnification and Minimization

These are complementary distortions whereby patients exaggerate negative evidence for depressing beliefs and minimize evidence for positive alternatives. Telescopes provide a useful metaphor for helping patients understand this particular distortion. It is as if they were looking through a telescope when assessing negative information, and turning the telescope around and looking at positive information from the other end.

Personalization

Personalization is a tendency to relate everything to the self, compare oneself with others, and downgrade one's self-worth (e.g., "They're not talking to me, so I must have said something wrong").

Filtering

Filtering involves focusing on one aspect of a situation to the exclusion of everything else (e.g., "I stammered a few times during my talk; I really blew it").

Black-or-White Thinking

Depressed patients often think about things in all-or-nothing terms instead of on a spectrum (e.g., "If I'm not perfect, then I'm a total loss").

Shoulding

Should statements are produced by rigid thinking about "right" and "wrong" thoughts or behaviors. They result in judgmental self-talk and considering oneself and other people bad or defective (e.g., "I shouldn't be so jumpy in social situations").

Emotional Thinking

This is a popular cognitive distortion that may even be advocated by some. The message is "If it feels true, it is true." There is no doubt that it is useful to pay attention to one's feelings, but it is equally true that something that feels right can be wrong. The cognitive distortion of emotional thinking is a depressogenic way of dealing with the head–heart split, which occurs when one feels that something is true while logically knowing that it is not. Its antithesis, rational thinking, is a way of countering negative self-suggestions.

Once patients have identified unrealistic thoughts that fall into these categories, they can learn to challenge them in straightforward, specific ways. For example, in the case of mind reading, patients can be challenged as follows:

> Therapist: Now go deep into your self-hypnosis and ask yourself the question, "Do you really believe you can read minds?" If you answered *yes*, then consider this: Can you often read the total cost of your purchase from the checker's mind in

a store or a pet's name from its master's mind? Can you usually tell when people are thinking about their friendly or generous feelings toward you? If you answered these questions in the negative, perhaps you are applying a different standard to yourself in such neutral and positive situations than you do when you fear negative evaluations. Recall that a tendency to believe that others are thinking ill of you is characteristic of social anxiety. Next time you find yourself engaging in mind reading, remind yourself that you no longer have to be limited by this mental trickery.

ADDITIONAL TECHNIQUES

Feeling one thing while logically knowing that something else is true plays a particularly important role in cognitive therapy. When a long-held belief is effectively challenged, there is often a transitional period in which there is a head–heart split. A patient knows he or she is not doomed to failure, but it still feels as if he or she is. At this point, the task of therapy is for the head to convince the heart of what it knows to be true.

The empty-chair technique is one way of facilitating this process. The patient is asked to speak only from the heart while sitting in one chair and only from the head while sitting in another. The two sides can then engage in a dialogue, each speaking in turn, with the therapist signaling a change of chairs when one side has finished for the time being.

Hypnotic suggestion is another way of facilitating resolution of head–heart splits. The context of hypnosis normalizes repetition, allowing the therapist to repeat the same idea many times. This repetition, of course, is a fundamental part of most hypnotic inductions. Hypnosis also permits a more emphatic tone of voice than is otherwise the norm, and it encourages a focus of attention on the suggestions that are being given. The patient's attention to emphatic repetitions of new cognitions may facilitate acceptance of them at a gut level.

Countering Low Self-Esteem

Depression is almost invariably accompanied by low self-esteem. One way of countering low self-esteem is to have patients list the qualities of people they admire—qualities that they would value in a friend. Next, the patient is instructed to place a check mark by each of those qualities that they themselves possess. Most people with low self-esteem are surprised to discover that they possess most of the attributes they most value in others. This list can then be used in and out of hypnosis to facilitate a more accurate and functional self-assessment.

Building Positive Expectations

The powerful placebo effect revealed in clinical trials of antidepressants (Kirsch & Sapirstein, 1998) underscores the role of expectancy in the treatment of depression. Given the centrality of hopelessness in depression (Abramson, Seligman, & Teasdale, 1978), this is not at all surprising. Hopelessness is an expectancy—an expectancy that a negative state of affairs will not get better, no matter what one does to alleviate it.

If you ask depressed people to identify the worst thing in their lives, many would tell you that it is their depression. They believe that their depression will continue, no matter what they do—a very depressing thought indeed. As Teasdale (1985) noted, these people are depressed about their depression. If this is the case, then the expectancy of improvement should produce improvement; that is, the belief that one will improve is the opposite of the hopelessness that may be maintaining the depression or at the very least is an important component of it. For this reason, countering negative expectations and building positive expectations are an essential component of the treatment of depression.

Michael Yapko (e.g., 1992, 1993, 2003) has delineated a sensible and straightforward process for building expectancy and treating depression with hypnosis. Yapko has developed what he terms a *hypnotic process* for building expectancy. He contends that depressed individuals have a stable cognitive deficit or attributional style that he calls a "disturbance of temporal orientation" (Yapko, 1989) in which negative life circumstances are not perceived as changeable. To give the patient hope, build positive expectancy, and chip away, if not demolish, this rigid way of approaching life, Yapko recommends initiating hypnosis as early as the first session. In a nutshell, Yapko's process involves interrupting patients' negative expectations for the future, facilitating awareness of personal resources, amplifying and guiding patients' motivation to change, and rehearsing new patterns and ways of coping with challenges in daily living. The linchpin of expectancy building is age progression in which the patient is "encouraged to experience positive future consequences now that arise from implementing new changes and decisions" (Yapko, 1993, p. 345). Yapko (1993) provided the following example of suggestions that are general yet sound specific and that can be given in the very earliest stages of treatment:

> You've described the discomfort that has led you to seek help . . . and you want to feel differently [sic] . . . and you really don't know yet that you can . . . but you'll discover quickly what you've known all along . . . that when you do something differently than you used to . . . the result will also be different . . . and so you can go forward in time . . . that it's been a while since our work together . . . and you can take a moment to be fully there . . . able to review decisions that you've recently

made . . . differently . . . and you can review the positive consequences of those decisions . . . on all dimensions within you . . . and what a pleasure to discover that you're so capable . . . of shifting thoughts and feelings . . . and that you can enjoy the relief you worked so hard for . . . and why not look forward to even more changes . . . that feel good . . . as you discover more and more ways of using what you've learned to continue growing stronger. (pp. 345–346)

These sorts of suggestions can be embedded in a more encompassing sequence of steps for expectancy building, as set forth by Yapko (2002, p. 67):

1. Identify the goal (expectancy regarding what specifically?).
2. Use induction to build a response set.
3. Use metaphors illustrating the inevitability of change.
4. Offer universal metaphors regarding future possibilities (e.g., there will be important changes and advances in medicine and technology).
5. Distinguish past events from future possibilities (It was almost impossible to predict that one day we would be friends with Russia).
6. Offer feedback regarding the appropriateness and feasibility of personal goals.
7. Highlight today's new actions that lead to tomorrow's improved possibilities.
8. Identify specific personal resources that can be used to realize specific goals.
9. Introduce distinctions between mood and action: Feelings do not have to drive actions.
10. Highlight action steps as transcending feelings of doubt or hopelessness.
11. Reinforce the willingness to experiment.
12. Generalize resources into future opportunities: Prompt the patient to use new skills in both general and specific situational contexts.
13. Use posthypnotic suggestions for generalization and integration into everyday life.
14. Disengage and terminate hypnosis.

Yapko's (2002) step-by-step approach that follows is designed to guide patients in exploring options and making "emotionally and intellectually intelligent decisions" (p. 104) as a counterweight to excessive rumination and passivity:

1. Initiate the induction process.
2. Build a response set regarding choice (e.g., "You can choose when to close your eyes . . . to notice which part of your

body is most relaxed . . . to read a book at home, or to cook a meal when you are hungry").

3. Describe possible frames of reference: There is no one frame of reference for making decisions. It is possible to discriminate what is easiest to achieve and what is best to achieve in terms of a particular goal.

4. Present alternative frames of reference salient to the problem context. Different viewpoints can be generated by the patient engaging in his or her own internal dialogue, imagining what others might say or do, or actually consulting others for their opinions.

5. Establish a goal orientation. Choices are best made in relation to specific goals. Encourage the patient to consider which frame of reference or viewpoint is most congruent with achieving the stated goal.

6. Identify personally plausible options: Focus the patient on selecting strategies to achieve goals that are sensible and effective.

7. Use age regression to explore each option's consequences. Yapko (2002) provides the following example similar in certain respects to the age progression suggestions previously described: "follow a decision to see where it takes you . . . and you can imagine in detail that it's been months since you chose a new path and began to follow it . . . notice how it feels to have decided . . . and what it has led you in these months to do differently . . . and what you like better in yourself now . . . and what it has allowed you to do that before you felt unable to do . . ." (p. 107).

8. Identify specific action steps associated with the selected option.

9. Associate action to context and reinforce. Provide suggestions that encourage the patient to evaluate different options, and decide on a sensible course of action that can be implemented in a stepwise fashion to achieve goals in everyday life.

10. Use posthypnotic suggestions. Yapko (2002) recommended the following kinds of suggestions: "You may be pleasantly surprised at how automatic it becomes to you . . . to make decisions according to what's best in the long run . . . and not what's easiest in the short run . . . and you can feel good about how quickly you seem to reach well-considered conclusions . . . and implement purposeful action that benefits you . . . and helps you feel so much better about yourself and your life." (p. 108)

Yapko's approach to the treatment of depression is entirely consistent with our contention that positive expectancies and adaptive response sets are instrumental to achieving personal goals, modifying habits, and regulating emotions. Yapko's program for the treatment of depression is sufficiently elaborated to permit controlled-outcome trials. In fact, a recently developed, commercially available audiotape/CD, *Focusing on Feeling Good*, offers seven hypnosis sessions, each targeting a different issue or symptom commonly associated with depression. This material can provide the basis for research comparing the effects of a self-help protocol for depression with no treatment, as well as comparisons of the procedures with and without a hypnotic induction.

Relapse Prevention: Mindfulness Training

One advantage of psychotherapy in the treatment of depression is that it reduces the rate of relapse, when compared with relapse following antidepressant medication (Hollon et al., 1991). Therapy often involves the learning of new skills for managing life's problems, so once a skill has been learned, its benefits remain. Having learned to drive a car, for example, one does not have to continue taking driving lessons to keep from forgetting. In contrast, antidepressant medication carries the implicit message that the depression will abate only so long as the medication is continued.

Emphasizing the skill acquisition component of treatment may ward off relapse. In particular, mindfulness techniques are particularly effective in preventing relapse (Segal, Williams, & Teasdale, 2002). Kabat-Zinn (2003) defined mindfulness as nonjudgmental awareness that emerges through purposeful attention to the unfolding of experience on a moment-by-moment basis. Mindfulness implies a radical and unvarnished acceptance of unpleasant as well as pleasant experiences. It teaches individuals to relate to thoughts and feelings in a wider, "decentered" perspective as "mental events," rather than aspects of the self or as necessarily accurate reflections of reality (Teasdale, Segal, & Williams, 2003). Meta-analyses (Baer, 2003) and qualitative research reviews (Walsh, 1999) provide evidence for the salutary effects of mindfulness techniques (e.g., meditation) across numerous measures of psychological functioning.

Mindfulness training can easily be incorporated into hypnotic treatment. We teach patients one or more of the following mindfulness exercises, which can be practiced for short periods throughout the day or while sitting quietly for longer periods of 10 to 30 minutes, after entering self-hypnosis. Our goal is to assist patients in accepting and becoming comfortable with evanescent emotional states and learning that there is no imperative to continue to react in habitual, maladaptive ways, including avoiding deep emotion. The following are among the mindfulness suggestions that can be given to patients in hypnosis and subsequently reinforced in self-hypnosis.

- Imagine that your thoughts are written on signs carried by parading soldiers (Hayes, 2002) or that thoughts "continually dissolve like a parade of characters marching across a stage" (Rimpoche, 1981, p. 53). Observe the parade of thoughts without becoming absorbed in any of them.
- Imagine that the mind is a conveyor belt. Thoughts and feelings that come down the belt are observed, labeled, and categorized (Linehan, 1994).
- The mind is the sky, and thoughts, feelings, and sensations are clouds that pass by; just watch them (Linehan, 1994).
- Imagine that each thought is a ripple on water or light on leaves. They naturally dissolve (Rimpoche, 1981, p. 44).

In controlled research, mindfulness techniques have been shown to be effective in preventing the relapse of depression (Segal, Williams, & Teasdale, 2002).

In conclusion, depression is the most widespread psychological disorder. It is a serious disorder that can have dire personal and social consequences. It is, fortunately, eminently treatable, as it responds to an exceptionally wide variety of treatments. The effects of cognitive and interpersonal therapies have been especially well documented and are highly recommended. Although the evidence is largely indirect, there is reason to suspect that, as in many other conditions, hypnosis can be a useful catalyst that might enhance the effectiveness of treatment. If nothing else, it provides a means of harnessing the placebo effect without the use of deception, an especially important task in the treatment of depression, where the placebo effect has been particularly large.

9

ANXIETY DISORDERS

When many people think of hypnosis, a picture comes to mind of a hypnotist waving a watch or shiny object in front of a person and saying, "Relax, relax." Although this stereotypic image does not begin to capture the multifaceted techniques and strategies at the disposal of modern-day practitioners of hypnosis, it does imply that hypnosis can replace anxious feelings with relaxation. And that is exactly the case, although ameliorating anxiety with hypnotic procedures is not quite that simple. In this chapter we illustrate how hypnotic methods can be integrated in a seamless manner with cognitive–behavioral principles and techniques that have demonstrated efficacy in the treatment of anxiety. We describe hypnotic and nonhypnotic self-control training procedures, cognitive therapy, and exposure techniques. The specific examples assume that the patient has been trained in basic self-hypnosis procedures, as described in chapter 4.

The fact that hypnosis is a useful adjunct in the treatment of anxiety is significant for this reason: Anxiety is pervasive and can be debilitating. More than 19 million Americans ages 18 to 54 suffer from one or more anxiety disorders each year (National Institute of Mental Health [NIMH], 2002), and an estimated 12.5 million people suffer so intensely from anxiety-related disorders that they seek mental health help (Narrow, Rae, & Regier, 1998). In a given year, the symptoms of panic (e.g., racing heart, dizziness, sense of unreality) afflict between one third and half of the people in the

United States (NIMH, 2001), and approximately 2.4 million people suffer from panic disorders, marked by recurrent panic attacks (Kessler et al., 1994).

Panic is part and parcel of many anxious conditions. In as many as three fourths of individuals with panic disorder, fears generalize to the point of agoraphobia, a condition in which people are terrified of situations where help might not be available in the event of panic or where escape might be difficult or embarrassing. Although agoraphobia occurs in no more than 5% of the population, fear renders some individuals homebound (Kessler et al., 1994).

More common social fears are generally not as debilitating as agoraphobia. However, excessive and unreasonable social fears burden the lives of an estimated 13.5% of the population, making it one of the most widespread phobias and anxiety conditions (Kessler et al., 1994). Fears of specific objects such as bugs or snakes or situations such as thunderstorms are also common and plague one of every nine people. For some people, anxiety is not focused on a particular place or thing but, rather, is tightly interwoven into the fabric of daily activity. Generalized anxiety disorder (GAD) consists of anxious thinking, physical and emotional tension, and feelings of apprehension that intensify around potential threats. The 9.2 million people nationwide who fully meet the diagnostic criteria for GAD as their primary or secondary psychiatric diagnosis worry for an average of 60% of each day, compared with 18% for the rest of the general population (NIMH, 2002).

REVERSE ENGINEERING: WHAT CAUSES ANXIETY?

The treatment of anxiety with hypnosis and empirically supported methods involves a process of reverse engineering—working backward, in effect, from the causes of anxiety reactions to the treatment of anxiety (Mellinger & Lynn, 2003). By working backward to figure out how to get a malfunctioning device functioning again, we can learn in the process what makes it tick. Reverse engineering helps keep things from children's bikes to artificial hearts running smoothly. When applied to anxiety disorders, reverse engineering involves analyzing catastrophic thinking, determining what went wrong when the danger prevention system stopped working properly, and using techniques designed to systematically reverse the damage and restore healthy functioning.

Catastrophic Thinking

To reverse-engineer anxiety, one must first understand what produces anxiety. Catastrophic thinking is a critical feature of many anxiety conditions (Beck, 1976; Ellis, 1962; Ellis & Dryden, 1997). Anxious people often predict that terrible events will happen, even though these events have a low probability of actually occurring. When phobic situations or objects are dangerous at all, the danger is by definition exaggerated: It is neither mortal nor imminent. Persons with phobias tend to exaggerate the negative impact of their particular phobic situations, and people who have GAD tend to exaggerate the likelihood of negative events occurring. Catastrophizing is a fundamental error of anxious thinking in which people exaggerate the negativity of an outcome that will result or has resulted from entering an anxiety-provoking situation. If a person thinks an elevator is unsafe and will crash to the ground, it is understandable that the person will experience an increase in heart rate in that situation. If the person expects to have an anxiety attack when entering an elevator, it is also understandable that panic ensues when the patient notices his or her heart rate accelerating as he or she presses the button.

Anxiety Expectancy

Anxiety expectancy—the apprehension of having an uncomfortable physiological stress reaction—is a self-confirming response expectancy that is at the heart of catastrophic thinking (Kirsch, 1985; Reiss & McNally, 1985). Goldstein and Chambless (1978) realized that patients with agoraphobia were not really afraid of the bridges, elevators, or shopping malls they were avoiding. Instead, they were afraid of the panic attacks that they anticipated experiencing in these situations. The expectation of a panic attack is frightening enough in itself to induce panic. Every attack seems to confirm the dangerous quality of phobic situations, because people with phobias are prone to being very vigilant for evidence that validates their fearfulness. In a similar fashion, socially anxious feelings are based on predictions that the individual will encounter negative experiences in "social evaluation situations"—situations in which other people can observe, interact with, and judge the anxious person (Heimberg & Juster, 1995). Common expectancies reported by people with social phobia include the following:

- People will think I look really silly.
- I am going to blow this.
- I will look ridiculous.
- They are going to laugh at me.
- They will realize how incompetent I am.
- Everyone here is better at this than I am.
- I won't know what to say. (Rapee, 1998)

The catastrophic images that fill the anxious person's mind are the direct consequence of unbidden automatic thoughts that arise when a person is negatively aroused by anxiety (A. T. Beck, 1964; J. S. Beck, 1995). As noted in chapter 8, automatic thoughts are spontaneously occurring dire predictions and images of possible physical, mental, or social harm. Automatic thoughts are often organized into anxiety propositions that describe the connection between specific anxiety-provoking events, situations, or activities and specific feared consequences. For example, a person may develop the anxiety proposition that he could tumble from a steep staircase where he feels dizzy and break every bone in his body, and this fear generalizes to other high places. Anxiety disorders thus appear to be self-confirming expectancy disorders: People who panic and are phobic have a fear of fear (Kirsch, 1985; Kirsch & Lynn, 1999).

Many people with anxiety disorders are characterized by anxiety sensitivity (AS)—the predisposition to experience anxious discomfort and develop anxiety disorders (Reiss & McNally, 1985). People with AS have a propensity to notice and attend to, rather than ignore, physical sensations and misinterpret normal bodily feelings as abnormal and thus react to them negatively with worry and distress. The tendency to transform harmless physical feelings into worrisome emotional feelings can lead to anxiety expectancies and avoidance of situations in which such feelings are instigated.

Avoidance

Research has shown that the stronger the anxiety expectancy, the stronger the avoidance (Kirsch, 1985; Kirsch & Lynn, 1999). When it is impossible to escape or avoid what is feared, a panic attack is an unwelcome yet likely eventuality. Because avoidance allows escape from what is feared, anxiety is reinforced and becomes more ingrained (Mowrer, 1960). Moreover, avoidance precludes the opportunity to learn from direct experience that fears are unrealistic or exaggerated. In this way, anxiety and hopelessness become stubbornly entrenched.

An interesting aspect of avoidance is that it is difficult, if not impossible, not to think about what is feared. Researchers have found that it is difficult to suppress anxiety-laden thoughts without them rebounding, or returning full force, when active attempts to suppress the thoughts cease (Wegner, 1994, 1997). Attempts to consciously suppress thoughts can make them all the more demoralizing when they recur, asserting their strong presence. In short, fears only grow stronger as they incubate. In learning to confront rather than avoid what is feared, a sense of effectiveness replaces hopelessness. Confronting fears in a step-wise, systematic, and controlled way and identifying, challenging, and changing the beliefs and expectancies that engender a sense of panic and fear make it possible to modify anxiety expectancies and contend with fear and anxiety (Mellinger & Lynn, 2003).

COGNITIVE–BEHAVIORAL APPROACHES

The cognitive–behavioral and hypnotic approaches we review are effective in reverse engineering anxiety disorders because they modify maladaptive thinking styles, discourage avoidance of what is feared, and foster perceptions of control and mastery over anxious thoughts and feelings. Cognitive–behavioral approaches are the most widely studied and effective interventions for anxiety disorders (Barlow, 2002; Chambless & Ollendick, 2001; Deacon & Abramowitz, 2004). In fact, no other approach to the treatment of anxiety rivals the effectiveness of cognitive–behavioral therapy (CBT). Over the past decade, seven meta-analytic reviews have documented the effectiveness of cognitive–behavioral interventions for panic with and without agoraphobia (see Deacon & Abramowitz, 2004). Over the same period, four meta-analytic reviews have supported the effectiveness of social phobia, revealing that treatment gains persist after treatment (Federoff & Taylor, 2001; Feske & Chambless, 1995; Gould, Buckminster, Pollack, Otto, & Yap, 1997; Taylor, 1996). Consistent with theses trends, three meta-analytic reviews indicate that CBT is effective for GAD (Borkovec & Wishman, 1996; Gould, Otto, Pollack, & Yap, 1977; Weston & Morrison, 2001).

Hypnosis and Cognitive–Behavioral Therapy

Research indicates that hypnosis can contribute to the efficacy of CBT. Schoenberger, Kirsch, Gearan, Montgomery, and Pastyrnak (1997) compared a cognitive–behavioral intervention that involved cognitive restructuring and in vivo (real-life) exposure for public speaking anxiety with a treatment that was identical in all respects except that relaxation was replaced with a hypnotic induction and suggestions. Participants were asked to give an impromptu speech, during which they rated their anxiety. Compared with no treatment, both treatments resulted in changes in anxiety; however, on both behavioral and subjective measures during the speech, only the hypnosis group was found to differ from the no-treatment condition. Moreover, anxiety dissipated more quickly when participants were hypnotized compared with the nonhypnotic cognitive–behavioral treatment. In a review of the literature on hypnosis and anxiety, Schoenberger (2000) concluded that cognitive–behavioral hypnotherapy is more efficacious than no treatment in the treatment of anxiety.

Because social phobia is the most common of all the phobias and is often accompanied by panic attacks, it serves as the focus for much of our discussion. However, the techniques and strategies we present are also applicable to panic and the entire range of phobic conditions. Specific strategies for the treatment of persistent worries (GAD) are presented as well. More detailed step-by-step descriptions of nonhypnotic procedures for the treatment of anxiety, similar to the methods described in the following section, can be found in Mellinger and Lynn (2003).

Assessment and Treatment of Panic and Phobic Anxiety

The treatment of anxiety can be conducted with most patients in 20 or fewer sessions, unless assessment reveals the presence of major depression or personality disorders, which complicate treatment and require more intensive intervention. Any anxiety disorder of which panic is a significant component can be tackled more directly once the panic is controlled or overcome. A careful assessment of panic symptoms and their role in the anxiety condition should be completed. Information should be obtained regarding family history of anxiety disorders, social support, and onset of symptoms. We further recommend that anxious patients receive a medical workup that includes an evaluation of thyroid or blood sugar imbalances, arrhythmias, Cushing's disease, transient ischemic attacks, hyperventilation, congestive heart failure, mitral valve prolapse (an often benign heart condition), inner ear conditions, and metabolic conditions such as vitamin B2 deficiency (see Ballenger, 1997). In cases of severe or recalcitrant anxiety, medications, especially antidepressant SSRIs, should be considered as adjunctive treatment (see Mellinger & Lynn, 2003, for a discussion of issues associated with medication). The ability to track changes in symptoms is facilitated by objective assessment including interview (e.g., Anxiety Disorders Interview Schedule—IV; T. A. Brown, DiNardo, & Barlow, 1994) and self-report measures (e.g., Anxiety Sensitivity Index; Reiss, Peterson, Gursky, & McNally, 1986; Generalized Anxiety Disorder Questionnaire; Roemer, Borkovec, Posa, & Borkovec, 1995; Penn State Worry Questionnaire; T. J. Meyer, Miller, Metzger, & Borkovec, 1990; Social Phobia Scale; Mattick & Clarke, 1998).

A behavioral or functional analysis of anxiety begins with identifying the patients' unique profile of physical symptoms of panic (e.g., frequency, intensity, variability), the situational antecedents of panic (e.g., cues that reliably trigger panic), and the catastrophic thoughts, anxiety propositions, and expectancies that come into play before, during, and after an episode of panic. Comprehensive assessment also includes examination of behavioral avoidance patterns as well as safety behaviors (e.g., reading a book, watching television, or a talisman) that constitute subtle avoidance maneuvers that maintain anxiety. This essential assessment phase can be accomplished by way of self-monitoring and record keeping in everyday life situations, a behavioral avoidance test (e.g., how close the patient can stand to a spider), and exploration following suggestions for self-hypnosis in which enhanced abilities to imagine feared events and detect feelings as they unfold are suggested, as in the example that follows:

Therapist: You have already described some of your social fears, but let's go deeper into them now. Let yourself enter the situation you fear in your imagination, knowing full well that it is only in your imagination. Imagine you see yourself onstage, and that you know exactly what you are thinking and feeling, first as you prepare to give your talk, and then during the talk. As you watch, you may feel some mild yet entirely manageable discomfort as you analyze carefully and accurately the reactions you observe on a moment-to-moment basis. As the images come into focus, be aware of the situation in which it occurs. Let it come into focus now. More and more clear. All the details of the scene coming into view. Note who, if anyone else, was there when the episode took place, and how long it lasted. How severe was the panic at the worst moment, and what specific physical panic symptoms does the person you observe feel?

Providing patients with a working model of anxiety and panic is vital to the treatment of this disorder. However, it is also imperative to describe the emergency response and impress on the patient the value of reinterpreting physical responses.

Therapist: [*The therapist continues speaking to the patient as follows.*] The physical portion of panic and anxiety attacks is known as the emergency response. The symptoms may be uncomfortable, but they are not at all dangerous. Note whether the person onstage wants to escape or avoid the anxious feelings. Is he able to soldier on despite his feelings? Again, realize that no matter how he feels, there is no immediate mortal danger, so the emergency response is really a false alarm. You can understand this very clearly now. Let this knowledge go deep within you—know that despite the anxiety you observe in the person onstage, you know, even if he doesn't know it, that there is no real danger. Don't confuse these physical symptoms with real danger. This is one of the tricks of anxiety! After you share with me what you experience, I will tell you more about the physical causes of each of the symptoms you identify in the person onstage.

Patient: [*The patient describes relevant cognitive activity and physical reactions.*]

Therapist: OK, stay focused on my words. Let them register and remain deep within you for when you may need them later. From this time forward, when you experience any of the physical symptoms you identified, you will be able to rapidly identify them as anxiety, and nothing more. They are just your response to what you are afraid of, but they are not dangerous in any way. I repeat, they are not dangerous in any way. You will be able to state the real cause of the symptom to yourself, and this will help you relax and feel comfortable. You will know the physical symptoms do not mean danger. Each time you recognize a cause of a physical sensation that troubles you, it will be your cue to enter self-hypnosis and to relax . . . relax. Go deeper now, and listen carefully.

You said you identified a tight chest and a strong heartbeat as physical symptoms of anxiety. Chest muscles and other muscles tighten in response to perceived danger. When chest muscles tighten, it forces rapid, shallow breathing. This is known as panic breathing. The tide of air causes the throat and mouth to feel dry and uncomfortable and creates the sensation of a lump in the throat. Panic breathing increases the body's supply of oxygen. To circulate the supercharged blood to the parts of the body where it is most needed, the heart beats extra strong. Scientific opinion holds that panic is frequently accompanied by altered breathing that usually results in an increased carbon dioxide level that can cause numbness, tingling, and lightheadedness. But I can reassure you that people do not faint during panic attacks. Numbness and tingling are also caused by the decrease in blood flow to the hands because blood tends to flow to the big skeletal muscles when a person is frightened. Sweating occurs because when the heart and lungs are all pumped up and muscles are tensed, it is hard physical work and the byproduct is heat. The body's cooling system offsets this by sweating. Muscle tensing also causes the feeling of heavy, achy muscles, trembling, and tremors. When the muscles around the throat tighten, it creates the feeling of choking. The sense of unreality, bright vision, and oversensitivity to noise is caused by the brain ramping up the senses of sight and sound. Pupils dilate and the volume control of the auditory nerves is set on high, leading to the sense that things are unreal. At the same time, the brain redirects energy from digesting food to coping with a sense of imminent danger, creating the feeling of butterflies and upset stomach.

Now, go deeper and register what I have told you, feeling comforted that you will be able to understand the true cause of physical symptoms and not confuse them for real danger. To ensure that you remember the important points, I will prepare a handout that explains the cause of each of the physical symptoms you identified. You can review this hand-out at your convenience after the session to assist your practice of self-hypnosis and gain the understanding you need to contend with panicky feelings.

Self-Control Relaxation Training

Modifying Breathing. Because shallow and rapid breathing and physical tension engender many anxiety-related symptoms (Fried, 1999), a core component of treatments for all anxiety disorders is self-control relaxation training (SCRT). SCRT helps alleviate anxiety-stimulated physical tension and quiet disturbing thoughts and impulses until they eventually dissipate. SCRT consists of training in diaphragmatic breathing, body-scan exercises and relaxation, and focus on present sensory awareness, as illustrated in the following example.

> *Therapist:* Today I will teach you a breathing technique that will enable you to consciously slow and regulate your breathing to remedy panic breathing. Go into your self-hypnosis and relax, relax completely. Breathe slowly, regularly. Place one hand on your solar plexus, the soft area near the top of the stomach, just beneath the upside-down V of the sternum bone, and rest it there lightly. Notice the motion as you breathe. As you breathe, pretend that your hand is resting on a balloon. The balloon inflates when you inhale and deflates when you exhale. The area beneath your solar plexus expands and thrusts out with each inflation, contracts and pulls in with each deflation. To help maintain a good rhythm in balloon breathing, count slowly back down from 10 to 1, inflating the balloon by inhaling with each count. Each time you are about to exhale, say the word *calm* or another calming word or phrase to yourself and deflate the balloon. Feel yourself relax as your breathing slows down and you give yourself suggestions to feel calm and at ease. Practice this exercise when you are not stressed at least five times a day. If you detect any stress, tension, or anxiety, focus on your breathing and inflate and deflate the balloon slowly and easily as you retain only as much physical tension in your body as you feel you need to accomplish the task at hand. Learn how little tension is necessary in your every-day life.
>
> Now let's try something different. Imagine you are in a mildly distressing situation that you fear. See it in your mind's eye. Begin to feel the fear creep in. Feel your breathing rate start to accelerate, if ever so slightly. Now notice how your fear releases its grip on you as you focus on your

breathing. Notice how the focus on breathing shifts your focus of attention, and deliberately, consciously begin to slow your breathing. Breathe as slowly, as easily, as rhythmically you can. If you breathe only seven or eight times a minute, that's all right. Feel yourself beginning to feel more at ease as you slow your breathing.

[Body scan] If you feel some tension in your body, note where it is. Locate it. Scan your body, that's it . . . carefully, from your head to your toes, and notice where there is any extra tension. Tension you don't need. Use the ability to relax we have practiced and rehearsed in earlier sessions. If any part of your body feels especially tense, release any and all of the tension you don't need. You may wish to tense that body part now, and then relax it slowly, feeling any tension replaced by a sense of calm and ease. If you are still anxious, register what it is you are telling yourself. What are you saying to yourself? After you open your eyes, you will be able to share your experiences with me. After you have learned to relax and slow your breathing at times when you are not tense, practice the imagination exercise I have taught you with a scene that is mildly to moderately but not terribly distressing. Stay in control and breathe through any discomfort. Continue the exercise until you feel comfortable and fully in control. We'll talk about how this works in our next session.

[Sensory awareness] I'd like to teach you another way to contend with anxiety. Focusing on sensory impressions will help you stay in the present, thus combating the tendency to fear the future. Be aware of thoughts, sensations, behaviors, and emotional feelings. Now let yourself be aware of sounds. Listen to the sounds from nearby, and from outside or in the distance. Notice low- and high-pitched sounds, their steadiness or intermittence, and the smoothness or roughness of the tones. Simply listen, expanding your attention to include all the sounds around you. Now notice the colors of whatever captures your attention, and the smells around you. Just be aware. Feel your body making contact with the surface it is resting on. Continue to breathe slowly and regularly. Bring yourself to the present; alert yourself to the present if you feel yourself slipping into anxious thoughts about the future. Remember to notice your breathing. If you feel any tension in the process, focus on slowing your breathing and use the relaxation tools you have learned.

[Cue-controlled relaxation] Repeated practice at times of minimal stress is important to hone breathing and awareness skills, but it is imperative to apply SCRT relaxation at selected times of stress. To prepare, start learning to relax on cue. Begin by practicing at will at times of minimal discomfort. Practice your self-hypnosis and cue yourself by mentally saying, "Relax!" "Calm!" or "Breathe through!" or use your anchor [see chap. 4] and then spend between ½ and 2 minutes trying to get maximum effect from your favorite SCRT relaxation technique. For instance, when you start to feel restless in the doctor's or dentist's waiting room, or you start to think about a talk you have to give, take a few calming breaths, tense and then relax your hands or jaws, or shift your focus to the sounds, sights, and aromas of the present. Try to resist the temptation of enlisting cue-controlled relaxation to contend with major episodes of panic or anxiety at this point in time. Between our sessions, practice, customize, and optimize the techniques you have learned.

Continue to practice and to customize your self-hypnosis practice for at least a couple of weeks, until you find that you can consistently lower your tension level shortly after beginning a session. Once you've attained this skill, continue regular, unstressed practices often enough to maintain it.

[*Subjective Units of Discomfort or SUDs ratings and practice*] To get a sense of how well you are able to lower your tension level, let me tell you about a widely used scale to rate your discomfort. It's called the Subjective Units of Discomfort or the SUD scale, for short. Zero represents *no panic at all*; 5 is *moderately panicky*, when the nervousness is definitely there and getting disturbing; and 10 is the *worst panic attack you've ever experienced*.

Be aware of when your anxiety is a 3 or over, and immediately practice self-hypnosis. Reinterpret any symptoms of anxiety, kick yourself into a relaxed mode by registering the deepest feelings of relaxation you have felt in our practice sessions, and recreate those feelings. With some practice, you will be able to do this quickly and easily. As close to the time you feel anxious as possible, write down what you were thinking when you became anxious and how you were able to calm yourself down. We will continue working until you can consistently keep your SUDs rating at 2 or lower.

Remember to rate your anxiety SUD at the beginning and end of every practice, so you can measure whether and how much it changes as a result of mini-practicing. As your level of confidence in cue-controlled relaxation gets stronger, try to use it in gradually more challenging situations.

[*Abbreviated practice*] After awhile, you may want to abbreviate your practices. After you have become skillful at relaxing, start shortening the sessions with each technique while aiming for the same calming effect. For instance, an initial trial of abbreviated relaxation practice might consist of two or three calming breaths, then focusing on actively relaxing only your arms, hands, and face. After a number of practices in which you devote your attention to the process of controlling and releasing your tension, you will probably be able to achieve results similar to those that result from extended practices (Mellinger & Lynn, 2003).

At this point, self-hypnosis training and practice may have quelled panic and phobic anxiety. SCRT is also useful across the spectrum of anxiety disorders and can be especially useful in treating GAD by using cue-controlled relaxation, and so forth, at the very earliest signs of nonproductive worrying. For many individuals, SCRT is usefully supplemented by additional cognitive restructuring and behavioral exposure as follows.

Modifying Catastrophic Thinking

Therapist: [*Two cognitive errors*] Sometimes people continue to feel anxious even after they learn SCRT because they continue to persist in worrying or conjure up frightening, catastrophic thoughts about what they fear. At this point, we can hopefully clear up two kinds of thinking errors. The first is that anxiety is the opening act to a terrible main event. Because you have already trained in understanding the real nature of panic and anxiety symptoms and controlling acute negative arousal, you already know that they don't portend heart attacks, respiratory arrest, public humiliation, or the onset of insanity. You have learned to effectively challenge these interpretations by countering them with accurate data and scientific explanations.

The second error is that once a panic attack begins, it will last a long time and be very severe. When you experienced self-hypnosis and imagined yourself onstage experiencing anxiety, although you were able to observe yourself feeling uncomfortable, the anxiety did end at some point. No one has ever experienced a panic attack that lasts forever. They always end. The next time you feel even somewhat anxious, deep in the back of your mind you will know that anxiety is only temporary. It always passes. Any time you need to, any time you want to, this thought will be available to you. Your moods and feelings change, and anxiety will pass and be replaced with a sense of calm and security.

Now let's talk about your last anxiety or panic attack. How long did it last? What did you tell yourself afterward? Did you remind yourself it was only a temporary mental state of affairs? Remember to remind yourself that your anxiety is only a very temporary state of affairs . . . let it come . . . and let it go . . . let it come and let it go (Mellinger & Lynn, 2003). [*Discussion ensues.*]

Reestimation. People who suffer from panic and phobic conditions tend to exaggerate the probability that things will come out badly when they are apprehensive. Participants in Borkovec's (1999) anxiety research program kept diaries of their worrisome negative predictions. Eighty-six percent of the time things came out better than they expected. The other 14% of the outcomes were not particularly good, but at least the worriers were satisfied with the ways they coped with what happened. Reestimation builds skill at modifying predictions that are flawed by anxiety.

Therapist: Go deeply into your self-hypnosis and visualize the event you fear when you feel most apprehensive. Rate how likely the event will turn out badly on the following scale: 0% if there's no chance of a bad outcome, 50% for a 50–50 proposition, 100% for a seemingly certain catastrophe. What is your rating? Now rethink your rating on the basis of the following considerations:

1. How often has this kind of situation come out this negative way before? Does what you are worried about usually happen?
2. What is your recent track record?
3. What evidence, if any, can you muster that the situation will have a negative outcome?
4. Ask yourself whether your objectivity is being impaired by all-or-nothing thinking. What if you drop all clear-cut demoralizing exaggerators from your self-talk, including *always*, *never*, and *total failure*?
5. Are there other ways of looking at the situation, or other explanations? For example, when you described how you felt when your friend did not pay attention to you, and how humiliated you felt, is it possible that she was distracted because her child entered the room?
6. Can you imagine any way in which your worry is helpful? Does your worry suggest a particular action to take to solve a problem, or is it unproductive and fruitless?

Now visualize the anxiety-producing event as if it is taking place onstage and the events are happening to someone else. Reestimate the realistic probability of the feared outcome for someone else. Will the situation necessarily turn out catastrophically? Now I'd like you to think of a preferable way to think about each of your concerns.

Discussion ensues about any discrepancies between the realistic probability of negative outcomes occurring in relation to the self versus another person. This discussion can lead to a greater appreciation of cognitive errors, automatic thoughts, and anxiety propositions that continue to evoke anxiety. The following two cognitive techniques can be useful in contending with remaining issues.

[Reconsider anxious thoughts] During the next week, as soon as you notice your apprehension building, ask yourself, "What am I afraid of?" Make a note of your fears and your specific anxiety propositions related to the automatic thoughts that trouble you regarding each fear you specify. Reconsider everything that provokes your anxiety to provide a basis for formulating a less fearful, more objective way of thinking about it. In a previous session, you identified the anxiety proposition that you would pass out before you gave a speech, as you were looking through your notes. Listen carefully to the following suggestions. Use them as a guide to what you tell yourself now and any time you have anxious thoughts along the lines you described. Your hyperventilation ensures that you will have plenty of oxygen, and your pounding heart circulates it throughout your body. Your lightheadedness is the byproduct of taking too much carbon dioxide into your body. Slow, regular breathing will relieve your physical anxiety. You will be able to reassure yourself that the last time you fainted was 10 years ago, and that it had nothing to do with anxiety. You never have fainted before a talk, during a talk, or after a talk. You feel apprehensive and panicky in these situations simply because of how you are talking to yourself, and your anxious mind mistakes your physical symptoms for real danger. You will experience great relief as you realize you can have a measure of control over your fears, and you will work hard to achieve this.

[What's the worst that can happen?] Let's try something else. Another anxiety proposition you identified earlier was that you would be at a party with your friends, and you would feel terrified that you were having a heart attack. Being flooded with these anxious thoughts was your worst-case scenario. But now let's take a closer look at the situation. Imagine you are at the party now and this happens. Get a sense of this happening to you . . . go deep into your self-hypnosis. Take some time to do this. Now ask yourself the question: Would your buddies resent you forever because you clutched your chest or treat you as an attention-seeker for begging someone to call the paramedics? No, you say, it's unlikely to happen? Often when you ask yourself, "What's the worst that can happen?" you realize that the realistic outcome is not what you feared. And if it did occur, wouldn't you be able to endure it? If necessary, couldn't you actually cope with the feared event? I think so. Get deeply in touch with your ability to cope effectively. Make a tight fist of determination now. Do this and get in touch with your strength that is within. Any time you need to remind yourself of this, simply make a fist or bring your fingers together, and you will quickly and easily have a sense of your personal strength that is within. Strength is within. Your strength is within, tap this strength now. Tap it and make it yours.

[*So what?*] If the worst case situation did happen, you also can say to yourself, "So what." If a powerful, pounding heartbeat played a part in your anxiety episode and made you feel acutely panicky, say to yourself that your heart is strong . . . strong. It can support immense exertion if truly necessary. You will know, deep within yourself, deep within yourself that you are only very fearful, nothing more serious than that, and that your buddies are more likely to offer their help in a caring way rather than to ignore and shun you. Even if your friends were a bit annoyed with you, would it mean the end of your friendship? Even if you felt it was necessary to call paramedics to help you through the worst of this panic and then left, so what? More and more you will be able to reassure yourself, calm yourself, and feel more confident that you can and will be able to contend with any anxiety you encounter. You are much, much more than any anxiety you experience. You are realizing that anxiety does not need to take charge of you; it does not define you. Get a sense of yourself being a person who is so much more than your anxiety, not defined any longer by what you fear, push open the possibilities, your horizons . . . get a sense of an expanded self, what you can and will be.

[*Posthypnotic suggestion*] And during the week, you will have flashes of the feeling of success. Perhaps you will find yourself thinking of times you successfully contended with anxiety, or times when things worked out much better than you feared. You may be surprised by how your thinking begins to change, how capable you are of transformation— transformation in the way you think, feel, and are as a person. And you will be able to enjoy this transformation as it occurs, as it unfolds.

[*The new you*] Now imagine that you have been transformed into what I will call *the new you*. Get inside the skin of this new you who embodies how you would like to think about the situation should it occur again. Think of it as a challenge. The old, socially anxious you probably tended to stress the really uncomfortable moments and dwell at length on their bad effects on your self-image. Get in touch with your strength, your creativity, your resolve to bravely contend with what you fear. In your imagination, place yourself in another situation where you felt very socially uncomfortable. How would you approach the situation? What would your self-talk be like? How would you cope with anxiety should it arise? Reconsider everything that provokes your anxiety in the situation to provide a basis for formulating a less fearful, more objective way of thinking about it. You will become more aware of the challenges you face and empowered to tackle the anticipated stressors more effectively. The new you will try out techniques that appear helpful and, as you begin socializing differently, adapt new, more positive perspectives on social situations. Now let this new you talk to me. [*Therapist–patient discussion ensues.*]

During the week, enter self-hypnosis when you need to and get in touch with this new you. Consult him [or her] to get a sense of how to think about situations you fear if they should occur again. List thoughts that raise your anxiety because they incorporate a prediction of negative or catastrophic outcome. Rate their anxious probability. After completing your reestimation homework, think about the realistic probability and note the considerations and rationale that led to your reestimation. How would you rather think about the situation? What does the new you think? Transform your anxiety propositions into realistic propositions. For example, to combat your fear of a catastrophic physical reaction, you can say to yourself, "This is just anxiety I'm having before my talk, not a heart attack, respiratory arrest, or acute psychosis." Tell yourself something along the lines of "It's not likely to last more than a few minutes, even at its worst, and I usually recover very quickly." Listen carefully, and let this register deep within you: You are much stronger—much, much stronger than your automatic thoughts depict you to be. From this moment on, you will engage in the process of decatastrophizing anxious thoughts, and remember to embrace the new you for assistance, if you desire. Be sure to practice your SCRT at least several times each day. Treat each incident of heightened anxiety as a challenge by coping with it strategically every time it occurs.

Imaginal and Behavioral Exposure

Imaginal Exposure. If SCRT and cognitive restructuring do not alleviate anxiety to the patient's satisfaction, the next step is to combine planned exposure with cognitive practices. Exposure may be imaginal or real. Imaginal desensitization, or imaginal exposure therapy (see Lazarus, 1973), is a good starting point for overcoming a state of severe avoidance, as in the example that follows.

Therapist: Today, we will begin to help you feel more comfortable being in social situations by learning how to practice imaginal exposure. The assumption underlying the procedure you will learn is that the things we fear in reality, we also fear in imagination; and the corollary is that the things we no longer fear in imagination will also not disturb us in the actual situation. [*More extensive discussion follows, and patient's cooperation is secured.*]

Go deep into your self-hypnosis now. Let the specific situation, or specific aspect of the situation you fear the most, come to your mind. Just let images and feelings come to you. You may find it interesting, but you will discover that you will be able to keep your anxiety manageable, quite manageable during this process. When you know what situation or aspect of the situation makes you the most uncomfortable, just begin to talk about it. And, without thinking, give it a SUD rating.

The patient gives a SUD rating and proceeds to talk about five to seven more situations that cover a range of ratings. After the patient is invited to open his or her eyes and come out of self-hypnosis, the therapist and patient talk about the situations and construct a hierarchy from the lowest to the highest levels of discomfort. The situations selected to work on initially should be accessible, involve a noticeable but manageable discomfort level, and give the patient the prospect of real satisfaction as a reward for mastering them.

Therapist: Now enter your self-hypnosis and go deep, go very deep . . . deep to the point that you let all of the tension you don't need drain out of your body. Now move, move in your mind's eye to your place of comfort and security. Let me know when you are there, when you have scanned your body, you are relaxed, and you are there. Good. Now begin to visualize the situation [X] you ranked lowest in discomfort. Focus deeply on it, and imagine the situation as vividly as possible, and signal me when you achieve a SUD rating of 4. Good. Now that you have achieved a rating of 4, mentally switch the scene off. Relax as deeply, no, even more deeply than you were before starting the exercise; go to your favorite place now, experience a sense of comfort and a sense of motivation to continue, to move forward in your life, to contend with whatever you need to in order to be the new you, the person you know you can be. Now let's do it again. The idea is to resume vividly visualizing the anxiety-provoking situation, then switching it off and relaxing deeply until you no longer feel any discomfort. After you spend some time in your place of comfort and security, then we will move on to the next item on your hierarchy. [*Therapy proceeds accordingly.*] You can practice on your own between sessions, but remember to tackle situations that are manageable for you, until we work our way to the most difficult situation.

Behavioral or Real-Life Exposure. Imaginal exposure has beneficial effects in its own right but may also serve as preparation and rehearsal for real-life exposure. As in imaginal exposure, a hierarchy of situations is selected and situations are chosen initially that are tolerably anxiety-provoking. Times and places for practice are arranged, and exposures are graduated—broken down into steps that cause a manageable level of anxiety, each of which should be practiced until the patient's anxiety decreases before going on to the next, more challenging step. Consider the example of an exposure hierarchy related to the patient's desire to feel comfortable studying in the library cafeteria (Mellinger & Lynn, 2003).

1. Walk into the cafeteria for a few minutes and make brief eye contact with several people.
2. Practice conversing briefly with the salesperson.
3. Wait in line and buy coffee.
4. Sit down at the table and drink coffee during nonpeak hours.
5. Do Step 4 when the place is busy.
6. Sit down near the exit, drinking coffee and studying for 15 minutes.
7. Same as above, but study for at least 45 minutes.
8. Sit in the middle of the cafeteria during a busy time.
9. Sit in the middle and study for at least 15 minutes.
10. Sit in the middle and study for at least 45 minutes.
11. During the daily exposures, which involve practice in one or more different situations or steps in the hierarchy, do the following: (a) enter a wakeful state of self-hypnosis; (b) practice SCRT, including cue-controlled relaxation; and (c) notice any automatic thoughts and anxiety propositions that can be examined, challenged, and restructured in individual therapy and replaced with flexible coping responses in daily life. It is important for the patient to remain in each situation until the SUD level has peaked and dropped.

Opportunistic Exposure. Certain phobias, such as social phobia, lend themselves to opportunistic exposures that arise in the context of everyday life. The following sample exposure plan is taken from Mellinger and Lynn (2003).

1. Make brief eye contact and smile at 50 people.
2. Greet at least 25 people whom you find attractive.
3. Ask 20 people directions to the restroom, the nearest pay phone, the nearest service station, or the nearest Italian, Chinese, Thai, or Mexican restaurant.
4. Introduce yourself to 25 people.
5. Purchase numerous small items at different stores. Pay with a check or credit card, so you can practice signing your name in front of other people.
6. Make brief neutral or positive comments to 25 people. For example, remark on the weather; the décor, ambience, or

efficiency of the staff in the place where you are or holidays approaching or just past.

7. Find out what is fascinating about 20 different people. Do so by watching them carefully and conversing with or about them.

8. Go out and collect rejections; push the envelope. People who have used this technique often find that they are rejected much less often and more gently than they anticipated, if they are rejected at all.

During weekly therapy sessions, the results of exposure practice sessions are reviewed. It is helpful for patients to record what they did, thought, imagined, and felt and how they were able to challenge anxious thoughts and arrive at a different perspective about their fears. The therapist should highlight success experiences and help the patient identify any remaining anxiety propositions and cognitive errors that require restructuring. This can be done by asking the patient to enter self-hypnosis, revisit the scene that aroused the most anxiety, and provide a commentary about the experience.

The scene can be reimagined, but this time, the patient can implement more effective ways of coping (e.g., challenge negative thinking, reinterpret physical symptoms) with and ultimately mastering the anxiety during the imaginal exposure practice session. Imaginal and behavioral exposure proceeds until all the steps in the hierarchy are completed with final SUDs ratings of 3 or less. In our experience, exposure provides relief in most patients in 5 to 10 sessions, unless the symptom picture is complicated by major depression, personality disorders, or other serious psychopathology, in which case more extensive treatment is required.

Techniques for Generalized Worry

The line between healthy and unhealthy worry can be fine. Healthy worry stimulates problem solving and planning, is generally of short duration, and creates only negligible emotional distress. When worry turns maladaptive, people exaggerate the possibility of negative events or outcomes, mental clarity and problem solving are compromised, and negative thoughts and images persist long after a problem is solved. Worry accompanies many anxiety disorders and can dominate the lives of people with GAD.

Early Worry Recognition

The treatment of GAD begins with early worry recognition followed by the implementation of strategies to curtail worry. Worry can be detected by noticing physical indicators of anxiety (e.g., fidgeting, muscle tension, sweating, rapid heartbeat) and anxious thoughts (e.g., "I'm overwhelmed," "I'm afraid of _____," or "What if _____?"). Borkovec (1999) recommended the technique of having patients monitor worries every time they pass through a doorway. We instruct patients to enter self-hypnosis for a few minutes on the hour and half hour, do a body scan and recognize anxious thinking and the source of such thinking ("What am I worried about?"), and then implement SCRT to counteract worry. If worry persists, the patient can use the following cognitive restructuring techniques discussed earlier: (a) reestimating the realistic probability of negative outcomes, (b) the worst-case scenario and so-what technique, and (c) identifying and disputing cognitive errors and maladaptive thinking. If the worry relates to a specific problem or event, the patient should brainstorm and devise a specific and detailed coping plan. Also useful are hypnotic suggestions that excessive worry does not improve decision making or prevent negative events; reminders that the patient has successfully negotiated many challenging situations in the past and that it is possible to learn from negative experiences; and suggested images such as placing lingering worries in a file, cabinet, drawer, or some other storage place.

Worry Periods

To achieve mastery over worry, patients may benefit from learning the behavioral techniques of worry periods and worry postponement. Worry monitoring will often reveal tenacious worries that recur during the course of daily living. The patient is instructed to schedule a definite time each day as a worry period, ideally a half hour or longer, during which time attention can be devoted to immediate, substantial concerns on an uninterrupted basis. A hierarchy of worries (least to most disturbing) can be developed, and patients can enter self-hypnosis and practice the cognitive–behavioral techniques (e.g., SCRT, cognitive restructuring) we have summarized. Patients observe that anxiety generally diminishes after a long enough contact with what is feared.

Worry Postponement

The technique of worry postponement involves the patient making a conscious decision to monitor and postpone worries for a period as short as a few seconds or as long as a part of a day. After lengthy postponements, worries should be scheduled for specific times. When the period of postponement has elapsed, the patient should either think about the anxious thought right then or decide to postpone it until a specific time once again. Worry postponement may be used repeatedly until the worry fades away.

Mindfulness and Acceptance

Mindfulness techniques, described in chapter 7, have also been found useful in the treatment of GAD (Borkovec, 2002). In our experience, these techniques are often especially useful with patients who do not respond to other interventions. Persons with GAD often scan the environment for threat and build fortifications against feeling and expressing strong emotions. The latest thinking about GAD is that it is necessary for the patient to accept and cope with painful emotions because the function of worry is to avoid deeper and more terrifying feelings (Borkovec & Newman, 1998). Avoidance may be somewhat effective in the short run. But the rub is that it precludes extinction of fear and perpetuates anxiety, which is ameliorated by exposure to feared emotions. In general, when people frequently use coping strategies that circumvent or suppress negative emotions or thoughts, clinical outcomes suffer (Hayes & Gifford, 1997; Hayes, Strosahl, & Wilson, 1999). One way of exposing individuals to the gamut of human emotions is the practice of mindfulness.

Emotional Processing of Interpersonal Feelings

Foa and Kozak (1986) identified the necessity for emotional processing of fear to overcome it. However, a very recent innovation in the treatment of GAD is the recognition of the importance of emotional processing of interpersonal feelings. More than any other topic, patients with GAD worry about interpersonal matters (Roemer, Molina, & Borkovec, 1997). In Newman, Castonguay, Borkovec, and Molnar's (2004) integrative therapy for GAD, patients are informed that they may be so bent on avoiding what they fear from others that they fail to pursue their interpersonal needs, inadvertently creating the very situations that engender not only anxiety but negative outcomes. For example, by protecting themselves from others by failing to disclose their needs and feelings, they may be perceived as unapproachable, disinterested, and cold. The goal is to shift the patient's focus "away from anticipating danger and toward openness, spontaneity, and vulnerability to others, as well as toward more empathic attention to the needs of others" (p. 329). Newman and her colleagues recommended combining CBT with a variety of emotional deepening techniques derived from other traditions (e.g., Gestalt therapy or experiential therapy two-chair technique). They further recommended in-depth exploration of relationships with significant people by way of the following questions: (a) "What event happened between you and another person?" (b) "What emotions did you feel?" (c) "What did you need or hope to get from the other person?" (d) "What did you fear from the other person?" (e) "What did you do?" (f) "What happened next between you and the other person?" and (g) continued exploration, returning to the question, "What emotions did you feel?"

Hypnosis can be integrated into this treatment framework by inviting the patient to enter self-hypnosis and observe his or her experience unfolding on a movie or video screen, while responding to the above questions. The patient is told that he or she has a start-and-stop control and a feeling control that can be turned both on and off. For the first run-through, the patient is instructed to describe what occurs while watching the action with the feeling knob turned off. This procedure is followed by another run-through during which the patient is instructed to turn the feeling knob on and stop the action whenever he or she senses his or her viewed self beginning to feel the slightest bit uncomfortable. At that point, the patient can "enter the movie," do a body scan, and examine exactly how his or her fear is related to catastrophic thoughts (e.g., ridicule, abandonment, rejection) and anticipations. The patient can then be asked to turn the feeling control to the point where he or she can feel the feelings as the scene unfolds, as he or she gains a better sense of what he or she needs, wants, and fears in relation to the target person while fully experiencing him- or herself in the moment with this person. At any time the therapist or patient wishes to have an intellectual discussion of the events, the patient can "step out of the movie" and turn the feeling knob off. The exercise can be repeated until the individual is able to tolerate and accept whatever feelings arise and gains a solid understanding of his or her avoidance patterns and the thoughts that support his or her emotional retreats. The therapist can also use the technique to foster empathy and insight by asking the patient to focus on the possible thoughts and feelings of the person he or she is interacting with, paying special attention to how the patient's behaviors may elicit interpersonal reactions that confirm fears and spark worries. Age regression can be used to explore childhood relationships with parents and other significant people to better understand the developmental antecedents of current avoidance patterns and interpersonal expectancies.

The treatment of anxiety is fundamental to interventions for many disorders and conditions that it accompanies. Many of the techniques and strategies for coping with anxiety can, therefore, be used in the comprehensive treatment of a variety of conditions including depression, eating disorders, and substance abuse. In the next chapter, we describe the treatment of posttraumatic stress disorder (PTSD), which is also considered to be an anxiety disorder and can be ameliorated with many of the hypnotic techniques we recommend for anxiety disorders. Indeed, exposure therapy is widely regarded as the first-line treatment for PTSD. Nevertheless, we present PTSD in a separate chapter because a distinct body of knowledge has coalesced around anxiety associated with trauma and intrusive imagery, and PTSD poses somewhat different challenges than does the treatment of nontrauma-related anxiety conditions and disorders.

10

POSTTRAUMATIC STRESS DISORDER

War, rape, crime, and natural disasters have plagued humankind from antiquity to the present. Indeed, most members of modern society are touched in some way by trauma. Kessler and his colleagues' (Kessler, Sonnega, Bromet, Hughes, & Nelson, 1995) study of nearly 6,000 men and women revealed that the majority of people sampled had experienced at least one traumatic event during their lifetime. To make matters worse, once one is traumatized, the risk of experiencing a second trauma is as high as 50% (Resnick, Kilpatrick, Dansky, Saunders, & Best, 1993). In one study of undergraduate college students (Vrana & Lauterbach, 1994), one third of the sample reported that they had experienced four or more traumatic events. Although many people—perhaps as many as 80%—are resilient enough to cope with a wide range of traumatic life events (e.g., violence, natural disasters, combat), 25% to 33% are not so fortunate and suffer serious, long-lasting repercussions including anxiety, depression, and posttraumatic stress disorder (PTSD; Meichenbaum, 1994; Yehuda, Resnick, Kahana, & Giller, 1993). By one estimate, the lifetime prevalence of PTSD is 5% in men and 10% in women (Kessler et al., 1995). In high-risk populations, such as Vietnam veterans, the rates skyrocket to as high as 30% (National Vietnam Veterans Readjustment Study; Kulka, Fairbank, Jordan, Weiss, & Cranston, 1990), although PTSD rates and negative traumatic reactions may be inflated (Dean, 1998).

FEATURES OF POSTTRAUMATIC STRESS DISORDER

In this chapter we illustrate how exposure-based techniques can be combined with hypnosis and cognitive interventions to ameliorate PTSD symptoms. For a diagnosis of PTSD to be made, the traumatic event must be life endangering and the person's response must involve intense fear, helplessness, or horror (American Psychiatric Association, 1994). It is also necessary for the symptoms to persist for at least 1 month; otherwise the condition is diagnosed as acute stress disorder. The symptoms of PTSD include stress and hyperarousal (e.g., sleep difficulties, exaggerated and distressing startle response), emotional numbing of responsiveness (e.g., restricted range of emotional experiences, feelings of detachment and alienation from others), and persistent avoidance of situations or reminders of trauma (e.g., efforts to avoid activities, places, or people associated with the event).

One of the hallmarks of PTSD is vivid memories, feelings, and images of traumatic experiences, widely known as flashbacks. These intrusive symptoms of PTSD can recur for decades after the original trauma and be reactivated by many everyday stimuli and stressful experiences. Tim O'Brien, author of the Vietnam novel *The Things They Carried*, in talking about his war experiences commented that "The hardest part, by far, is to make the bad pictures go away. In war time, the world is one big long horror movie, image after image, and if it's anything like Vietnam, I'm in for a lifetime of wee-hour creeps" (1990, p. 56). Flashbacks have been associated with chronic somatic distress, anxiety, depression, dissociation, avoidance of situations linked with their emergence, paranoid thinking, and sleep disturbance (Baum, Cohen, & Hall, 1993; Bremner et al., 1995; Jones & Barlow, 1990; Nolen-Hoeksema, 1990) and should be given a high priority in treatment, as illustrated in the discussion that follows.

HYPNOSIS AND POSTTRAUMATIC STRESS DISORDER

Many published clinical reports, dating back nearly 200 years to the use of hypnosis by Dutch physicians (Vijselaar & Van der Hart, 1992), document the potential effectiveness of hypnosis in the treatment of an assortment of posttraumatic conditions related to combat, sexual assaults, anesthesia failure, and car accidents (see Cardena, 2000). In addition, a randomized control study (Brom, Kleber, & Defare, 1989) indicated that hypnosis in the context of behavior therapy, desensitization, and psychodynamic psychotherapy was more effective than a waiting-list control group—at the end of treatment and at 3-month follow-up. Although no one treatment emerged as clearly superior, intrusion symptoms (e.g., flashbacks) responded best to hypnosis and desensitization, whereas avoidance symptoms responded best to psychodynamic therapy.

On the basis of a comprehensive review of the literature on hypnosis in the treatment of posttraumatic conditions, Cardena, Maldonado, van der Hart, and Spiegel (2000, p. 270) contended that there are compelling reasons and clinical observations to recommend the use of hypnosis as an adjunct for the treatment of PTSD. As mentioned earlier, hypnotic procedures can serve as a useful adjunct to cognitive–behavioral and exposure therapy. The fact that exposure therapy has been found to be effective in all 12 studies of the treatment of PTSD in which it was used (see Rothbaum, Meadows, Resnick, & Foy, 2000) and that cognitive–behavioral treatments for PTSD are also highly effective (Deacon & Abramowitz, 2004; Van Etten & Taylor, 1998) makes hypnosis a promising adjunctive intervention for ameliorating the suffering of trauma victims. This impression is reinforced by the fact that patients with posttraumatic conditions seem to be more hypnotically suggestible than are most other patient populations (D. Spiegel, Hunt, & Dondershine, 1988; Stutman & Bliss, 1985) and are therefore likely to benefit from hypnotic procedures (see Cardena, 2000; Cardena et al., 2000).

ASSESSMENT AND TREATMENT OF POSTTRAUMATIC STRESS DISORDER

The treatment of posttraumatic conditions begins with the assessment of the traumatized individual. Unless questioned specifically, some patients are reluctant to disclose a trauma history because of shame, self-blame, and the tendency to avoid disturbing topics (Kilpatrick, 1983). It is thus imperative that the therapist ask straightforward and direct questions to obtain a well-rounded history of trauma. According to a consensus conference regarding the assessment of PTSD (Keane, Solomon, & Maser, 1996), it is advisable to obtain the following data: (a) information from standardized clinician-administered diagnostic interviews (e.g., SCID–PTSD module, DSM–IV; American Psychiatric Association, 1994; First, Spitzer, Gibbon, & Williams, 1996); (b) ratings of trauma-related impairment and disability; (c) aspects of the event including age, perceived life threat, injuries, harm, frequency, and duration; and (d) findings from self-report instruments (e.g., Impact of Event Scale—Revised; D. S. Weiss & Marmar, 1997) with established validity and reliability.

In addition, we advise gathering information regarding personal attributes, as well as behaviors, feelings, and thoughts that occurred before, during, and after the traumatic experience including (a) personal resources and limitations (e.g., capacity for insight, ability to tolerate and accept negative emotions, memory problems) and social support; (b) comorbid psychological disorders and previous trauma history; (c) changes in the person's sense of self (e.g., "I'm worthless because I didn't resist the sexual assault") and worldview ("I can't trust any man") in response to the traumatic event; (d) current triggers of posttraumatic reactions; (e) the content of flashbacks and reports of concomitant psychophysiological and emotional reactivity; (f) successful (if any) and unsuccessful strategies used to control flashbacks; (g) memory problems; and (h) the ability to form a working alliance with the therapist.

Finally, the need for pharmacotherapy should be evaluated. Many people with PTSD benefit from selective serotonin reuptake inhibitors (SSRIs; e.g., Prozac, Zoloft), which have the added bonus of treating depression and panic disorder that are frequently comorbid with PTSD (M. J. Friedman, Davidson, Mellman, & Southwick, 2000).

Treatment of Flashbacks and Posttraumatic Stress Disorder: Exposure Therapy and Hypnosis

Rationale for Exposure Therapy

Exposure therapy may be effective for several reasons. Traumatic experiences are thought to lead to the establishment of fear structures or networks in memory (see Foa & Rothbaum, 1998; Foa, Steketee, & Rothbaum, 1989) that are activated in response to reminders of trauma and lead to escape and avoidance. Exposure may therefore be a direct route to accessing and modifying fear structures and minimizing avoidance. Repeated exposure to what is feared in a safe environment results in habituation and adaptive changes in the fear structure. Exposure may also be effective because observing fears wax and wane in the safe and controlled treatment milieu engenders positive self-suggestions and expectancies (e.g., "I am in control," "I can turn fear on and off") that both reduce anxiety and change maladaptive beliefs that maintain avoidance (e.g., "I'm weak and vulnerable"). Exposure also provides an opportunity for the person to reevaluate the event and his or her reaction to it. For example, during exposure victims of sexual assault may have the opportunity to focus on their resistance to the assault and realize that they did their best to avert it. As Meichenbaum (1994; Meichenbaum & Fong, 1993) has observed, the entire narrative in which the traumatic event is embedded can change with retelling or reexperiencing in the direction of greater self-acceptance and a more realistic assessment of the dangerousness of the environment and the likelihood of retraumatization (see also Foa & Kozak, 1986).

Affect Management

It is imperative to prepare the patient for exposure therapy. A candidate for exposure therapy ideally should experience psychophysiological reactivity to specific, reexperienced traumatic memories (Litz, Blake, Gerardi, & Keane, 1990). At the same time, anxiety and panic symptoms can be an unwelcome byproduct of exposure treatment (Pittman et al., 1991). Accordingly, a cardinal rule of treating PTSD is that a degree of symptom stability, along with the ability to tolerate emotionally charged imagery, is prerequisite to embarking on exposure therapy.

Exposure should be instituted only after a good rapport with the patient has been established, the nature of PTSD and the benefits of exposure have been explained, and self-hypnosis and relaxation skills have been mastered in-session. A menu of affect management strategies, including SCRT (self-control relaxation training; see chap. 7), should be at the patient's disposal. In the face of reminders of trauma, cue-controlled relaxation and the use of individualized cognitive and physical anchors (see chap. 4) often prove indispensable. Self-suggestions such as "That was then and this is now," "You survived and are a survivor," and "You did what you could do," as well as reassuring words and phrases such as "I'm going to be all right," "This feeling will pass," and "I am strong and good" can be empowering. Patients can engage in self-hypnosis and imagine a place of comfort and safety to soothe themselves or cultivate pleasant and distracting memories, images, and sensations in diverse sensory modalities (e.g., the smell of flowers) to replace traumatic memories. Visualizing scenes related to feeling accepted, loving and caring for another person, being needed, and feeling competent can also comfort some individuals.

The gesture of bringing the thumb and forefinger together can be used as a cue or anchor to induce self-hypnosis or relaxation. In the case of flashbacks associated with temporally distant events, patients can carry a newly minted coin and examine the date as a way of grounding their experience in the present. An object such as a small, smooth stone that is imbued with special meaning and "power" can be touched, on cue, to create a semblance of emotional constancy across situations and a sense of being centered in the present. Another portable strategy is for patients to place a hand near their heart; count slow, deep breaths; notice details of their present surroundings; and say to themselves, "I am safe in the present."

Preparation for Exposure

To lay the proper groundwork for exposure therapy, we inform patients that though they may never have thought of flashbacks in this way, they reflect a talent that can be exploited as an advantage during hypnosis. The talent is the ability to imagine and recreate events "as real as real" that are not actually happening in the present. The occurrence of a flashback implies above-average and perhaps high suggestibility insofar as the patient comes to believe, if only temporarily, that the imagined event is taking place and experiences concomitant physical effects, as one might when absorbed in a hypnotic suggestion. If the patient can imagine negative events vividly, it is possible to harness imaginal skills and suggestibility to create a variety of pleasant and adaptive hypnotic and nonhypnotic experiences. To foster positive expectancies, therapists can inform patients that research indicates that many persons who suffer from PTSD are highly suggestible, and that a high level of suggestibility is helpful but not required to learn to separate the past from the present, feel safe in the now, and move forward in life.

Suggestions along the following lines can be given during self-hypnosis, prior to implementing exposure techniques, to interrupt and defuse traumatic memories:

It is understandable and normal to experience stress and a disruption in your life after experiencing a traumatic event that, by definition, is outside the realm of normal experience and engenders fear and avoidance. The fact that thinking about the event still has the power to upset you a great deal, and that you have flashbacks, indicates that you have not yet processed what happened to the point that you can peacefully coexist with your past and let your guard down and feel safe and secure in the present. Reminders of what happened are still painful, but you can discover that they will lose their power to affect you as you come to realize, at all levels of your being, that there is no immediate threat in the present. . . . The event is past . . . you can begin to let it go . . . because it is safe now . . . and you can move on with your life . . . move on . . . as your experience unfolds, moment by moment. By experiencing the event repeatedly and vividly in your imagination, in the exposure exercises we will do together, you will discover that you are in control, you will realize that when the event replays, it is nothing more than a mental tape . . . a tape that runs in your own mind and not in reality. As this tape's malign power to threaten and frighten you discharges, you become increasingly free . . . free to live your life, to make choices, to breathe each breath . . . unshackled by the past. More and more you will take away from what happened important learnings. As your confidence returns . . . you appreciate your ability to bounce back, your resilience . . . you will get in touch with a new appreciation for what you need to do to take care of yourself, be good to yourself, soothe yourself. . . . As you practice your self-control relaxation training, your breathing exercises, and your cue-controlled relaxation at the first signs of stressing out, you remind yourself that any discomfort you experience will pass, and you will be able to increasingly take charge of your mind, your body, and ultimately the direction of your life.

Elevator Exercise

The elevator technique is a way of generating treatment goals and tasks and priming positive thinking about the benefits of overcoming phobic avoidance of trauma-related situations and coping with flashbacks by way of exposure.

> Before we start exposure, let's examine together how your life will be different when you are no longer troubled by reexperiencing the automobile accident. You have an opportunity to rebuild your life from the ground floor up. You can do this. So what I'd like you to do is go deeper into your self-hypnosis, deeper and deeper, as you like. Imagine you are on an elevator, and on the first or ground floor. I'd like you to press the button that says *2* and feel yourself being elevated to the next level . . . to the next level as you rise to the second floor. When you step off the elevator, you will have a strong sense of the first thing you need to do after you are no longer troubled by reexperiencing the automobile accident. Perhaps you will have images of what you need to do. . . . You will be aware of decisions to be made, how you need to think about yourself, actions or risks to be taken, ways in which you might see yourself and the world differently. Okay, now have a good strong sense of what you need to do, and imagine you have done exactly what you need to do, and you are transformed in the process. Now press the button for the next floor, number 3, aware that your life has changed for the better before you step out. Now step out and get a sense of what you need to do next. . . . What is it you need to do now? After you have a sense of what you need to do, imagine that you have done it and that your life has changed, changed for the better. This building has one more floor, and you will do the same thing you have done, to get to the pinnacle of where you need to go, what you need to achieve. Go to the top floor now, with an awareness of how your life has changed, and get a sense of what you need to do to be completely healed, to feel more calm and at ease, relaxed and safe with yourself and with others. More comfortable living in the world . . . flowing with experience. Okay, now get this sense of what you need to do, and exactly how you will be changed . . . changed for the better. Good, now when you open your eyes, you will be able to share it with me. I'd appreciate that very much.

Initiating Exposure

Before exposure is initiated, we ask the patient to discuss the target event in a matter-of-fact way, to gauge the ability to describe what occurred while remaining relatively calm and relaxed. We recommend conducting exposure only after the patient can tolerate emotions instigated by a relatively superficial or cursory discussion of the event. Each scene should be discussed in advance of exposure, and the patient should decide at what pace to proceed and the amount of anxiety she is prepared to tolerate, as indexed by a Subjective Units of Discomfort (SUD) rating. We recommend starting with scenes of moderate intensity, in the range of 4 through 7 on the 10-point SUD scale. At first, an entire session may be devoted to exposure with the most upsetting details omitted or not verbalized. However, after one or two sessions, it is often possible to go through each scene in detail and repeat the scene several times, after a detailed rendition of the scene is processed. Self-hypnosis and relaxation should follow each exposure trial, along with a discussion of how upsetting the scene was at different points (SUD ratings), what themes emerged (e.g., loss, anger, fear of death, guilt), and how the experience can be fodder for learning how to master fear.

Because talking about, much less reliving traumatic memories, can be stressful, we recommend that exposure proceed at a pace that patients can tolerate, both physically in terms of arousal level and emotionally in terms of feeling in control and not feeling overwhelmed. If SUD ratings indicate a level of stress beyond 5 or 6, or patients appear visibly agitated after self-hypnosis and relaxation procedures have been implemented, we ask patients specifically if they wish to proceed or if they wish to take a breather and discuss their residual anxiety and not proceed until their discomfort subsides. Under these circumstances, we do not press forward until the patient indicates a willingness to do so. This tact will help alleviate patients' understandable reluctance to engage in exposure therapy (Rothbaum et al., 2000) and minimize the possibility of negative sequelae (e.g., intense shame and guilt, intolerable arousal) following reexposure to traumatic events (Davidson & Baum, 1993). Nevertheless, exposure should be conducted with great caution or avoided entirely in cases in which patients experience ongoing crises and suicidality, have a substance abuse problem, have made a recent claim for compensation for trauma-related damages, exhibit treatment resistance, or have difficulty generating imagery (Litz et al., 1990).

> Now that you have a better understanding of what you will gain by learning to contend with flashbacks and learning to accept your past, it is time to practice exposure to learn how to coexist with and ultimately master the disturbing memories and images that have their roots in your past. Go deeper now into your hypnosis, knowing at the deepest levels of your being that you will be safe in this room, even though your mind tricks you into relating to the past as if it were present. On this deep level, you will know that that was then, and this is now. And it is safe in the now. Each time you practice exposure, it will get easier for you to experience what you fear. Like when you watch a tape of a scary movie the first time, at the scariest part you may feel like jumping out of your skin. But if you were to watch it over and over, your fear would diminish with each viewing. When it's time, you will turn the

imaginary tape on by imagining you are watching the scene on a video on your mental TV. You can imagine dials that can be used to control the degree of emotion you feel during the scene, and you can zoom in to observe details you wish to focus on. If the emotion gets to be too much for you, simply dial it down, take a deep breath, and be sure to remind yourself you are safe in the present. But keep the emotional intensity turned up as high as you can tolerate it. Soon I will ask you to let the mental tape unroll and play the scene from beginning to end. I'd like to hear all about your experience, in the first person and in present tense, all the details you wish to share at this point . . . what the scariest moment is . . . what you are thinking and feeling. If you go a bit too fast, I will tell you to roll the tape in slow motion. You can control the speed with a remote control . . . fast . . . slow . . . but let's keep it as slow as you can go, so you experience everything to the fullest extent you are capable of at this point in time. Create it, feel it, live it, but deep within yourself, all the while you know that it is you who is letting the tape roll . . . you who is doing it, and you who will control it. And you will know that the event is not actually occurring in the present, but in your mind and nowhere else. At the end of the tape, you will go deeper and deeper into your hypnosis, letting yourself relax completely, relax completely, calm and at ease, taking away from the scene what you can, what you will, learning what you can . . . growing as a person in subtle or perhaps not-so-subtle ways. Learning and growing. Learning to feel comfortable with your experience of life, what is pleasant and what is not so pleasant. Now let's let the scene roll. If I tell you to stop the scene, you will be able to stop it immediately. Quickly and easily. Negative emotions associated with the scene will break up, dissipate, like clouds in the wind, as you let them go.

This procedure is repeated, typically for three to nine sessions, until the scene can be experienced with a SUD rating of no more than 2. Other traumatic scenes sometimes emerge, such as childhood sexual abuse in the case of sexually assaulted adult women, which can be targeted in subsequent exposure sessions. If the patient is phobic of places or situations associated with a traumatic event, in vivo exposure can be implemented, as explained in our discussion of exposure to phobic situations (see chap. 9).

Flashback Periods

Like worry periods in the treatment of generalized anxiety disorder (GAD), flashback periods can be used in the case of relatively well-stabilized PTSD patients. In this technique, time is set aside to enter self-hypnosis, relive the event for an initial period of approximately 20 minutes (marked by timer or alarm clock) and, at the end of the period, achieve a state of deep relaxation and calm. Two such periods should be scheduled each day, with the second period lasting no longer than 5 to 10 minutes. Each day, for at least a week, the longer period should be decreased by 2 minutes, affording the patient the opportunity to experience control over the memory that becomes increasingly condensed and circumscribed over trials. The patient or therapist can make tapes of the traumatic event to enhance involvement in exposure.

Mindfulness

Because experiential avoidance is inherent in many posttraumatic reactions, the mindfulness techniques presented in chapter 8 may well prove to be a useful adjunct to both formal exposure and worry periods. The practice of mindfulness requires nothing more than sitting quietly and adopting a nonjudgmental, accepting attitude toward whatever thoughts and feelings arise. The premium placed on acceptance of negative (as well as positive) experiences, rather than avoidance; the idea that even anxious feelings can be tolerated and morph, in time, to positive feelings; and opportunities for exposure and habituation with respect to trauma-related fears may all contribute to the effectiveness of mindfulness practice in treating PTSD.

Working With Memories

Techniques that involve titrating affect and affirming the patient's control over mental imagery can be used to supplement exposure, or as techniques in their own right. Although the strategies we recommend have not been empirically evaluated, we have found them to be very helpful with our clientele. Suggestions can be given for patients to (a) have their inner self watch events from a distance or from a different perspective or mental point of view (e.g., commenting on insecurity of person beating the child in the scene); (b) interrupt the mental tape, make it run backward from different points, then fast forward and give the scene a different ending; (c) watch events first from the viewpoint of a dispassionate observer, before entering the scene; (d) make the scene become brighter, dimmer, or out of focus; (e) change the characteristics of key persons (e.g., become smaller or larger—feet can grow to ridiculous proportions like a clown's) so that their threatening aspects are neutralized; (f) stop and start the tape repeatedly; (g) restructure the memory until different feelings develop or actively cultivate different feelings (e.g., anger vs. fear) while watching the tape; (h) shuttle back and forth between the traumatic incident and a memory of an incident in which the patient felt in control, safe, and secure; and (i) contain disturbing memories between sessions in a file drawer, locked vault, or in a special holding room.

Age Progression and Regression

Age progression can be achieved in most patients by giving suggestions for walking along a road to recovery to a time in which the memory has been processed and is no longer distressing. We instruct patients to notice all of the small changes in thoughts, feelings, and actions that occur along the road, and to specify how they were able to achieve these changes. If they are not able to identify specific changes, patients can be reassured that they can enter a self-reflective state of hypnosis at least once each day to learn how to stay grounded in the present and that as their wisdom grows, they will notice small changes that ordinarily escape notice and gain a deeper understanding about what they need to do to achieve a complete recovery.

Age regression to joyful times can be an antidote to despair when patients forget that they experienced moments of happiness and contentment before a traumatic event turned their lives topsy-turvy. Reminders of happier days, juxtaposed with age progression to a time when the event is successfully processed, can be used to isolate the traumatic event and elicit positive treatment expectancies. In addition, posthypnotic suggestions can be given for patients to have positive flashbacks in which they remember very positive experiences in vivid detail; these flashbacks provide reassurance that they will be able to achieve psychological equilibrium. Times when the patient felt strong, confident, and resourceful can also be recalled, with instructions to amplify and use these feelings in the present, as needed.

In cases of complex trauma or dissociative disorder in which recent traumatic experiences resonate with earlier, prolonged sexual and physical abuse, for example, patients may not be able to locate times during childhood when they felt joyful, carefree, and truly happy. In such cases, it is very important prior to any attempted regression to ascertain whether age regression is an appropriate procedure and to identify specific targets of age regression suggestions that have a high likelihood of activating positive associations and expectancies.

Cognitive Restructuring

Traumatic events can jar a person's sense of self and challenge cherished worldviews. According to a cognitive view of PTSD, it is not the event so much as the meaning that is ascribed to it and related statements about the self that drive posttraumatic reactions (A. T. Beck, 1976). Simple reassurance may suffice if flashbacks are interpreted as a loss of control or a sign of psychological decompensation. Although patients can be informed that a myriad of reactions occur in the face of a traumatic event, they can also be reassured that fears and flashbacks are understandable when emotional reactions to a stressor are especially intense and overwhelming.

More problematic is when patients interpret the event to mean that the world is no longer safe, people cannot be trusted, and life is completely unpredictable. Meichenbaum (1994) contended that individuals who experience PTSD tend to get stuck in the following narrative: "Why me?" "It's so unfair." "How much control can I ever have?" "Whom can I count on?" and so forth. Questions of this sort, Meichenbaum noted, reduce the likelihood the person will accept, resolve, or find meaning in the loss or traumatic event. We have observed that flashbacks can serve the purpose of reminding people, in a superstitious way, that if they are frightened, are vigilant, and believe the world is unsafe, then danger can be averted. In such cases, flashbacks may persist until the person feels safe and strong enough to contend with everyday challenges without them.

Cognitive restructuring, along the lines described in the previous chapter, may be necessary to assist the person in reconciling what occurred with his or her (pretrauma) belief system, especially in cases in which emotions like self-blame, guilt, and shame are part of the symptom picture. Cognitive therapy examines and challenges patients' automatic, dysfunctional thoughts (e.g., "Nowhere is safe," "Trust no one") that emanate from the event, and replaces negative thought patterns with more adaptive ones (e.g., people have to earn my trust). Resick's (Resick, 1992; Resick & Schnicke, 1992) cognitive processing therapy (CPT) is designed to treat sexual assault survivors and combines exposure with cognitive therapy. The cognitive component involves challenging self-blame and other overgeneralized beliefs that have their origin in specific *stuck points*, that is, times during the assault that engendered conflict with entrenched beliefs and thereby created anxiety and distress.

The Split-Screen Technique

Cardena et al. (2000) argued that an important aspect of cognitive restructuring is to make traumatic memories "more bearable" (p. 257). To make the traumatic event more bearable, Cardena et al. (2000; see also D. Spiegel, 1981, 1992) recommended a split-screen technique in which the patient projects images of memories of the trauma on the left side and something he or she did to protect themselves or someone else (e.g., fight back, scream, protest, lie still) on the right side. If patients blame themselves for a sexual assault, for example, or feel they did not resist enough, they can be told that not resisting is an automatic and common survival strategy in the face of mortal danger that is entirely understandable in such instances. As Cardena et al. (2000) stated, "The image on the right may help patients realize that while they were indeed victimized, they were also attempting to master the situation and displayed courage during a time of overwhelming threat" (p. 257).

Comforting the Child Technique

The following technique can be used to glean meaning from a child-hood traumatic event by viewing it from an adult perspective. In light of the risk of suggested memories and confabulation we alluded to earlier, the target event should be one that is well remembered and discussed prior to using this technique.

> Now you can see yourself watching a movie . . . a movie of something from your past . . . something that we have talked about before, but you want to know more about . . . to learn more about . . . to reclaim your past . . . to learn from it. . . . You can watch this scene . . . an old traumatic scene . . . the scene of _____ . . . something you remember but want to learn more about. . . . You can watch it from beginning to end . . . and learn from it . . . learn how it affected you . . . learn what decisions you made as a result of it . . . and learn how you can move beyond . . . perhaps to love and wholeness . . . perhaps to understanding . . . and forgiving [as appropriate to the patient] . . . learn more about you . . . and what you can be now, in the present. . . . What is really interesting about this movie is that you can float right into the picture . . . or walk right into it. . . . You can comfort the child . . . you can reassure the child . . . you can communicate with the child on many levels . . . you can touch the child . . . or hold the child . . . embrace the child . . . or just look lovingly at the child . . . with the eyes of wisdom and knowing . . . and forgiveness . . . and protection and care . . . whatever you want to say or do is entirely up to you . . . but you have a feeling . . . a sense that you know what is right to do . . . what is the next best thing to do. . . .
>
> If the child made some decisions at the time of the event . . . talk to the child about them. . . . You are more experienced than the child . . . you have more understanding . . . you have more empathy . . . you have more insight. . . . The child is wise too . . . and can understand . . . yet the child needs your nurturing and your guidance, your adult perspective. . . . Talk to him [or her] . . . let the child know how you feel . . . what you think.
>
> Soon you will be ready to let go of this scene. . . . Yet to hold onto the child and feel it hold onto you . . . just right . . . so tight . . . you need to care for this child . . . it needs to let you know how it feels . . . what it thinks. . . . You can do this . . . take some time to do this now . . . [allow 60 seconds]. Now you can step out of the scene, take with it what you want. . . . The drama of life will continue with you richer for the learning . . . for the witnessing . . . wondering in what small ways you will be enriched . . . so much still to learn . . . so much time . . . so much time.

Another option is for the patient to project into the movie the therapist, the wise inner self, a benign or caring parent, or the person he or she will become after the repercussions of trauma have been resolved (the new you). Some patients may be unable to comfort themselves during these sorts of exercises. If this is the case, it suggests that affect regulation techniques should be instituted before exposure is implemented. In addition, scenes involving an inner child should be used with caution or avoided in treating highly dissociative patients who might have a tendency to reify such imagery.

An Example

The following example illustrates how age regression, memory alteration techniques, and images of a supportive parent can be used to contend with flashbacks triggered by a combination of situational cues. The patient, Mary, reported that her sexual relations with her spouse were disrupted on a number of occasions when she experienced an unbidden, anxiety-evoking image of her grandfather. After the situation was carefully monitored, it became evident that this reaction occurred on nights when the couple visited a friend who smoked a cigar. The cigar smell reminded the patient of her grandfather, who sexually molested her at age 8. He always smoked a cigar when he visited and molested her. The intrusive imagery occurred only when both sets of cues were present: engaging in sexual relations with her husband and the memory of the smell of cigars.

When flashbacks disrupted her sexual relations, Mary tried to focus on other thoughts and ignore the image of her grandfather, generally with little effect. At the therapist's suggestion, she was able to achieve some relief during these episodes by opening her eyes and noticing differences between her husband and her grandfather and the house she grew up in and her current home. Mary also asked her husband to understand what she was experiencing at those times and to terminate sex and remind her of where she was and who he was. Because these measures helped but were not sufficient to dispel her anxiety on a consistent basis, other techniques were used to alleviate her distress. During self-hypnosis, the patient was asked to create a realistic image of her paternal grandfather. She was reluctant to do this, so she was asked to watch herself on a mental video monitor as an 8-year-old child, small and vulnerable in the soothing presence of her mother. She responded well to this, and she was asked to observe her mother, who somehow learned what had happened, confront her grandfather, make him stop molesting her, and reassure her that it was over and she would be safe, and tell her in no uncertain terms that he no longer had the power to hurt her in any way. This imagery helped Mary relax. Then she was asked to turn the video monitor off and create an image of her grandfather and make it dimmer and smaller. She was able to make increasing modifications in the image, eventually to the point where it was invisible. The procedure was repeated the next session, and she reported a SUD level of only 2 when she tried to imagine her grandfather. Finally, she was invited to create this image the next time she had sexual relations with her husband and to turn it on and off at will, if she was able to conjure the image of her grandfather at all. During the next session, she reported that she attempted to visualize him, but she was unable to do so. She was able to discern only a faint image of him "in which he looked old, wizened, and harmless," and she reported that she had a satisfying sexual experience with her husband. At 1-year follow-up, she reported she was flashback free. Moreover, Mary did not experience untoward reactions after she visited her friend who smoked a cigar.

In this case, it bears mention that had Mary not had a supportive relationship with her mother and had the therapist proceeded intrepidly without knowledge of the mother–child relationship, the therapy session could have gone awry. For example, Mary might have been retraumatized if her mother was callous or had mistreated or abused her in some way during childhood. It is clear that a sensitivity to the family dynamics and knowledge of the patient's feelings about significant people in her life are imperative when age regression, video-monitor viewing techniques, or exposure procedures are implemented.

Hypnosis is a promising albeit far from definitively proven technique for ameliorating posttraumatic symptoms. More research on hypnosis, hypnotic suggestibility, and PTSD is urgently needed. A useful starting point would be to conduct studies that compare exposure therapies with and without hypnosis, as well as research on PTSD in which flashbacks and dissociative symptoms are especially prominent versus cases in which such symptomatology is less salient (Lynn, Kirsch, Barabasz, Cardena, & Patterson, 2000).

11

PAIN MANAGEMENT, BEHAVIORAL MEDICINE, AND DENTISTRY

An Institute of Medicine (2004) study reached a significant conclusion: "No physician's education would be complete without an understanding of the role played by behavioral and social factors in human health and disease, knowledge of the ways in which these factors can be modified, and an appreciation of how personal life experiences influence physician-patient relationships" (p. 60). Hypnosis is a tool that offers considerable leverage in changing behaviors and experiences related to pain and the treatment or management of a variety of medical conditions (Chaves, 1993, 1997b; DuBreuil & Spanos, 1993; Pinnell & Covino, 2000). This chapter begins with a discussion of how to select patients for hypnotic treatment of pain and how to prepare them for the use of hypnosis. As there are differences in the way chronic and acute pain are managed hypnotically, sample inductions and suggestions are given separately for each. Additional suggestions that can be used in the treatment of pain are also given. Hypnosis can also be used in other medical and physical health contexts. For example, hypnosis has been shown to be helpful in the preparation and treatment of surgical patients and in the treatment of postoperative nausea, irritable bowel

---

This chapter was coauthored with Danielle G. Koby.

syndrome (IBS), asthma, and warts, each of which are discussed in this chapter. Finally, we consider the use of hypnosis in dentistry.

The property of hypnosis that has the greatest potential for social good arguably resides in the ability of participants to radically reduce, or in some cases eliminate, both chronic and acute pain (Lynn, Kirsch, Barabasz, Cardena, & Patterson, 2000). Tales of seemingly miraculous relief of pain from physical injury, debilitation, and disease have been associated with hypnosis from antiquity to the present time, and with the claims of luminaries such as Mesmer and de Puysegur (Gauld, 1996). As we observed in chapter 1, 19th-century claims of painless surgery with mesmeric procedures were overblown, impressive reductions in pain can be achieved in the absence of hypnosis, and hypnosis-related pain reductions are not the product of a unique or special state of consciousness. However, a steady stream of case reports and anecdotal observations has supported many of the early optimistic assessments of hypnosis in the medical arena. Beginning in the 1980s, well-controlled studies empirically evaluated the role of hypnosis in the treatment of medical conditions and began to provide convincing evidence for the efficacy of hypnosis-based interventions (Lynn et al., 2000; Pinnell & Covino, 2000).

Hypnosis has been used successfully to ameliorate an array of physiological disorders, from hypertension to warts to asthma (see Pinnell & Covino, 2000, for a review). However, the complex nature of pain is perhaps best suited to psychological management. Indeed, a meta-analysis of controlled trials of hypnotic analgesia indicates that hypnosis can provide substantial relief for 75% of the population (Montgomery, DuHamel, & Redd, 2000). The effect is largest among patients who are highly suggestible but is relatively large also for moderately suggestible people, and a comprehensive review of the clinical trial literature indicates that it is effective in the treatment of both chronic and acute pain (Patterson & Jensen, 2003). Hypnotic suggestion has been found to reduce acute pain associated with labor during childbirth (Harmon, Hynan, & Tyre, 1990), burns (Patterson, Everett, Burns, & Marvin, 1992; Patterson, Questad, & DeLateur, 1989; Wakeman & Kaplan, 1978; Wright & Drummond, 2000), and various surgical and radiological procedures (Faymonville et al., 1997; Kuttner, 1988; Lang, Joyce, Spiegel, Hamilton, & Lee, 1996; Liossi & Hatira, 1999; Syrjala, Cummings, & Donaldson, 1992; Wakeman & Kaplan, 1978; Weinstein & Au, 1991) in both medical and dental settings (see Pinnell & Covino, 2000). Among the chronic pain conditions that have been found amenable to hypnotic treatment are cancer (D. Spiegel & Bloom, 1983), fibromyalgia (Haanen et al., 1991), and headache (Anderson, Basker, & Dalton, 1975; Andreychuk & Skriver, 1975; H. Friedman & Taub, 1984; Schlutter, Golden, & Blume, 1980; Zitman, Van Dyck, Spinhoven, & Linssen, 1992).

Pain is a subjective experience, and self-reports of experience are subject to a variety of biases. For that reason, it is especially impressive that hypnotic pain reduction has been verified with both behavioral and physiological measures. In addition to reporting less pain, pregnant women given hypnotic training have been reported to have shorter labor, more spontaneous deliveries, and babies with higher Apgar scores (Harmon et al., 1990) and patients given suggestions for pain relief have been found to use less pain medication (Faymonville et al., 1997; Haanen et al., 1991; Harmon et al., 1990; Syrjala et al., 1992; Wakeman & Kaplan, 1978; Weinstein & Au, 1991; Wright & Drummond, 2000). In addition, self-reports of hypnotic analgesia are accompanied by corresponding changes in the brain (Hofbauer, Rainville, Duncan, & Bushnell, 2001; Rainville, Duncan, Price, Carrier, & Bushnell, 1997). The recognition of the role of hypnosis in pain management by the National Institutes of Health Consensus Task Force (Anonymous, 1996) accords with Montgomery et al.'s (2000) observation that hypnotic pain reduction should now be regarded as a well-established, empirically validated treatment.

In addition to a basic biological element, the experience of pain includes subjective and cognitive components that lend themselves to hypnotic modification. The pain experience has a sensory component and an affective component. The sensory component pertains to the intensity of the pain experience. The affective component concerns the unpleasantness of the pain, that is, the individual's subjective level of distress, which may be driven by cognitions and which may fluctuate substantially over time. Each individual's tolerance for pain is different, and that tolerance may change in response to affective state. What may be extremely distressful to one patient may not even register as painful to another, and it is less the objective measure of how much it should hurt than the subjective component of how much is does hurt that matters for treatment. Brain imaging studies indicate that hypnotic suggestions can affect both components, depending on the specific wording of the suggestions (Hofbauer et al., 2001; Rainville et al., 1997).

One of the variables affecting pain is the expectancy of its occurrence. As a result, there is a substantial placebo effect in the treatment of pain. Compared with untreated controls, people given placebo analgesia report less pain, tolerate more intense levels of stimulation, and have a higher threshold for reporting that a stimulus is painful (e.g., Baker & Kirsch, 1993; Camatte, Gerolami, & Sarles, 1969; Gelfand, Ullman, & Krasner, 1963; Liberman, 1964). Placebo administration can be thought of as an indirect suggestion for improvement. Patients are led to believe that they may be ingesting an active substance that is believed to ameliorate the condition from which they are suffering. This practice, however, is deceptive, and, as we noted in chapter 3, the use of deception is a barrier to clinical application of the placebo effect. Hypnosis may provide a means of overcoming this barrier. Hypnotic suggestion may entail more than just a placebo effect, but the placebo effect is certainly one of its components (Baker & Kirsch, 1993; McGlashan, Evans, & Orne, 1969). The importance of the placebo effect is also illustrated by significant correlations between hypnotic analgesia and changes in pain expectancies (e.g., Milling, Kirsch, Allen, & Reutenauer, 2005; Milling, Kirsch, Meunier, & Levine, 2002). So at the very least, hypnotic suggestion can be used as a nondeceptive alternative to this deceptive indirect suggestion.

Chaves and Brown (1987) were among the first to contend that maladaptive thinking is a central mechanism in pain management. The reduction of catastrophizing may be a factor that is common to both hypnotic and placebo pain reduction. Catastrophizing is one of the most robust and reliable psychological predictors of pain and adjustment to painful chronic states (Geisser, Roth, Bachman, & Eckert, 1996; Keefe et al., 1999; Turk & Rudy, 1992). A relation between catastrophizing and pain has been demonstrated in prospective studies, and catastrophizing has been shown to account for pain-related outcomes better than have medical status variables (Keefe, Brown, Wallston, & Caldwell, 1989; Martin, Bradley, Alexander, & Alarcon, 1996; Sullivan & Neish, 1998) as well as measures of fear of pain and state and trait anxiety (Stroud, Thorn, Jensen, & Boothby, 2000). In addition, the association between pain and catastrophizing is partially mediated by response expectancy (M. J. Sullivan, Rodgers, & Kirsch, 2001). Chaves (1997b) claimed that hypnotic procedures for pain reduction are likely to be most effective with patients who are catastrophizers because hypnosis supplies them with a kind of cognitive prosthesis, that is, a strategy for "engaging in effective coping using thoughts and images consistent with the therapeutic goal" (p. 16). Chaves' observation underlines the importance of evaluating the patient's tendency to catastrophize and of framing suggestions that lead to its minimization.

Another aspect of the cognitive component of pain that is important to evaluate is the meaning of the pain, that is, its significance for the patient. For example, in the case of an otherwise healthy child with a sports injury, the pain may mean that he or she has to sit out the rest of the season, or at least until sufficient healing has occurred. In this case the child's attitude may be quite good, and he or she may be highly motivated to reduce pain and to engage in therapeutic exercise and other forms of treatment. In contrast, an adult with chronic pain may feel quite different about attempting hypnotic intervention. Chronic and debilitating pain often means that individuals cannot do many of the things they once enjoyed—that they are unable to hold the type of job they want, that their day-to-day experience of life is extremely restricted. Although this patient may also be highly motivated to reduce his or her pain, feelings of hopelessness, depression, insecurity, and low self-esteem may limit the overall effectiveness of the intervention.

Hypnosis is an ideal instrument in the treatment of pain because through the generation of imagery, patients in essence learn to design their own treatment plan in response to their current levels of pain. Thus, hypnosis for pain management offers both the flexibility and the opportunity for finely tuned adjustments that manual or pharmacological forms of treatment cannot provide. On another level, hypnosis may include a very emotionally therapeutic component, allowing patients to experience moments of peace, rest, and relaxation that they have not enjoyed for some time. In the case of patients with chronic pain, reduction in pain via hypnosis may also impart to them a sense of mastery over their pain and their experience, and thereby a sense of hope and self-efficacy in general.

As noted in earlier chapters, hypnosis is generally considered an adjunct to treatment, rather than a treatment in and of itself. For that reason, merely saying that someone has been treated with hypnotherapy is not very informative. Instead, a therapist might use cognitive–behavioral hypnotherapy, psychodynamic hypnotherapy, or patient-centered hypnotherapy. In each case, hypnosis is being used as a catalyst to enhance the efficacy of a treatment that is effective even without the addition of hypnosis. Hypnotic pain management may be an exception to this rule. Simple hypnotic suggestions for pain relief reduce pain to a degree that is equivalent to that produced by more complex psychological procedures (e.g., stress inoculation; Milling et al., 2002).

PATIENT SELECTION AND PREPARATION

Almost any patient might benefit from the use of suggestion for pain reduction. Although high levels of hypnotic suggestibility may be required for extremely challenging applications—such as the use of hypnosis as a sole anesthetic or to influence localized blood flow during surgical procedures—moderately suggestible people also show substantial levels of pain reduction in response to hypnotic suggestion (Montgomery et al., 2000). Hypnotic pain management can be viewed as a skill that can be learned and improved on with practice. Because hypnotic pain control includes a placebo component, even low suggestible patients can experience a reduction in pain through suggestive techniques. Indeed, hypnotic analgesia seems to be more reliably correlated with expectancy than with hypnotic suggestibility (Milling et al., 2005). However, low suggestible patients may require a change in the treatment protocol. These patients often have negative attitudes and expectations about hypnosis, which can interfere substantially with treatment outcome. One way around this problem is the use of nonhypnotic suggestion with these patients. Clinical and experimental studies have shown that suggestions for pain relief can be effective without mention of hypnosis (Lang et al., 2000; Lang et al., 1996; Spanos, 1986).

The preparatory phase and specific implications for pain management are detailed below and followed by specific therapeutic suggestions for the relief of chronic versus acute pain. Deepening procedures may be used to further enhance pain reduction, although among highly suggestible patients there may be no need to use a deepening technique, as these patients may respond to hypnosis with relative ease.

Patients who are in extreme pain, such as that arising from extensive burn damage, may not be able to concentrate to the extent that a deepening technique warrants, and thus suggestions for pain relief may be given immediately following the induction. In contrast, some patients may not be able to experience relief without the use of deepening suggestions, and thus this issue should be discussed with the patient both before and after the first few inductions, to determine which approach will bring about the most relief. Examples of deepening techniques are discussed in chapter 4 and include having the patient envision him- or herself walking down a flight of stairs, envisioning the light in a room going from extremely bright to extremely dim, or imagining him- or herself in a familiar and relaxing place. Deepening techniques may be facilitated by tailoring the imagined scene to the individual patient; thus, making the suggestions as specific as possible is ideal. In the case of a set of stairs, for instance, having the patient identify one staircase in particular is best; in the case of a favorite place, have the patient identify familiar sights, sounds, and smells associated with that place.

As with the use of hypnosis in any context, each patient's previous experiences, ideas, and expectations surrounding hypnosis should be addressed, and any misperceptions should be corrected prior to treatment. Positive expectations regarding the use of hypnosis should be supported and incorporated into the treatment whenever possible, provided they are not grossly unrealistic and will thus likely lead to disappointment and disillusionment. Patients must both be invested in the treatment and have a firm yet realistic expectation about the extent to which they will be able to affect positive change. Clinicians and patients should discuss favored imagery prior to the treatment and, if possible, should use only imagery that is specific to the patient's experiences. The selection of images is another aspect of the treatment in which each individual component of pain should be considered, as previously discussed.

Although several specific images are suggested in the next section for the treatment of acute versus chronic pain, it is important to consider the patient's emotional and cognitive state when selecting an imagery plan. Patients with acute, localized, and short-term pain may realize the most benefit from a more aggressive or active imagery sequence, in which they visualize themselves taking specific action to reduce their pain. Patients with chronic pain or with extensive, pervasive pain may instead benefit more from images involving relaxation and suggestions of vague, soothing sensory experiences. Regardless of the imagery chosen, patients should be encouraged to give feedback after each session, and the imagery should be adjusted according to the patient's recommendations.

Finally, audiotapes play an import role in the hypnotic treatment of pain. Audiotapes facilitate the use of self-hypnosis, so that pain can be managed outside of the hypnotic session. Thus, hypnotic pain management is best thought of as a self-control technique, in which patients are taught to ameliorate and cope more effectively with their pain.

SUGGESTIONS FOR CHRONIC, PERVASIVE, AND EXTREME PAIN

The hypnotic induction and suggestions that follow are aimed specifically at reducing extreme and pervasive pain, such as that experienced by patients with rheumatoid arthritis, fibromyalgia, or related pain disorders. The nonspecific nature of the imagery, as well as the relatively nondetailed images that patients are asked to produce, makes this and related scripts ideal for patients who are in a great deal of distress and who may not have the attention span, patience, or presence of mind to create an elaborate visual image. The goal of the induction is to reduce as much as possible the overall level of distress, by encouraging global relaxation and deep breathing.

Patients who are in a great deal of physical pain may hold their posture rigid in an attempt to avoid any unnecessary movement or impact, and this constant muscular tension may increase their distress as well as hinder efforts to manage pain. Thus, the first goal of the hypnotic session is to encourage as much relaxation as possible and to give patients a safe space in which to let down their guard and give their muscles a chance to relax. Encouraging patients to take this initial step will often give them a measured amount of pain relief, in addition to some mental or emotional release, and may strengthen their investment in hypnosis.

Depression is frequently concomitant with chronic pain. For that reason, techniques used in the treatment of depression (see chap. 8) are also useful in the management of chronic pain. In particular, the automatic thoughts and self-suggestions that foster a sense of hopelessness can be identified, challenged, and replaced with more adaptive self-statements.

The following script includes an induction and suggestions for pain-reducing imagery, tips for modifying the images for specific populations, and supplementary images that are discussed at the end of this section. The patient should be relaxed, lying down if possible, and in the most comfortable position possible.

Relaxation

If you are comfortable doing so, I would like you to close your eyes and begin listening to the sound of my voice. . . . I realize that you are in a lot of distress right now, and that you are in a lot of pain. . . . You and I are going to work together to let some of that pain go, so that you might feel a little bit better.

If you are comfortable doing so I'd like you to take some slow, relaxed breaths in and out, and to focus on your breathing, as you begin to let go of everything going on around you. . . . Sometimes it's easier to let go of other things if you focus your attention on your breathing. . . . Some people find it helpful to breathe in a specific pattern, to a specific rhythm, as they enter hypnosis—I wonder if this might help you to feel more relaxed? If you like, you may find it helpful to breathe in on a count of four, to hold your breath for a count of four, and to breathe out on a count of six. . . . You can breathe in (two, three, four), and hold it (two, three, four), and let your breath go (two, three, four, five, six). . . .

Repeat twice more and observe if patient is attempting to follow this breathing pattern. If so, repeat several more times, adjusting your speed to the patient's observed level of comfort or distress; repeat until the patient appears to have mastered the breathing or seems to become disinterested (e.g., begins breathing at a completely different rate, fidgets, sighs).

As you continue to breathe and relax, feel yourself letting go of some of the tension in your muscles. . . . With every breath you exhale, you can feel a little bit of that tension leaving your body—feel your muscles start to shift and find a position that is most comfortable for them right now. . . . With every breath you exhale, you can feel a little bit of the tension draining out of your fingertips, leaving your body with your breath, draining out of the tips of your toes. . . . With every breath in, you are replacing that tension with a feeling of relaxation and calm surrender, allowing yourself to be quiet and safe, to let go of the stress you have been carrying. . . . Let your muscles shift and find their most comfortable position—it's all right if they want to shift slightly through-out hypnosis; this is a time to let your body and your mind relax in any way they want to. . . .

As you focus on your muscles and your breath and your mind, begin to let go of anything going on around you. . . . You may hear sounds and know that other things are going on around you, but as you focus your mind inward you are less and less interested in outside things. . . . Continue to breathe and relax, relaxing more with every breath, allowing yourself to fall into a deep and peaceful state of hypnosis, of relaxation. . . . As you continue to focus your mind inward, to hear your breath and the sound of my voice, you may feel the outside world starting to slip away, just a little, allowing you to become more relaxed, and more at peace. . . . As you relax, you may feel your body becoming softer, more fluid, more flexible, and more completely relaxed on the couch [or bed, table, etc.] where you are resting. With every breath you exhale you can feel yourself letting go of your body, of the points where your body meets the couch. . . . You may feel yourself sinking into the couch a little bit more with every breath you exhale. . . . You may not be able to feel every point where your body rests now—the line between where your body ends and the couch begins is becoming blurry, as you relax more and more and go deeper and deeper into hypnosis. . . . [Continue until the patient is visibly more relaxed, is breathing more deeply and regularly, or is at least somewhat absorbed in the experience of relaxation.]

Pain Reduction

As you continue to breathe and relax, you may start to feel a different, and completely relaxing, completely wonderful sensation coming over your body. . . . You may feel it starting in your toes; you may feel your fingertips begin tingling, or the very top of your head start to tingle and feel slightly numb. . . . As you relax and breathe, and let go of all the tension in your body, you may start to feel a very faint, very gradual numbness come over the tips of your toes . . . washing over the tips of your toes as though you are standing on the beach and letting the waves lap over them. . . . The numbness may ebb and flow over the very tops of your toes, coming and going, maybe tingling, maybe tickling them ever so slightly. . . . As you breathe and relax and let go of all that is going on around you, you will feel this numbness come and stay over the tips of your toes, and begin to work its way slowly, very slowly, over the tops of your feet, and along the soles of your feet. . . . And as this numbness grows, slowly, slowly at first, it is like nothing you have ever felt before, and it is so wonderful, so peaceful, so remarkable, that it captures all of your attention, and the rest of your body starts to slip away from consciousness. . . . You are focused on the tops of your feet, as a gentle numbness begins to crawl up over them, leaving behind a nothingness that is peaceful and completely relaxing. . . . Feel this numbness moving its way slowly across the soles of your feet, and over the tops of your feet, toward your ankles. . . . Feel it coming up over your heels and encircling your ankles, and hold that feeling for a moment . . . examine it . . . allow it to happen. . . .

As you relax and try to feel your feet, you feel only nothingness and complete relaxation—as though your feet were no longer there—you have let them go and let yourself relax without them. . . . You might picture this numbness as a pair of socks being pulled slowly over your feet—invisible socks—once they are pulled on, your feet feel completely numb and completely invisible. . . . Or you may picture your entire body, a drawing of your entire body—lying calm, in a state of relaxation—and as you study your body an eraser appears, and begins gently erasing your feet, so that in the drawing you have no feet and no feeling in your feet—only numbness—total and complete relaxation. . . .

And as you embrace and surrender to this feeling of relaxation, the feeling becomes stronger and begins to move slowly from your ankles toward your legs, leaving only numbness and nothingness behind. . . . Feel the numbness moving slowly up each of your legs, feel your muscles being slowly erased, feeling the invisibility slowly swallowing your calves as the numbness moves toward each of your knees. . . . If you mentally examine your feet and your lower legs now, you find that you cannot move them, and that you cannot picture them. . . . You cannot tell where they are in space and you cannot feel anything at all. . . . And this feeling is so relaxing, so peaceful, so calm. . . . You may see more and more of your body erased, or you may feel that more and more of you is becoming invisible, as the numbness comes up and over each of your knees—feel the muscles along the backs of your legs completely disappearing . . . feel any tension completely disappear as your muscles are erased. . . . Yet knowing you are safe inside your body.

Feel the numbness moving up each of your thighs, toward your hips, moving slowly up the sides of your legs and toward your spine. . . . Take a moment and enjoy the entire lower half of your body being completely numb—no tension, no feeling, no sensation at all. . . . Feel the numbness moving up over your hips, across your abdomen and along your lower back, slowly and completely erasing every muscle fiber, every place where tension was held. . . . Feel the numbness moving slowly up your spine, across your stomach, along your side—moving slowly upward, leaving only peaceful relaxation and nothingness behind. . . . Feel the numbness move across your chest, across your upper back and shoulder blades, across your collarbone and out toward your shoulders. Feel the numbness come up over your shoulders and move down your arms, slowly moving past your elbows, toward your wrists and across the tops of your hands. . . . Feel any remaining feeling and tension being pushed out of your fingertips as the numbness completely swallows your fingers, leaving nothing behind. . . . Allow the numbness to move upward along your neck, feeling it massaging the back of your neck like tiny, invisible fingers, wiping out feeling and tension. . . . Feel the front of your neck become completely numb . . . perhaps the most relaxing part of this entire process—feel the numbness inch slowly along the back of your head, moving upward ever so slowly, allowing muscles in your scalp and forehead to start to relax and give themselves over to being invisible. The numbness moves slowly up and over your jaw, relaxing and erasing all of the muscles in your face, the muscles around your mouth and your eyes, and meeting the numbness that is moving across your forehead. . . . Feel the numbness encircle both of your eyes and massage away any tension and feeling in the muscles around your eyes, and just let go.

Allow your mind to float over any topic, any image, any idea it wishes. . . . Your mind is completely free from your body and from any constraints, and you may stay in this state for as long as you wish—feeling no pain, feeling no stress, feeling completely relaxed and invisible and at peace. Allow yourself to rest, to feel rejuvenated by the relaxation you are now feeling. . . .

And know that you may achieve a state of relaxation whenever you wish. . . . You can achieve this relaxation by simply closing your eyes, taking some slow, relaxed breaths in and out, focusing on your breathing, and letting go of everything that may be going on around you. . . . And then you can let go of your body, a little at a time . . . beginning with your feet, reminding yourself to let them become numb . . . and then moving the numbness upward, until your mind is completely free from your body.

Some patients may prefer a shorter and less detailed suggestion for pain relief—particularly if they are unable to remain still for more than 15 minutes or so. In this case a suggestion of feelings of floating may be beneficial, if the patient has had positive experiences with being in the ocean or floating in water. Floating may be especially suited to patients who are unable to remain still, as small movements take place continually while one floats in water and would not be distracting or discouraging. In addition, in the case of burn victims, a suggestion of soothing aloe on the skin may be as or more beneficial than a suggestion of numbness: As aloe cools, it produces feelings of analgesia.

LOCALIZED, ACUTE PAIN

In cases of chronic pain, the subjective experience of inflammation may be so overwhelming as to give the patient the sense that his or her entire body is in distress and that nothing may be done to combat it and produce relief. In contrast, injuries and minor to moderate pain (e.g., postoperative pain) are generally understood to be both temporary and amenable to therapeutic management—a point that carries important treatment implications at every stage of the hypnotic experience. In addition to the physiological differences between acute, localized and more diffuse, chronic pain, the cognitive and affective representations of that pain may be quite different. For example, patients with chronic pain may exhibit symptoms of depression and exhaustion as a result of continually dealing with pain they do not see improving. In contrast, anxiety is a dominant emotion during acute pain. For this reason, many of the techniques described in chapter 9 can be usefully applied to the treatment of patients with acute pain. In particular, identification of the catastrophizing thoughts that contribute to pain-related anxiety is an important part of treatment for acute pain. The replacement of these thoughts with minimizing alternatives can reduce the unpleasantness of the pain experience.

Patients may view localized pain as more of an annoyance than a debilitating condition, and may feel frustration and even outright anger in response to their experience. In the context of hypnotic pain management, a patient's anger and resolve serve as fuel for the imagery used; the greater the cognitive and affective isolation of pain, the greater the relief one may expect to achieve through hypnosis. Overall levels of focus, concentration, and perceived self-efficacy are also assumed to be higher in patients with injuries than in patients with chronic or pervasive pain, and thus, one may invoke more specific, active, and detailed images in these cases.

To complement and build on the subjective experience of acute, localized pain it may be most efficacious to use imagery to target and isolate the affected area. As in the case of more pervasive and chronic pain, significant muscle tension may be present throughout the body, particularly in the large muscle groups surrounding the affected area, as they attempt to compensate for and protect the injured tissue. As a consequence, suggestions for overall bodily relaxation should constitute a large portion of the initial induction, after which more specific techniques may be used to reduce pain in the target area(s). As underlying muscle tension and rigidity are reduced, the injured region is isolated and thus left exposed to the effects of hypnotic imagery and suggestion. The primary aims at this point are (a) to allow the patient to fully appreciate and experience his or her level of pain, (b) to gain a sense of mastery over the size and intensity of that pain, and (c) to work toward reducing or eliminating the pain entirely.

These points are illustrated and elaborated in the following script, which is to be implemented immediately after hypnosis has been induced. The specific images may be tailored to fit each patient's personal experiences and preferences, but should always include distinct and easily visualized elements.

> Now that you are feeling more relaxed and comfortable with hypnosis, I want you to picture an image that we will use to reduce your pain. Are you ready?
>
> I would like you to imagine a perfectly round bubble, perhaps about the size of your palm . . . any bubble you like, any image you may have seen, in real life or on TV or in the movies. Perhaps your bubble looks like the kind that little kids play with . . . perhaps it looks like one of those blown-glass Christmas tree ornaments. . . . Maybe it even looks like a crystal ball. . . . Any image you see will be fine—any image that

is round, like a sphere ... clear, and colorless, so that you can see through it and see all around it. Perhaps it is floating in the air right in front of you, or perhaps you can hold it in your hand and look through it.

Picture this sphere, picture its shape and its size, and then slowly, very slowly, picture your bubble floating toward the site of pain on your body. Perhaps you are moving your sphere slowly toward your pain, perhaps the bubble is beginning to float toward that pain by itself, but it will soon come to rest on top of the site where you feel the pain.

As you continue to relax and breathe, picture that bubble sitting right over the spot where you are feeling pain. ... Picture the bubble next to your skin, see it completely covering the area where your pain is now. ... Picture the bubble moving over and around your pain, as though it's even able to move below the surface of your skin, through your body, into your muscles, to completely surround the pain you are feeling. Picture that bubble completely surrounding and enveloping your pain, so that the pain is completely contained within the sphere, and you are able to hold it in place and look at it, study it, feel it ...

And as you look at the bubble, maybe its round, perfect shape becomes even more clear, and the edges become slightly sharper, crisper, more distinct—almost as if the entire bubble has a black outline to it. Maybe it even looks a little like a magnifying glass now, whose glass is completely encircling and covering the area of your pain. Perhaps you can start to change the feeling of your pain inside the sphere—perhaps you can make it sharper or duller ... perhaps you can make it hotter or cooler. ... Or maybe it's as though you're looking at it through a microscope and you're simply adjusting the focus back and forth. You can change the picture within the sphere, even if only slightly—and the pain is still there, but you're changing its texture and quality—you can affect how it feels, you can magnify the pain or make it less intense, simply by changing the way it looks inside the circle.

And as your pain is completely held within the sphere, you can sit back and see the sphere overlapping that part of your body where there is pain. The pain is kept completely within the circle—trapped, held firmly—so that you can sit back and relax and not worry about it moving at all. Picture your whole entire body, as you lie back, relaxed, breathing deeply, in a comfortable state of deep hypnosis and relaxation. ... And as you continue to relax, you are able to see the sphere move ever so slightly. ... First just a little, just a tiny little bit. ... Perhaps it's moving up away from your body, perhaps it's moving out to the side away from your muscles—but the most amazing thing is that your pain is still firmly within the sphere. ... You can see your pain swirling inside the sphere, swirling like liquid ink inside the bubble, as it begins to move away from you. ... The bubble moves as slowly as you would like it to. Perhaps it moves extra slowly if it was embedded deep within your muscles or a certain part of your body, but it starts to move, with your pain, away from that area of your body and into the air around you.

Perhaps you envision the bubble being carried away by the wind—you may feel light currents of air passing over the surface of your body, picking up the bubble and blowing it, carrying it away. Perhaps you are able to see the sphere floating in front of you; maybe you are able to hold it in your hand. . . . And as you do this, notice how your body is feeling in the spot where your pain was. . . . Notice the feeling of calm and relaxation in the area where there was so much pain, notice the area feeling quiet and relaxed, as your pain is locked within the bubble and moving, floating ever so slowly away. You can almost reach out and touch this bubble, as it carries away your pain and leaves you feeling quiet and relaxed.

As you continue to relax and scan your body, perhaps your muscles and your mind feel tired, and if so, just let them relax as you enjoy this state of hypnosis. . . . Continue to breathe and relax, and know that you can erase your pain any time you wish by imagining a bubble, letting it completely surround your pain, and letting it carry that pain away, leaving you relaxed and calm and in a quiet state of relaxation. . . .

The patient may bring him- or herself out of hypnosis at any point after this, or may choose to spend additional time enjoying and committing to memory the reduction in pain that has been achieved. With practice, patients will be able to successfully recall this state of relaxation and pain relief, thereby speeding the reduction of their pain during subsequent sessions. An important element of this script is the opportunity for personalization. Talking with the patient before and after the session and getting feedback and ideas for imagery is helpful in achieving maximum pain relief. For example, one patient using this imagery used her memories of the movie *The Wizard of Oz* to picture specific kinds of bubbles. In the movie, before the good witch appears to Dorothy, she is preceded by a clear, pink bubble, which gradually gets larger and larger until she magically presents herself. Though every patient may have a unique set of images that come to mind, some of them quite amusing, this example illustrates that the best imagery is based on the patient's salient memories and experiences.

To the same end, encouraging patient creativity is also extremely beneficial, and clinicians and patients should discuss what imagery might work best and what images come to mind during the sessions. Finally, although for the purposes of learning and acquiring self-hypnosis skills it may be most beneficial for the patient to be lying down with eyes closed, it is not at all necessary—many if not all pain reduction images may be invoked while the patient is upright and fully alert. With practice it may be possible to reduce pain during activities that normally generate it, and perhaps even before a patient engages in these activities, as a preventative measure.

ADDITIONAL SUGGESTIONS

The two sets of suggestions described in detail in the previous section contain a number of identifiable components that are frequently used in hypnotic pain management. These include dissociation (the sense that the mind has become separated from the body), numbness, transformation of the specific qualities of the pain sensation, relaxation, thermal imagery, and distraction (by focusing on breathing or on specific images and by allowing one's mind to float to any topic or image it wishes). In this section, we present some additional suggestions that can be used independently or incorporated into the suggestions already presented.

Transformation

I wonder if you can let yourself see your pain. Imagine what it looks like. What shape is it? Does it have smooth edges or sharp jagged edges? How large is it? What is its shape? I wonder how much its shape can change. Can it slowly become smaller? Smaller and smaller. . . . Can the sharp edges begin to smooth out? Maybe the edges can even begin to get fuzzy?

What color is your pain? [*Typically hot colors such as red, yellow, and orange are described.*] Let's see if that color can change. I wonder what color you might like it to be . . . maybe a soft powdery pink . . . or perhaps a fluffy baby blue. Maybe the color will change on its own. . . . What does the color look like now?

Reinterpretation

I wonder if you can describe the sensation you are feeling. Is it more like an intense pressure? Is it hot or cold? Does it tingle or throb? [*Elicit an answer from the patient. Then focus on understanding the sensation as something other than pain. In the continuation of this example, we are assuming that the patient has described the pain as pressure.*] I'd like you to focus on that pressure. It is a sensation, like so many other sensations you have experienced . . . and as you become more aware of it as a sensation, it becomes less and less like a pain.

Distraction

To experience anything consciously, one must attend to it, and people have only a limited scope of attention. Because of this, distraction is one of the most powerful tools for pain control. Almost everyone has experienced this (e.g., becoming unaware of a headache or toothache while absorbed in an interesting movie), which makes it a useful tool for hypnotic pain relief. Indeed, distraction and relaxation should work independently of the person's level of suggestibility. The following is an example of distraction as might be used with a young child.

Therapist: What is your favorite TV show?

Patient: *Sesame Street.*

Therapist: And who is your favorite character on *Sesame Street*?

Patient: Oscar.

Therapist: The grouch?

Patient: Uh-huh!

Therapist: And would you like to be on *Sesame Street* right now?

Patient: Yes.

Therapist: You can do that, you know. Let's pretend we're on *Sesame Street* right now. Look! There's a garbage can right in front of you, and there's someone in the garbage can . . . someone small and fuzzy. I wonder who it is.

Patient: Oscar.

Therapist: That's right, it's Oscar! And look, he's waving hello to you! . . .

POSTHYPNOTIC PROCEDURES

The final phase of clinical hypnosis for pain relief includes posthypnotic suggestions and instructions. Techniques such as anchoring may be used to remind the patient of his or her hypnotic experiences between sessions. Patients can be told specifically that particular objects or individuals that they encounter daily will serve as cues that will remind them of the sense of well-being they have experienced during hypnosis. Internal cues (such as focusing on a particular word) and physical gestures, as described in chapter 3, can be linked to relaxation and pain relief. In addition, patients can be taught self-hypnosis or given an individually prepared audiotape that can be used at home daily. An emphasis may be placed on the process of pain management and on the need for continued patience and practice to achieve relief.

ADDITIONAL APPLICATIONS
IN BEHAVIORAL MEDICINE AND
HEALTH PSYCHOLOGY

As noted at the outset, hypnosis has many applications in the field of behavioral medicine and health psychology that extend well beyond the treatment of pain. In the remainder of this chapter, we review medical conditions, disorders, and treatment contexts in which hypnosis holds special promise for the amelioration of suffering and illness.

Irritable Bowel Syndrome

Hypnosis has demonstrated efficacy in the treatment of IBS, a disorder commonly encountered in medical practice (Mitchell & Drossman, 1987). An important study of IBS (Whorwell, Prior, & Faragher, 1984) involved the treatment of severe IBS that failed to respond to prior treatment for at least a year. Patients were randomly assigned to one of two treatments: hypnosis or placebo medication plus psychotherapy. Hypnosis reduced both pain reports and abdominal distention relative to the psychotherapy treatment at 12 weeks. These gains were maintained at follow-up a year and a half later (Whorwell, Prior, & Colgan, 1987). However, the most impressive study of IBS was a prospective one in which 204 patients treated with hypnotherapy were followed for as long as 6 years, and nearly three quarters (71%) of the patients maintained their initially positive response to treatment. Of those patients who benefited, fully 81% improved over time, and the remainder reported only a slight deterioration in their condition. Measures of quality of life and depression also improved, and medication use and medical consultation decreased, as a function of treatment (Gonsalkorale, Miller, Afzal, & Whorwell, 2003).

Asthma

Studies of the hypnotic treatment of large numbers ($N = 252$) of patients with asthma (Research Committee of the British Tuberculosis Association, 1968), patients with mild and moderate asthma (Ewer & Stewart, 1986), and exercise-induced asthma (Ben-Zvi, Spohn, Young, & Kattan, 1982) have provided a modicum of evidence for the effectiveness of hypnotic procedures. However, in one study (Ewer & Stewart, 1986) the benefits of hypnosis (e.g., pulmonary function, use of bronchodilator) were limited to highly suggestible patients, and in another study (Ben-Zvi et al., 1982), women reported greater symptom reduction than did men.

Warts

DuBreuil and Spanos' (1993) careful review of the research on the psychological treatment of warts concluded that hypnotic suggestions can produce wart remission that cannot be attributable to spontaneous remission or placebo effects. Spanos, Stenstrom, and Johnston (1988) have provided the following suggestions as examples of how wart loss can be accomplished:

> Notice that the skin on and around the warts on your hand is beginning to feel warm and a little tingly. The skin around the warts on your hand is beginning to tingle. Notice the sensations around the warts on your hand; you can feel the tingling, prickling sensation around the warts on your hand, you know that this sensation will cause the warts on your hand to disappear. . . . As you feel these sensations you can see the warts on your hand shrinking in size and dissolving away, shrinking in size and dissolving away. (Spanos et al., 1988, as quoted in DuBreuil & Spanos, 1993, p. 628)

It is interesting that DuBreuil and Spanos (1993) contended that direct suggestion for wart removal, rather than hypnosis per se, is responsible for wart disappearance (Spanos et al., 1988; Spanos, Williams, & Gwynn, 1990). Imagery is also associated with wart loss. In one study (Spanos et al., 1988), the participants who lost the most warts were those who had both high expectations for treatment success and higher suggested imagery vividness. Vivid suggestion-related imagery may be responsible for wart loss. However, another possibility is that imagery measures index treatment motivation and beliefs that participants are able to control physiological processes. At any rate, imagery and hypnosis appear to be cost-effective methods of reducing or eliminating warts.

Preparation and Treatment of Surgical Patients

A number of methodologically sophisticated studies have examined the effectiveness of hypnotic suggestions in the preparation and treatment of surgical patients (Lambert, 1996; Lang et al., 1996; Lang et al., 2000). In Lang et al.'s (1996) randomized control treatment study, for example, a brief self-hypnosis and relaxation intervention during interventional radiologic procedures was associated with fewer interruptions in the procedure, seven times fewer drug units, and fewer self-administrations of analgesic medications than with a nonhypnotic control procedure. The intervention included suggestions for deep breathing, feelings of spreading relaxation, and feelings of numbness, warmth, or coolness in the face of painful procedures. Other studies of a more preliminary nature suggest that hypnotic suggestions may play a role in reducing blood loss and in enhancing postoperative recovery (Blankfield, 1991; Enqvist, von Konow, & Bystedt, 1995).

In a meta-analytic study of 20 research reports of patients' responses to a variety of surgical procedures, Montgomery, David, Winkel, Silverstein, and Bovbjerg (2002) found that 89% of hypnosis patients fared better than did patients assigned to the control groups.

Postoperative Nausea and Emesis

Hypnosis and imaginative suggestions have been used to control postoperative nausea and emesis in randomly controlled trials in samples of (a) surgical patients who receive general anesthesia (Enqvist, Bjorklund, Engman, & Jakobsson, 1997) in a randomly controlled trial; (b) children who receive cancer treatments (Jacknow, Tschann, Link, & Boyce, 1994; Zeltzer, Dolgin, LeBaron, & LeBaron, 1991); and (c) bone marrow transplant patients who receive chemotherapy (Syrjala et al., 1992). In all of these studies, patients who received suggestions experienced less nausea or pain than did patients who were assigned to control conditions.

HYPNOSIS IN DENTISTRY

A survey (Clarke, 1996) of dental schools in North America (United States and Canada) revealed that 26% offered at least one course in clinical hypnosis, and that nearly a third (30%) provided students with a 1- to 2-hour introduction to hypnosis. This level of interest reflects the fact that hypnosis has a wide range of application in dentistry. Chaves' (1997b) comprehensive review of the spectrum of such applications indicates that in addition to helping patients relax in the face of stressful dental procedures and quieting phobic anxiety about dental injections, hypnosis can play an important role in the following areas of dental practice: (a) improved tolerance for orthodontic or prosthetic appliances; (b) modification of maladaptive oral habits; (c) reduction of the use of chemical anesthetics, analgesics, and sedation; (d) supplementation or substitution for surgical premedication; (e) control of salivary flow and bleeding; (f) therapeutic intervention for chronic facial pain syndromes such as temporomandibular disorders; (g) a complement to the use of nitrous oxide, and (h) enhanced compliance with personal oral hygiene recommendations.

In each of these areas, anecdotal and, in some cases, empirical studies lend support to the use of hypnosis in dentistry, although hypnosis should not be considered a substitute for local anesthesia. The most research support has been garnered for the use of hypnosis in inducing relaxation, treating discrete phobias, and alleviating chronic pain syndromes. Relatively less empirical support and attention has been accorded to the use of hypnosis to improve tolerance for orthodontic or prosthodontic appliances and as a supplement or substitute for surgical premedication, although additional research in these areas is justified by the available evidence.

Unfortunately, research (see Lynn, Neufeld, & Mare, 1993) has provided little basis for optimism regarding the effectiveness of rapid induction analgesia (RIA), which was hailed as a hypnotic breakthrough when it was introduced 25 years ago (J. Barber, 1977). For example, Gillett and Coe (1984) were unable to replicate J. Barber's stunning finding of the achievement of successful analgesia in 99 out of 100 unselected dental patients, although sizable numbers of patients in Gillett and Coe's research did seem to benefit from RIA. Claims for the effectiveness of RIA have been tempered by a steadily accumulating body of evidence that has failed to confirm the initial impression that a magic bullet for pain was discovered.

Procedures

Finkelstein (2003) offered a number of brief inductions that he found useful in treating dental patients and that can be completed in 5 minutes or less. Following is a summary of each of the inductions recommended by Finkelstein.

Relaxation

Patients are asked to bring relaxation to various body parts, including the arms, hands, shoulders, chest, stomach, hips, upper legs, knees, ankles, and feet, with instructions to breathe out and "relax very deeply." Patients are then instructed to imagine being on the fifth floor of a lovely building with an elevator with an "interesting property" of permitting the patient to double his or her relaxation with each descent to a lower floor. Patients are also given a choice of relaxing with an "escalator with a comfortable chair" and a "wide carpeted stairway with lovely pictures on the walls and windows through which you can see a lovely day outside." Instructions are then given to exit the building and enter an "absolutely wonderful" place of refuge where "nothing can bother or disturb you." Posthypnotic suggestions are given to feel refreshed and feel "terrific, because you are a terrifically wonderful person" (Finkelstein, 2003, pp. 82–83).

Cloud Induction

Patients are asked to imagine that they are comfortably supported by a cloud. The cloud keeps them warm and secure while they "breathe normally and without discomfort." This induction, and the ones in the next section, can be supplemented with other "ego strengthening" suggestions for comfort, relaxation, and well-being (Finkelstein, 2003, p. 83).

Breathing Induction

Patients are instructed to take three deep breaths, hold them, and relax as they exhale, becoming more deeply relaxed and comfortable with each breath.

Somatic Awareness Induction

This induction facilitates somatic awareness by way of a series of questions such as the following: (a) "Can you notice how your relaxation increases when you exhale?" (b) "Does the right hand feel as if it is lying on your leg or does it feel as if it is supported by the leg?" (c) "Do your right and left legs feel the weight of your hands equally or is there a difference?" and (d) "Is it time for you to go to your special place, changing it whenever you want, with the people you want and only those, changing them whenever you wish, or would you prefer being by yourself?" (Finkelstein, 2003, p. 83).

Eye-Roll Induction

Patients are asked to hold their heads steady, look up as far as they can, slowly close their eyelids, relax the muscles around the eyes, take deep breaths, and with each exhalation feel increasing relaxation (Finkelstein, 2003, p. 84).

Acceptance of Procedures

Calm appraisal of situations, feelings of personal well-being, enjoyment of support and love, feeling protected and wonderful, safety and security, inner strength, and deep relaxation are suggested, followed by suggestions for progressive relaxation. Deepening of the experience of hypnosis is achieved by an image of being safely surrounded by wider and wider transparent, concentric spheres of luminous serenity.

Finkelstein (2003) recommended assessing patient motivation, positive treatment expectancies, and the need for ego strengthening, reassurance, and positive reinforcement, as well as capacity for imagery in all five senses before hypnosis is initiated. The complete inductions are available (Finkelstein, 2003), which will facilitate research on the effectiveness of brief, cost-effective hypnotic inductions in dental settings. We concur with Chaves' (1997b) conclusion that the field of dentistry affords tremendous research and training opportunities in health care.

Randomized controlled trials, which compare hypnosis with established treatments and well-designed placebo control treatments, are not yet the norm. So it is premature to claim that hypnotic procedures, rather than relaxation and other nonspecific factors, for example, are responsible for the treatment gains reported in many studies of medical and dental conditions. Nevertheless, it is clear that hypnosis can ameliorate pain and suffering and perhaps play an important role in the treatment of a variety of health-related conditions.

12

QUESTIONS AND CONTROVERSIES

From the days of Mesmer to the present, hypnosis has not been far from the swirl of controversy. Provocative debates that range from the question of whether hypnosis is an altered state of consciousness or trance to the role of hypnosis in memory recovery have sparked our personal fascination with hypnosis for the past 25 years, and will no doubt continue to do so. To be a serious student of hypnosis is to grapple with questions that extend well beyond hypnosis to the fundamental nature of consciousness, and how words and deeds can mitigate human suffering. And it is to a number of these questions that we now turn, reminding the reader that our perspective on each of these topics is but one of many accounts that have been advanced.

IS HYPNOSIS AN ALTERED OR TRANCE STATE OF CONSCIOUSNESS?

Most contemporary theories of hypnosis are rooted in the work of Robert W. White (1941). White concluded that because of their overly mechanistic nature, neither the theory of dissociation nor the theory of ideomotor action (reviewed in chap. 1) could adequately explain hypnotic responding. He argued that hypnotic behavior was goal-directed social action, and that hypnotic participants responded in terms of their ideas about what the hypnotist wished them to do. At the same time, however, White continued to believe that hypnotic behavior occurred during an altered state of consciousness that was characterized by subtle cognitive changes, a view also embraced by Martin Orne (1959).

Following White (1941), a number of different altered-state theories (e.g., Edmonston, 1981; Hilgard, 1965; D. Spiegel, 1998; H. Spiegel & Spiegel, 1978) and a number of different nonstate theories (e.g., T. X. Barber, 1969; Kirsch, 1991; Lynn & Rhue, 1991b; Sarbin, 1991; Spanos, 1986; Wagstaff, 1991) have been proposed, along with a number of theories that do not clearly belong in either camp (e.g., Hilgard, 1986; Kihlstrom, 2005; McConkey, 1991; Sheehan, 1991). Besides these specific positions, it is possible to identify a generic altered state (GAS) conception of hypnosis and a generic nonstate (GNS) view. These are not really theories. Rather, the GAS conception consists of the commonalities among the altered-state theories and the GNS conception consists of those assumptions and opinions that various nonstate theorists share. These are the shared commitments that allow the grouping of these theories under common labels (see Kuhn, 1971).

Common tenets of altered-state theories include that hypnosis involves an altered state of consciousness, generally designated as a trance. Kallio and Revonsuo (2003) identified the central question regarding hypnosis as an altered state of consciousness: "Is there a special hypnotic state . . . that serves as a background and gives rise to altered experiences produced by suggestion?" (p. 125). It is also believed by many altered-state proponents that enhanced suggestibility is one of the features of trance, and that trance is required for at least some hypnotic phenomena to occur. In contrast to these views, nonstate theorists hold that the feeling of an altered state is merely one of the many subjective effects of suggestion and that it is not required for the experience of any other suggested effects.

During the 1960s, hypnosis theorists and researchers were grouped into two warring camps that differed on the question of whether hypnosis could best be understood as an altered state of consciousness. During the 1960s and 1970s, the altered-state issue was acknowledged to be the most contentious issue in the field (Sheehan & Perry, 1976). Despite various pronouncements of convergence in the altered-state debate (Hilgard, 1973; Kirsch & Lynn, 1995; Spanos & Barber, 1974), the controversy has continued. For instance, Gruzelier's (1996) review of the psychophysiological concomitants of hypnosis concluded that "We can now acknowledge that hypnosis is indeed a 'state' and redirect energies earlier spent on the state–nonstate debate" (p. 315). Others weighed in and, for a variety of reasons, were not willing to pronounce the altered-state debate dead (see Chaves, 1997a; Hasegawa & Jamieson, 2002; Kihlstrom, 1997; Rainville & Price, 2003; Wagstaff, 1998). Kallio and Revonsuo (2003) recently proposed an altered state of consciousness hypothesis that postulates that true hypnosis is a rare phenomenon experienced only by hypnotic virtuosos (i.e., very highly suggestible participants) who are capable of experiencing hallucinations without voluntary effort.

The best evidence of an altered state would be the detection of physiological markers of the trance state. Gruzelier's (1996) review marshalled evidence to document different neurophysiological effects on high and low suggestible individuals following a hypnotic induction. The typical design in many of these studies involves screening for high level of hypnotic suggestibility, inducing trance, and suggesting a particular change in experience. There are at least two problems with the interpretation of these data as support for the trance hypothesis. First, in many of these studies, trance induction and the target suggestion (e.g., pain reduction or altered visual perception) are confounded. The same target suggestion (with the same wording) is rarely given to highly suggestible participants without the induction of hypnosis. For example, one should not tell hypnotized participants that they will see something but tell nonhypnotized participants to imagine something (e.g., Kosslyn, Thompson, Costantini-Ferrando, Alpert, & Spiegel, 2000). The confounding of suggestion with induction precludes any conclusions about the altered-state hypothesis.

Second, even if the same suggestion were given with and without the induction of trance, the data would be only indirectly pertinent to the altered-state hypothesis. At best, they might show that the experimenters had failed to detect physiological data supporting the reported experiential changes of participants who had not been hypnotized. In principle, this is not different from the substantial data showing that inductions do make a difference, albeit a small one, in responsiveness to suggestion (e.g., T. X. Barber, 1969; Braffman & Kirsch, 1999; Hilgard, 1965).

Direct evidence of an altered state of consciousness would require finding physiological markers of response to the suggestion to enter trance, without any further suggestions (what has been termed *neutral hypnosis*) and also finding that these markers were necessary prerequisites for response to at least some suggestions. As far as we know, evidence of this sort has not yet been found (see also Dixon & Laurence, 1992; Hasegawa & Jamieson, 2002; Sarbin & Slagle, 1979; Wagstaff, 1998; Weitzenhoffer, 1985). To assert that the trance state involves "major alterations in both the content and pattern of functioning of consciousness" (Tart, 1983, p. 19) but that it has no physiological representation in the brain is beyond the bounds of science. If there are physiological markers of neutral hypnosis, but they are the correlates of mundane subjective states (e.g., attention, absorption, interest, cognitive effort, expectancy), as some have suggested (e.g., Wagstaff, 1998), then neutral hypnosis is not an altered state of consciousness.

Actually, there is little debate that hypnotic suggestions can affect brain functioning. In fact, studies of the neurophysiology of hypnosis (see

Hasegawa & Jamieson, 2002) point to the anterior cingulate area of the brain as playing an important role in alterations in conscious experience during hypnosis (e.g., Faymonville et al., 2000; Kropotov, Crawford, & Polyakov, 1997; Rainville et al., 1997; Szechtman, Woody, Bowers, & Nahmias, 1998). Nevertheless, while undeniably interesting, these findings "do not indicate a discrete state of hypnosis" (Hasegawa & Jamieson, 2002, p. 113). The search for such a state is arguably one of the most fascinating and important endeavors in the field of hypnosis, which will no doubt be abetted by increasingly sophisticated brain imaging methodologies (Ray & Oathies, 2003). Whether or not a consensus is reached regarding the existence of a discrete state of hypnosis, research on the neurophysiological concomitants of both hypnotic and nonhypnotic experiences promises to illuminate many important aspects of human consciousness (see Hasegawa & Jamieson, 2002).

Should Hypnosis Be Used to Recover Memories in Therapy?

The notion that hypnosis can permanently alter memories was known to 19th-century luminaries (e.g., Freud, Bernheim, Janet, Forel) in the field of hypnosis and psychology (Laurence & Perry, 1983a, 1988). Indeed, many examples of hypnotically induced false memories—*pseudomemories*—can be found in the literature dating back more than 100 years. But over the past 20 years or so, the controversy regarding the possibility that memory recovery techniques can tamper with recall has riven hypnosis researchers, as it has polarized psychotherapists. Much of the hoopla can be attributed to questions about the accuracy of memories recovered in the course of child abuse investigations, the possible creation of multiple or dissociated personalities by the use of hypnosis and other suggestive procedures, and sensationalized popular media accounts on both sides of the controversy (see Lynn & McConkey, 1998).

Hypnosis has been at the front and center of this controversy, in no small measure because it is the most widely researched and widely used memory recovery technique. Survey research (Poole, Lindsay, Memon, & Bull, 1995) reveals that approximately one third (29%–34%) of psychologists in the United States who were sampled reported that they used hypnosis to help patients recall memories of sexual abuse. Despite increased awareness of the problems of false recall associated with hypnosis, our experience indicates that even today, therapists known to be experienced in the use of hypnosis are called on by potential patients or their therapists to assist in the retrieval of forgotten or repressed memories. Compliance with this request can lead to the production of new material that becomes part of the memory structure of the patient. However, knowledge of the nature and malleability of memory indicates that this risky procedure may result in the iatrogenic production of false memories (Lynn & McConkey, 1998; Lynn & Nash, 1994).

The Research Base

Today, there is a consensus among contemporary cognitive scientists that everyday memories are fallible, quirky, and reconstructive in nature (Lynn & McConkey, 1998), even if consensus is lacking regarding whether hypnosis is a more risky procedure than nonhypnotic recall enhancement procedures. Not only is memory fallible, but some people place an inordinate degree of confidence in their remembrances, even to the point of being convinced that events that did not take place actually did occur (Laurence & Perry, 1983b; McConkey, Barnier, & Sheehan, 1998).

Even in the absence of a hypnotic induction, it is possible to create complex memories of events that never occurred. Studies with college students have shown that approximately 20% to 50% report experiencing such fictitious events as (a) being lost in a shopping mall (Loftus & Pickrell, 1995); (b) being hospitalized overnight for a high fever and a possible ear infection, accidentally spilling a bowl of punch on the parents of the bride at a wedding reception, and evacuating a grocery store when the overhead sprinkler systems erroneously activated (Hyman, Husband, & Billings, 1995); (c) experiencing a serious animal attack, serious indoor accident, serious outdoor accident, a serious medical procedure, and being injured by another child (Porter, Yuille, & Lehman, 1999); (d) being bullied as a child (Mazzoni, Loftus, Seitz, & Lynn, 1999); and (e) taking a ride in a hot air balloon (Wade, Garry, Read, & Lindsay, 2002).

Hypnosis in no way obviates the hazards of memory distortion. To the contrary, hypnosis may exacerbate the problem (Lynn & Nash, 1994), as the following points make plain (see Lynn et al., 2003).

- Hypnosis increases the sheer volume of recall, resulting in more incorrect as well as correct information. When response productivity is controlled, hypnotic recall is no more accurate than nonhypnotic recall (Erdelyi, 1994, review of 34 studies; Steblay & Bothwell, 1994, review of 24 studies) and results in increased confidence for responses designated as guesses during a prior waking test (Whitehouse, Dinges, Orne, & Orne, 1988).
- Hypnosis produces more recall errors, more intrusions of uncued errors, and higher levels of memories for false information relative to nonhypnotic methods (Steblay & Bothwell, 1994).
- False memories are associated with hypnotic responsiveness. Although highly suggestible individuals tend to report more false memories than do low hypnotizable persons, even

relatively nonhypnotizable participants, including witnesses of live and videotaped events, report false memories (Lynn, Myers, & Malinoski, 1997).

- Research (see Spanos, 1996; Steblay & Bothwell, 1994) indicates that hypnotized participants are at least as likely as non-hypnotized participants to be misled in their recall by leading questions and sometimes exhibit recall deficits compared with nonhypnotized participants. There also are indications that high hypnotizable persons are particularly prone to memory errors in response to misleading information.
- In general, hypnotized individuals are more confident about their recall accuracy than are nonhypnotized individuals (Steblay & Bothwell, 1994). Furthermore, an association between hypnotizability and confidence has been well documented, particularly in hypnotized participants (Steblay & Bothwell, 1994). Confidence effects are not always present and are not universally large. However, hypnosis does not selectively increase confidence in accurate memories. At times, hypnotized participants can be very confident in false memories.
- Even when participants are warned about possible memory problems associated with hypnotic recollections, they continue to report false memories during and after hypnosis, although some studies indicate that warnings have the potential to reduce the rate of pseudomemories in hypnotized and nonhypnotized individuals (Lynn, Lock, Loftus, Lilienfeld, & Krackow, 2003).
- Some writers (D. P. Brown, Scheflin, & Hammond, 1998; Hammond et al., 1995) have advocated the use of hypnosis to recover memories of emotional or traumatic experiences. Contrary to this position, seven studies (see Lynn et al., 1997) that compared hypnotic versus nonhypnotic memory in the face of relatively emotionally arousing stimuli (e.g., films of shop accidents, depictions of fatal stabbings, a mock assassination, videotape of an actual murder) yielded an unambiguous conclusion: Hypnosis does not improve recall of emotionally arousing events nor does arousal level affect hypnotic recall.
- Hypnosis does not necessarily yield more false memories than do nonhypnotic procedures that are highly suggestive or leading in nature (Lynn et al., 1997). Indeed, any procedure that conveys the expectation that accurate memories can be easily recovered is likely to increase the sheer volume of memories and bolster confidence in inaccurate as well as accurate memories. Scoboria, Mazzoni, Kirsch, and Milling's (2002) research re-

vealed that the induction of hypnosis and using leading interview procedures each had a negative effect on participants' recall.

- Although hypnosis is often used to facilitate the experience of age regression, it can distort memories of early life events. Nash, Drake, Wiley, Khalsa, and Lynn (1986) attempted to corroborate the memories of participants who had been part of an earlier age-regression experiment. This experiment involved age regressing hypnotized and role-playing (control) participants to age 3 to a scene in which they were in the soothing presence of their mothers. During the experiment, participants reported the identity of their transitional objects (e.g., blankets, teddy bears). Third-party verification (parent report) of the accuracy of recall was obtained for 14 hypnotized participants and 10 control participants. Hypnotic participants were less able than control participants to identify the transitional objects actually used. Hypnotic participants' hypnotic recollections matched their parents' reports only 21% of the time, whereas control participants' reports were corroborated by their parents 70% of the time.

    Sivec, Lynn, and Malinoski (1997) age-regressed participants to the age of 5 and suggested that they played with a Cabbage Patch Doll if they were a girl or a He-Man toy if they were a boy. (These toys were not released until two or three years after the target time of the age-regression suggestion.) Half of the participants received hypnotic age-regression instructions and half received suggestions to age regress that were not administered in a hypnotic context. Whereas none of the nonhypnotized persons were influenced by the suggestion, 20% of the hypnotized participants rated the memory as real and were confident that the event occurred at the age to which they were regressed.

- The search for traumatic memories can extend to well before birth (see Mills & Lynn, 2000). Past-life regression therapy is based on the premise that traumas that occurred in previous lives contribute to current psychological and physical symptoms. For example, psychiatrist Brian Weiss (1988) published a widely publicized series of cases focusing on patients who were hypnotized and age regressed to go back to the origin of a present-day problem. When patients were regressed, they reported events that Weiss interpreted as having their source in previous lives.

What are we to make of vivid and realistic reports of past lives? Is the information recovered from a past life reliable? If so, it would constitute strong evidence that hypnosis was an effective age-regression technique and that past lives were indeed a reality. However, the research bears out neither possibility. Spanos, Menary, Gabora, DuBreuil, and Dewhirst (1991) determined that the information participants provided about specific periods during their hypnotic age regression was almost invariably incorrect. For example, one participant who was regressed to ancient times claimed to be Julius Caesar, emperor of Rome, in 50 BC, even though the designations of BC and AD were not adopted until centuries later, and even though Julius Caesar died decades prior to the first Roman emperor. Spanos et al. (1991) informed some participants that past-life identities were likely to be of a different gender, culture, and race from that of the present personality, whereas other participants received no prehypnotic information about past-life identities. Participants' past-life experiences were elaborate, conformed to induced expectancies about past-life identities (e.g., gender, race), and varied in terms of the prehypnotic information participants received about the frequency of child abuse during past historical periods. In summary, hypnotically induced past-life experiences are fantasies constructed from available cultural narratives about past lives and known or surmised facts regarding specific historical periods, as well as cues present in the hypnotic situation (Spanos, 1996).

Why Does Hypnosis Increase False Memory Risk?

A free flow of imagination and fantasy is a common response to a hypnotic induction. In fact, one of the central demands of hypnosis is to fantasize and imagine along with suggested events and to relinquish a critical, analytical stance in favor of the direct experience of suggested events (Lynn, Martin, & Frauman, 1996). Guided imagery, even when hypnosis is not used, warrants concern because people frequently confuse real and imagined memories, particularly when memories are initially hazy or unavailable (Hyman & Pentland, 1996). A sizable body of research has shown that simply having participants imagine an event can lead to the formation of false memories. Confidence in the occurrence of fictitious events typically increases after those events have been imagined. This phenomenon is called imagination inflation and has been demonstrated repeatedly (reviewed in Garry & Polaschek, 2000).

In addition to imagination, people's beliefs about hypnosis likely play a role in false memory formation. The information that is remembered during hypnosis is typically reported in a context of implicitly and explicitly communicated acceptance of its accuracy. People's beliefs have always shaped their hypnotic experiences. When people believed that convulsions were the sine qua non of mesmerism, they convulsed. When they thought it required a trance, they went into a trance. Catalepsy and spontaneous amnesia have been signs of hypnosis, but only among people who believed that these were to be expected. Many people believe that hypnosis enhances memory, and this belief leads them to accept more of their confabulation as memory (Whitehouse et al., 1988). The combination of increased fantasy and decreased objectivity, along with the commonly held belief that hypnosis enhances recall, may promote the confusion of fantasy and historical reality and the tenacious belief that imagined events actually occurred.

Professional Societies

Our pessimistic assessment of hypnosis for recovering memories has been echoed by professional societies, including divisions and task forces of the American Psychological Association (APA, 1995) and the Canadian Psychiatric Association (CPA, 1996). The American Medical Association (AMA, 1994) has asserted that hypnosis be used only for investigative purposes in forensic contexts. However, hypnosis should be used in forensic contexts only when it is possible to corroborate any memories elicited by hypnosis, and only when strict procedures are used to ensure that proper, nonleading investigative procedures have been implemented.

It is sometimes argued that the actual truth of a memory may be unimportant and what matters is its narrative truth. According to this view, if the recovery of a memory is therapeutic, it does not matter if it is true. The idea that the recovery of a memory is therapeutic is an untested and questionable assumption. But the proposition that a false memory can have negative effects is unquestionable. Among other things, it can lead to the disruption of family bonds. Thus, the use of hypnosis to enhance or recover memory is rarely justified. If exceptional circumstances lead to the decision that hypnotic exploration of suspected forgotten memories is warranted, it should be undertaken only with the following precautions:

- As part of informed consent, educate patients about the risk of memory distortion and the inadvisability of acting on what they remember outside of the treatment context (e.g., legal proceedings). The patient should be told that far from guaranteeing the veracity of a memory, hypnosis might lead one to be overly confident in misinterpreting a fantasy as a memory. Without independent corroboration there is no way to assess the veracity of an apparent memory. The patient should be further informed that being hypnotized to obtain or refresh a memory may disqualify a person from being able to testify about it in court in some states.

- Warn patients that recalling traumatic events from childhood will not automatically—or even easily—resolve their difficulties.
- Scrupulously avoid leading and suggestive questions.
- If a patient recovers a memory during hypnosis or apart from the hypnotic context, evaluate the credibility of the memory. Consider the patient's suggestibility and the nature of the procedures used to uncover the remembrances. (Lynn, Kirsch, & Rhue, 1996)

As an alternative, the therapist might recommend tentatively adopting the view that a suspected event did in fact occur in some particular matter, while knowing full well that this hypothesis is unproven. If it were true, how does this change the person's current life? What can he or she do about it? How does it hinder or facilitate resolving and coping with current problems? These questions may be followed by temporary adoption of the hypothesis that the event did not occur or that it occurred differently. What are the consequences of this hypothesis for the patient's current dilemmas? A process of this sort may obviate the need to establish what actually occurred. Yet if highly implausible memories surface, the therapist should not hesitate to corroborate them by way of collateral informants and other means, although we recognize that this may be impossible or clinically unadvisable in many instances. The bottom line is that using hypnosis for memory recovery is a gamble. We are hard pressed to envision a situation in which the gamble is worth the risk.

SHOULD CLINICIANS TEST FOR HYPNOTIC SUGGESTIBILITY?

A survey conducted some 15 years ago suggested that most therapists (54%) do not routinely test their patients for hypnotic suggestibility by any means, and less than a third use standardized suggestibility scales to assess suggestibility (Cohen, 1989). We would wager that if the survey were re-administered today, the numbers would not be much different. Many clinicians we know share Diamond's (1989) view that suggestibility assessment is a risky venture that is potentially a "misleading, intrusive, and transference-contaminating obstacle to the therapeutic work ahead" (p. 12). Many clinicians also question the clinical usefulness of hypnotic suggestibility scores (J. Barber, 1989), an understandable concern given our earlier observation that high suggestibility is not required to respond to many useful suggestions and high scores do not necessarily predict treatment outcome. We would add yet another concern: The failure to pass suggestibility tests could dampen positive treatment expectancies and motivation and therefore beget treatment failure.

These reservations aside, at least some knowledge of the patient's degree of suggestibility is easy to obtain and poses little or no risk to the therapeutic enterprise. In chapter 3, we discussed using the Chevreul pendulum to provide a rough assessment of waking suggestibility, along with a fail-safe induction that involved reinforcing suggestions of either lightness (arm/hand raising) or heaviness (arm/hand lowering). These simple yet powerful demonstrations increase the patient's expectations of responsiveness in hypnotic situations. We would add a third tactic: Administer suggestions in a waking rather than a hypnotic context. As patients who respond to waking imaginative suggestions are very likely to respond in kind, if not more so, to suggestions preceded by a hypnotic induction (T. X. Barber, 1969; Braffman & Kirsch, 1999), administering waking suggestions can provide an excellent indication of hypnotic suggestibility. If there is little or no response to waking suggestions, then there is probably little to gain in administering a hypnotic induction (E. Meyer & Lynn, 2004), unless the therapist is invested in training the low suggestible patient to be more responsive. You will recall that there is considerable evidence that individuals who initially test as low suggestible can often increase their responsiveness to suggestions (Gfeller, 1993) with the establishment of adequate rapport with the hypnotist, support and encouragement to imagine along with suggestions, and instructions in how to interpret suggestions (e.g., assume an active role in responding to suggestions, don't wait passively to respond). However, this approach does have a cost in terms of time and effort and therefore may not be a viable option. A positive response to waking suggestions can often bolster positive treatment expectancies and can be framed as an indicator of potentially high hypnotic suggestibility.

If therapists require additional information about patients' suggestibility, they must decide whether to use formal, standardized tests or nonstandard tests of responsiveness carefully tailored to the treatment at hand (Bates, 1993; D. P. Brown & Fromm, 1986). Formal, standardized measures are preferred in research settings or when reporting of clinical studies is anticipated. In clinical situations, informal approaches will suffice with most patients when treatment involves basic relaxation and ego-strengthening suggestions, visualization exercises, and many of the suggestions and scripts we have provided for your consideration. If treatment centers on one particular suggestion, such as for age regression, amnesia, or pain relief, then the decision to confine assessment to a specific, treatment-relevant suggestion is defensible. Highly suggestible individuals are generally more responsive to analgesia suggestions than are low suggestible individuals. However, it would be foolhardy to use hypnosis as an anesthetic in the dental chair, even with a person who is, in general, highly suggestible, without first establishing the ability to respond to anesthesia suggestions in the clinician's office. It is interesting that some individuals who do not achieve pain reduction when analgesia suggestions are couched in hypnotic terms do achieve significant pain relief when the same suggestions are presented with no hint that hypnosis is involved (see Spanos, 1991, for a review). This is probably the case because some patients have counterproductive and recalcitrant attitudes and expectations about hypnosis that interfere with their responsiveness to the analgesia suggestion. In such cases, it is wise to administer analgesia suggestions with no mention of hypnosis. Knowing something about the response to hypnosis can thus guide treatment decisions in this area of application (Lynn, Kirsch, Neufeld, & Rhue, 1996).

The argument has been advanced that assessment is to be eschewed because it is inefficient, costly, and time consuming (Diamond, 1989). However, H. Spiegel (1989) has contended that suggestibility can, in fact, be quickly and easily assessed and can provide a metric to gauge not only suggestibility but also the degree to which a person is malleable and can "focalize concentration and internalize and control a new perspective" (p. 16). Spiegel's Hypnotic Induction Profile (H. Spiegel & Spiegel, 1978) is a sensible choice for a short assessment instrument. Nadon and Laurence (1994), however, have strongly recommended the much longer Stanford Hypnotic Susceptibility Scale, Form C (Weitzenhoffer & Hilgard, 1962) or a tailored version (Hilgard, Crawford, Bowers, & Kihlstrom, 1979) "primarily because of its stringency and its broad sampling of hypnotic suggestions" (p. 91). The advantage of a tailored version is that it can provide information about specific responses relevant to treatment (Lynn, Kirsch, Neufeld, & Rhue, 1996).

If the clinician decides to implement formal testing, Frankel and Orne (1976) recommend that the patient be told that the purpose of standardized testing is to tailor the individual's treatment more effectively. They suggest that the patient be told, "Knowing how you respond will enable us to modify the technique so that it can fit in with the needs of your treatment" (pp. 1259–1260).

Even though there is not a tight relation between hypnotic suggestibility and treatment gains, suggestibility is not completely irrelevant to outcome. In no study we located is high hypnotic suggestibility associated with a negative treatment outcome. The link between analgesia suggestions and hypnotic suggestibility is well established; however, even medium suggestible individuals can often derive considerable benefit from hypnotic analgesia. The findings regarding suggestibility and treatment outcome are mixed yet at least somewhat promising for smoking cessation, obesity, warts, anxiety, somatization, conversion disorders, and asthma (Lynn, Shindler, & Meyer, 2003). In fact, in a study of the hypnotic treatment of conversion disorder, hypnotic suggestibility was a better predictor of outcome than were expectancies (Moene, Spinhoven, Hoogduin, & Van Dyck, 2003). As implied earlier, the fact that many studies indicate little or no relation between hypnotic suggestibility and treatment outcome may reflect the fact that typical hypnotic interventions rely on relatively easy suggestions (e.g., relaxation, guided imagery, imaginative rehearsal) that require little hypnotic or imaginative abilities to pass.

When trauma resolution work is contemplated, clinicians should have at least a rough estimate of the patient's suggestibility. You will recall that a consistent finding in the literature is that pseudomemories are most likely to occur in participants who are at least moderately suggestible (see Lynn & Nash, 1994). Vigilance for suggestive influences is demanded in any psychotherapy; however, patients with at least moderate hypnotic abilities are especially vulnerable. Moreover, because suggestibility is associated with pseudomemory rate even in nonhypnotic contexts, it might be worthwhile to test for suggestibility in nonhypnotic contexts when trauma work is on the agenda. Although each therapist must weigh the costs and benefits of assessment with each patient, at the very least, an informal evaluation of hypnotic suggestibility can often yield valuable information.

DOES HYPNOSIS PRODUCE NEGATIVE EFFECTS?

Practitioners might shy away from hypnosis because they are afraid they will encounter a reaction to hypnosis that they may be unable to handle. After all, if hypnosis produces profound alterations in consciousness, perceptions, and sensations, might things get out of control during the session? We suspect that most clinicians have heard of one or more untoward reactions that occurred during hypnosis. Indeed, negative effects, as they are termed, can and do happen on an occasional basis—therapists need to be alert to the fact that a minority (i.e., 8%–49%) of individuals report mostly transient negative posthypnotic experiences (e.g., headaches, dizziness, nausea, stiff necks, mild cognitive distortions). However, there is more to the story. Over the years, the great majority of the participants tested in our experimental studies—in the neighborhood of 80% (Lynn, Martin, & Frauman, 1996)—described their experience of hypnosis as very positive (e.g., relaxing). Our clinical experience leads us to conclude that most patients appraise their experience of hypnosis in equally positive terms.

On the basis of a number of reviews (Coe & Ryken, 1979; Lynn, Brentar, Carlson, Kurzhals, & Green, 1992; Lynn, Martin, & Frauman, 1996) of the research on hypnosis and negative effects, it is clear that negative reactions also occur following nonhypnotic treatments. Yet hypnosis evokes no more negative experiences than do mundane activities such as sitting with eyes closed, taking a college examination, attending a college class, and college life in general. Yet because of common misconceptions concerning hypnosis (e.g., trance, loss of control) and the timing of negative posthypnotic reactions, patients mistakenly attribute negative reactions to a hypnotically induced altered state of consciousness.

Nevertheless, the possibility of negative or unanticipated reactions merits careful attention by the therapist. We have encountered a number of such negative reactions in our own practice. Most of the negative reactions occurred in the early years of our work with hypnosis. In one instance, a patient received a suggestion to walk to a beach and count waves as a deepening technique. Within a minute of receiving this suggestion, the patient burst into tears and when roused from hypnosis indicated that she had, in fact, gone to a lake the previous week and contemplated suicide at the water's edge. In another instance, a patient with a diagnosis of borderline personality selected an island as her favorite place and, though she initially reported feeling comfortable and relaxed, became quite anxious as she imagined that killer sharks were coming toward her on the beach, approaching her with foot-like appendages. What these examples imply is that preexisting psychological problems or recall of unpleasant experiences can be associated with psychological distress, but this is likely to be related to the content of the memory or spontaneous imagery rather than the use of hypnosis per se (Lynn, Martin, & Frauman, 1996).

It is fortunate that many negative effects can be prevented or minimized (see also Crawford, Hilgard, & MacDonald, 1982; MacHovec, 1986; Page & Green, 2002), and we recommend the following steps to ensure the most positive experience of hypnosis possible. A number of these recommendations recapitulate and reinforce earlier themes regarding the need to educate patients and build therapeutic response sets to maximize hypnotic suggestibility and treatment gains.

1. Carefully assess (pre- and posttreatment) each patient's medical and psychological history (e.g., fears, phobias, social problems), psychological defenses, and coping skills. Note any secondary gains or reinforcement contingencies that maintain or exacerbate current symptoms. Try to anticipate negative reactions. As you recall from our earlier discussion, obsessive–compulsive, borderline, paranoid, and psychotic individuals may be poor candidates for clinical hypnosis or require special treatment considerations.

2. Carefully assess patients' expectancies, attitudes, and beliefs about hypnosis. Ask about prior experiences with hypnosis, and listen for signs of previous negative reactions and their source (e.g., poor therapist technique versus discussion of sensitive issues that evoked anxiety). Disabuse patients of the

view that hypnosis is a quick fix or a road to the unconscious. Demystify hypnosis and correct any misconceptions about hypnosis. Portray hypnosis as a therapeutic tool that can promote relaxation and increase personal control.

3. If despite concerted efforts to educate the patient, he or she is still very concerned about being dominated or out of control, consider defining hypnotic procedures as imagery work, goal-directed fantasies, or self-hypnosis.

4. Determine what role hypnosis will play in treatment and discuss this role with the patient. Thoroughly prepare him or her for hypnosis, structure realistic expectations, and retain a high degree of flexibility and openness to reconceptualize not only the focal problem but also the role of hypnosis in psychotherapy.

5. Obtain the patient's informed consent to participate in hypnosis. This is particularly important when past issues are explored. In such cases, patients should be aware of the potential of hypnosis to increase confidence in inaccurate as well as accurate memories, as previously discussed. However, do not draw attention to the possibility of negative aftereffects (e.g., headaches) before hypnosis, during hypnosis, or after hypnosis. This tactic may be unduly suggestive. Nevertheless, review the patient's experience of hypnosis and make it plain that if he or she wishes to discuss any aspect of the experience to feel free to contact you after the session.

6. Work hard to establish a resilient working alliance with the patient as a deterrent against negative or idealized transference reactions (Lynn, Kirsch, & Rhue, 1996).

7. Be permissive. Present and respect choices as therapeutic double binds, so that either choice promotes improvement and minimizes resistance. Notice what the person does "right," and comment on it. By focusing on patients' small changes in respiration, for example, and linking these small changes with statements to the effect that it demonstrates the person is beginning to relax in a way that facilitates the experience of hypnosis, the therapist can convey the idea that change begins with changes so small they may escape notice. This technique allows small increments, such as those produced by random fluctuations, to be interpreted as signs of therapeutic success (Lynn, Kirsch, & Rhue, 1996).

8. The dictum "never treat anything with hypnosis that you are not trained or equipped to treat in nonhypnotic therapy" is an indispensable hedge against unmanageable reactions.

For example, abreactions associated with cognitive–behavioral exposure techniques, when managed with skill and sensitivity, can have therapeutic benefit. However, therapists should have training in using such techniques (with or without hypnosis) before incorporating them into their clinical practice.

9. When the therapist is aware of having particularly strong positive, sexualized, or hostile feelings toward the patient or feels a need to control the therapeutic encounter with little regard for the patient's well-being, consultation, supervision, or individual psychotherapy for the therapist is called for.

10. In general, avoid direct suggestions to relinquish symptoms in the absence of a foundation of adequate psychological defenses and coping skills (Lynn, Martin, & Frauman, 1996). Consider the patient's readiness to try something new or to make requisite life changes. How would the person's life be changed if the symptom were no longer present? What would have to change in the person's life for him or her to be symptom-free? Suggestions for symptom reduction may be safer and more effective than suggestions for symptom elimination, and permissive wording can forestall a sense of failure and respect the patient's intuitive sense of timing. A suggestion like the following, for example, might be preferred to a direct suggestion that pain will no longer be felt:

> Pain is an important danger signal, and the pain you experienced once served a useful function. But I wonder if you still need the degree of discomfort that you have experienced in the past. As you are learning to pay closer attention to your body's wise signals, your need for intense pain diminishes—getting less and less—until just enough discomfort remains to remind you to treat your back with respect.

11. After hypnosis, ensure that the patient is fully alert and does not feel sleepy or drowsy or have any other unintended effects of suggestions when he or she leaves the office.

If you follow these recommendations and exercise good clinical judgment, we are confident that you will optimize your patients' experience of hypnosis and minimize the possibility of adverse reactions to the hypnotic procedures we have recommended in the course of our discussion.

CONCLUSIONS

Hypnosis has been formally recognized as a therapeutic procedure by the American Medical Association and American Psychiatric Association. Its use has been supported by strong empirical data demonstrating its effectiveness in many clinical conditions. For example, it appears to be the most efficient psychological technique in the management of pain, and it can double the effectiveness of treatments for obesity. Nevertheless, many clinicians are reluctant to use hypnosis in their practices. We hope that this book will contribute to reversing that reluctance.

The reluctance to use hypnosis has its roots in history. In particular, it is related to misperceptions of hypnosis as an arcane and esoteric practice associated with magic, mysticism, and myth. At times, these unfortunate and inaccurate conclusions have been strengthened by irresponsible claims by proponents. However, modern research and theory paint a very different picture. Hypnotic phenomena are normal human processes, governed by the same psychological factors that shape nonhypnotic experience and behavior.

The techniques and procedures described in this book are based on sound clinical and laboratory research. Many are empirically derived and well validated. Many can also be used without formal induction or mention of hypnosis, and this method may be indicated for patients whose apprehensions about hypnosis render them poor candidates for hypnotic treatment. The clinician, however, should not share those unwarranted apprehensions. Though the idea of hypnosis may be an obstacle to treatment for a minority of patients, it can significantly enhance treatment for most.

Between us, we have practiced and researched hypnosis for 50 years. And yet, our curiosity is not satisfied. We are as fascinated with hypnosis as we were when we witnessed our first demonstration of hypnotic procedures many years ago. We hope we have succeeded in sharing our enthusiasm for the value of using hypnosis in the context of evidence-based principles and practices, and in whetting your appetite for learning more about the questions and controversies we have presented for your consideration.

REFERENCES

Abramson, L. Y., Seligman, M. E. P., & Teasdale, J. (1978). Learned helplessness in humans: Critique and reformulation. *Journal of Abnormal Psychology, 87*, 49–74.

Agras, W. S., Walsh, B. T., Fairburn, C. G., Wilson, G. T., & Kraemer, H. C. (2000). A multicenter comparison of cognitive–behavioral therapy and interpersonal psychotherapy for bulimia nervosa. *Archives of General Psychiatry, 57*, 459–466.

Alden, P. (1995). Back to the past: Introducing the bubble. *Contemporary Hypnosis, 12*, 59–67.

American Medical Association, Council on Scientific Affairs. (1994). *Memories of childhood abuse* (CSA Report 5-A-94). Chicago: Author.

American Psychiatric Association. (1980). *Diagnostic and statistical manual of mental disorders* (3rd ed.). Washington, DC: Author.

American Psychiatric Association. (1994). *Diagnostic and statistical manual of mental disorders* (4th ed.). Washington, DC: Author.

American Psychiatric Association. (2000). *Practice guideline for the treatment of clients with eating disorders (Revision)*. Washington, DC: Author.

American Psychological Association, Division 17 Committee on Women, Division 42 Trauma and Gender Issues Committee. (1995, July 25). *Psychotherapy guidelines for working with clients who may have an abuse or trauma history*. Washington, DC: Author.

American Psychological Association, Division 30. (2004, Winter/Spring). Hypnosis: A definition. *Psychological Hypnosis: A Bulletin of Division, 30*, 13.

Andersen, A. E. (1995). Eating disorders in males. In K. D. Brownell & C. G. Fairburn (Eds.), *Eating disorders and obesity: A comprehensive handbook* (pp. 177–187). New York, NY: Guilford Press.

Anderson, J. A., Basker, M. A., & Dalton, R. (1975). Migraine and hypnotherapy. *International Journal of Clinical and Experimental Hypnosis, 23*, 48–58.

Andreychuk, T., & Skriver, C. (1975). Hypnosis and biofeedback in the treatment of migraine headache. *International Journal of Clinical and Experimental Hypnosis, 23*, 172–183.

Anonymous. (1996). Integration of behavioral and relaxation approaches into the treatment of chronic pain and insomnia. NIH technology assessment panel on integration of behavioral and relaxation approaches into the treatment of chronic pain and insomnia. *Journal of the American Medical Association, 275*, 887–891.

Baer, R. A. (2003). Mindfulness training as a clinical intervention: A conceptual and empirical review. *Clinical Psychology: Science and Practice, 10*, 125–143.

Baker, E. (1981). An hypnotherapeutic approach to enhance object relatedness in psychotic patients. *International Journal of Clinical and Experimental Hypnosis, 24,* 136–147.

Baker, E. (1987). The state of the art of clinical hypnosis. *International Journal of Clinical and Experimental Hypnosis, 35,* 203–214.

Baker, S. L., & Kirsch, I. (1993). Hypnotic and placebo analgesia: Order effects and the placebo label. *Contemporary Hypnosis, 10,* 117–126.

Ballenger, J. C. (1997). Panic disorder in the medical setting. *Journal of Clinical Psychiatry, 58,* 13–17.

Bányai, É. I. (1991). Toward a social–psychobiological model of hypnosis. In S. J. Lynn & J. W. Rhue (Eds.), *Theories of hypnosis: Current models and perspectives* (pp. 564–598). New York: Guilford Press.

Bányai, É. I., & Hilgard, E. R. (1976). A comparison of active-alert hypnotic induction with traditional relaxation induction. *Journal of Abnormal Psychology, 85,* 218–224.

Barabasz, A. F., Baer, L., Sheehan, D., & Barabasz, M. (1986). A three-year follow-up of hypnosis and restricted environmental stimulation therapy for smoking. *International Journal of Clinical and Experimental Hypnosis, 24,* 169–181.

Barabasz, M. (2000). Hypnosis in the treatment of eating disorders. In L. M. Hornyak & J. P. Green (Eds.), *Healing from within: The use of hypnosis in women's health care* (pp. 233–254). Washington, DC: American Psychological Association.

Barber, J. (1977). Rapid induction analgesia: A clinical report. *American Journal of Clinical Hypnosis, 19,* 138–147.

Barber, J. (1989). Predicting the efficacy of hypnotic treatment. *American Journal of Clinical Hypnosis, 32,* 10–11.

Barber, T. X. (1969). *Hypnosis: A scientific approach.* New York: Van Nostrand Reinhold.

Barber, T. X. (1985). Hypnosuggestive procedures as catalysts for psychotherapies. In S. J. Lynn & J. P. Garske (Eds.), *Contemporary psychotherapies: Models and methods* (pp. 333–376). Columbus, OH: Charles E. Merrill.

Barber, T. X. (1999). A comprehensive three-dimensional theory of hypnosis. In I. Kirsch, E. Cardena, & S. Amigo (Eds.), *Clinical hypnosis and self-regulation: Cognitive–behavioral perspectives* (pp. 21–48). Washington, DC: American Psychological Association.

Barber, T. X., & Calverley, D. S. (1964). Toward a theory of "hypnotic" behavior: Effects on suggestibility of defining response to suggestion as easy. *Journal of Abnormal and Social Psychology, 68,* 585–592.

Barber, T. X., Spanos, N. P., & Chaves, J. F. (1974). *Hypnosis, imagination, and human potentialities.* New York: Pergamon Press.

Barkley, R. A., Hastings, J. E., & Jackson, T. L. (1977). The effects of rapid smoking and hypnosis in the treatment of smoking behavior. *International Journal of Clinical and Experimental Hypnosis, 25,* 7–17.

Barlow, D. H. (2002). *Anxiety and its disorders. The nature and treatment of anxiety and panic.* New York: Guilford Press.

Basker, M. A. (1985). Hypnosis in the alleviation of the smoking habit. In D. Waxman, P. C. Misra, M. Gibson, & M. Basker (Eds.), *Modern trends in hypnosis* (pp. 269–276). New York: Plenum Press.

Bates, B. L. (1993). Individual differences in response to hypnosis. In J. Rhue, S. Lynn, & I. Kirsch (Eds.), *Handbook of clinical hypnosis* (pp. 23–54). Washington, DC: American Psychological Association.

Baum, A., Cohen, L., & Hall, M. (1993). Control and intrusive memories as possible determinants of chronic stress. *Psychosomatic Medicine, 55,* 274–286.

Beck, A. T. (1964). Thinking and depression: II. Theory and therapy. *Archives of General Psychiatry, 10,* 561–571.

Beck, A. T. (1976). *Cognitive therapy and the emotional disorders.* New York: International Universities Press.

Beck, A. T., Rush, A. J., Shaw, B. F., & Emery, G. (1979). *Cognitive therapy for depression: A treatment manual.* New York: Guilford Press.

Beck, A. T., Steer, R. A., & Garbin, M. G. (1988). Psychometric properties of the Beck Depression Inventory: Twenty-five years of evaluation. *Clinical Psychology Review, 8,* 77–100.

Beck, J. S. (1995). *Cognitive therapy: Basics and beyond.* New York: Guilford Press.

Beecher, H. K. (1955). The powerful placebo. *Journal of the American Medical Association, 159,* 1602–1606.

Benivieni, A. (1954). *De abditis nonnullis ac mirandis morborum et sanationumcausis.* [On the hidden and marvelous causes of disease and healing]. Springfield, IL: Thomas.

Ben-Zvi, Z., Spohn, W. A., Young, S. H., & Kattan, M. (1982). Hypnosis for exercise-induced asthma. *American Review of Respiratory Disease, 125,* 392–395

Bernheim, H. (1887). *Suggestive therapeutics: A treatise on the nature and uses of hypnotism* (C. A. Herter, Trans.). Westport, CT: Associated Booksellers. (Original work published 1886)

Bikel, O. (Producer). (1995). *Divided memories* [Television series episode]. *Frontline.* Washington, DC: Public Broadcasting Service.

Binet, A. (1892). *Alterations of the personality.* Paris: Felix Alcan.

Binet, A., & Féré, C. (1888). *Animal magnetism.* New York: Appleton.

Black, D. R., Coe, W. C., Friesen, J. G., & Wurzmann, A. G. (1984). Minimal interventions for weight control: A cost-effective alternative. *Journal of Addictive Behaviors, 9,* 279–285.

Blankfield, R. P. (1991). Suggestion, relaxation, and hypnosis as adjuncts in the care of surgery patients: A review of the literature. *American Journal of Clinical Hypnosis, 33,* 1782–1786.

Bliss, E. L. (1984). Hysteria and hypnosis. *Journal of Nervous and Mental Disease, 172,* 203–206.

Bohart, A. C., Elliott, R., Greenberg, L. S., & Watson, J. C. (2002). Empathy. In J. Norcross (Ed.), *Psychotherapy relationships that work: Therapist contributions and responsiveness to patients* (pp. 89–108). London: Oxford University Press.

Bolocofsky, D. N., Spinler, D., & Coulthard-Morris, L. (1985). Effectiveness of hypnosis as an adjunct to behavioral weight management. *Journal of Clinical Psychology, 41,* 35–41.

Borkovec, T. D. (1999, March). *New developments in the treatment of worry.* Paper presented at the advanced practice symposium at the national conference of the Anxiety Disorders Association of America, San Diego, CA.

Borkovec, T. D. (2002). Life in the future versus life in the present. *Clinical Psychology: Science and Practice, 9,* 76–80.

Borkovec, T. D., & Newman, M. G. (1998). Worry and generalized anxiety disorder. In P. Salkovskis, A. S. Bellack, & M. Hersen (Eds.), *Comprehensive clinical psychology: Vol. 6. Adults: Clinical formulation and treatment* (pp. 439–459). New York: Pergamon Press.

Borkovec, T. D., & Wishman, M. A. (1996). Psychosocial treatment of generalized anxiety disorder. In M. Mavissakalian & R. Prien (Eds), *Long-term treatments of anxiety disorders* (pp. 171–199). Washington, DC: American Psychiatric Press.

Bowers, K. S., & Davidson, T. M. (1991). A neodissociative critique of Spanos's social–psychological model of hypnosis. In S. J. Lynn & J. W. Rhue (Eds.), *Theories of hypnosis: Current models and perspectives* (pp. 105–143). New York: Guilford Press.

Braffman, W., & Kirsch, I. (1999). Imaginative suggestibility and hypnotizability: An empirical analysis. *Journal of Personality and Social Psychology, 77,* 578–587.

Braid, J. (1843). *Neurypnology, or the rationale of nervous sleep considered in relation with animal magnetism.* London: Churchill.

Bremner, J. D., Randall, P. K., Southwick, S. M., Krystal, J. H., Ignis, R. B., & Charney, D. S. (1995). Stress-induced changes in memory and development. *American Psychiatric Association and Syllabus Proceedings Summary, 148,* 112.

Brom, D., Kleber, R. J., & Defare, P. B. (1989). Brief psychotherapy for post-traumatic stress disorder. *Journal of Consulting and Clinical Psychology, 87,* 607–612.

Brown, D. P. (1992, October). *The bubble induction.* Handout and technique demonstrated at the Workshop of Acute and Chronic Pain, SCEH Annual Scientific Meeting, Washington, DC.

Brown, D. P., & Fromm, E. (1986). *Hypnotherapy and hypnoanalysis.* Hillsdale, NJ: Erlbaum.

Brown, D. P., Scheflin, A. W., & Hammond, D. C. (1998). *Memory, trauma treatment, and the law.* New York: Norton.

Brown, P. (1993). Hypnosis and metaphor. In J. W. Rhue, S. J. Lynn, & I. Kirsch (Eds.), *Handbook of clinical hypnosis* (pp. 291–308). Washington, DC: American Psychological Association.

Brown, T. A., DiNardo, P., & Barlow, D. H. (1994). *Anxiety Disorders Interview Schedule for DSM–IV*. San Antonio, TX: Psychological Corporation.

Camatte, R., Gerolami, A., & Sarles, H. (1969). Comparative study of the action of different treatments and placebos on pain crises of gastro-duodenal ulcers. *Clinica Terapeutica, 49,* 411–419.

Canadian Psychiatric Association. (1996). Position statement: Adult recovered memories of childhood sexual abuse. *Canadian Journal of Psychiatry, 41,* 305–306.

Cancer doctors urge focused war against tobacco. (2003, May 31). *Yahoo News.* Retrieved August 23, 2005, from http://62.149.229.227/forcesarc/10f1/money-mouth.htm

Cardena, E. (2000). Hypnosis in the treatment of trauma: A promising, but not fully supported, efficacious intervention. *International Journal of Clinical and Experimental Hypnosis, 48,* 225–238.

Cardena, E., Maldonado, J., van der Hart, O., & Spiegel, D. (2000). Hypnosis. In E. B. Foa, T. M. Keane, & M. J. Friedman (Eds.), *Effective treatments for PTSD* (pp. 247–279). New York: Guilford Press.

Chambless, D. L., & Hollon, S. D. (1998). Defining empirically supported therapies. *Journal of Consulting and Clinical Psychology, 66,* 7–18.

Chambless, D. L., & Ollendick, T. H. (2001). Empirically supported psychological interventions: Controversies and evidence. *Annual Review of Psychology, 52,* 685–716.

Charcot, J. M. (1889). *Clinical lectures on the diseases of the nervous system: Vol. 3.* London: New Sydenham Society.

Chaves, J. F. (1989). Hypnotic control of clinical pain. In N. P. Spanos & J. F. Chaves (Eds.), *Hypnosis: The cognitive–behavioral perspective* (pp. 242–272). Buffalo, NY: Prometheus Books.

Chaves, J. F. (1993). Hypnosis in pain management. In J. W. Rhue & S. J. Lynn (Eds.), *Handbook of clinical hypnosis* (pp. 511–532). Washington, DC: American Psychological Association.

Chaves, J. F. (1997a). The state of the "state" debate in hypnosis: A view from the cognitive–behavioral perspective. *International Journal of Clinical and Experimental Hypnosis, 45,* 251–265.

Chaves, J. F. (1997b). Hypnosis in dentistry: Historical overview and critical appraisal. *Hypnosis International Monographs, 3,* 5–23.

Chaves, J. F. (2000). Hypnosis in the management of anxiety associated with medical conditions and their treatment In D. I. Mostofsky & D. H. Barlow (Eds.), *The management of stress and anxiety in medical disorders* (pp. 119–142). Needham Heights, MA: Allyn & Bacon.

Chaves, J. F., & Barber, T. X. (1976). Hypnotic procedures and surgery. A critical analysis with applications to "acupuncture analgesia." *American Journal of Clinical Hypnosis, 8,* 217–236.

Chaves, J. F., & Brown, J. (1987). Spontaneous cognitive strategies for the control of clinical pain and stress. *Journal of Behavioral Medicine, 10,* 263–275.

Clarke, J. J. (1996). Teaching clinical hypnosis in U.S. and Canadian dental schools. *American Journal of Clinical Hypnosis, 39,* 89–92.

Coe, W. C., & Ryken, K. (1979). Hypnosis and risks to human subjects. *American Psychologist, 34,* 673–681.

Coe, W. C., & Sarbin, T. R. (1991). Role theory: Hypnosis from a dramaturgical and narrational perspective. In S. J. Lynn & J. W. Rhue (Eds.), *Theories of hypnosis: Current models and perspectives* (pp. 303–323). New York: Guilford Press.

Cohen, S. B. (1989). Clinical uses of measures of hypnotizability. *American Journal of Clinical Hypnosis, 32,* 4–9.

Coker, S., Vize, C., Wade, T., & Cooper, P. J. (1993). Patients with bulimia nervosa who fail to engage in cognitive behavior therapy. *International Journal of Eating Disorders, 13,* 35–40.

Colletti, G., Supnick, J. A., & Payne, T. J. (1985). The smoking self-efficacy questionnaire (SSEQ): Preliminary scale development and validation. *Behavioral Assessment, 7,* 249–260.

Comey, G., & Kirsch, I. (1999). Intentional and spontaneous imagery in hypnosis: The phenomenology of hypnotic responding. *International Journal of Clinical and Experimental Hypnosis, 47,* 65–85.

Cooley, E., & LaJoy, R. (1980). Therapeutic relationship and improvement as seen by clients and therapists. *Journal of Clinical Psychology, 36,* 562–570.

Cooper, M. J., & Fairburn, C. (1987). The Eating Disorders Examination: A semi-structured interview for the specific pathology of eating disorders. *International Journal of Eating Disorders, 6,* 1–8.

Cooper, M. J., Todd, G., & Wells, A. (2000). *Bulimia nervosa: A cognitive therapy program for clients.* London: Jessica Kingsley.

Covino, N. P., Jimerson, D. C., Wolfe, E., Franko, D. L., & Frankel, F. H. (1994). Hypnotizability, dissociation, and bulimia nervosa. *Journal of Abnormal Psychology, 103,* 455–459.

Craighead, L. W. (2002). Obesity and eating disorders. In M. M. Antony & D. H. Barlow (Eds.), *Handbook of assessment and treatment planning for psychological disorders* (pp. 300–340). New York: Guilford Press.

Craighead, W. E. (2002). Psychosocial treatments for major depressive disorder. In P. E. Nathan & J. E. Gorman (Eds.), *A guide to treatments that work* (2nd ed., pp. 245–262). New York: Oxford.

Crasilneck, H., & Hall, J. (1975). *Clinical hypnosis.* New York: Grune & Stratton.

Crawford, H. J., Hilgard, J. R., & MacDonald, H. (1982). Transient experiences following hypnotic testing and special termination procedures. *International Journal of Clinical and Experimental Hypnosis, 30,* 117–126.

Davidson, L. M., & Baum, A. (1993). Predictors of chronic stress among Vietnam veterans: Stressor exposure and intrusive recall. *Journal of Traumatic Stress, 6,* 195–202.

Deacon, B. J., & Abramowitz, J. S. (2004). Cognitive and behavioral treatments for anxiety disorders: A review of meta-analytic findings. *Journal of Clinical Psychology, 60,* 429–444.

Dean, E. T. (1998). *Shook-over hell: Posttraumatic stress, Vietnam, and the Civil War.* Cambridge, MA: Harvard University Press.

de Shazer, S. (1985). *Keys to solution in brief therapy.* New York: Norton.

Devine, D. A., & Fernald, P. S. (1973). Outcome effects of receiving a preferred, randomly assigned, or nonpreferred therapy. *Journal of Consulting & Clinical Psychology, 41,* 104–107.

Diamond, M. J. (1989). Is hypnotherapy art or science? *American Journal of Clinical Hypnosis, 32,* 11–12.

Dillard, J. (1991). The current status of research on sequential-request compliance techniques. *Personality and Social Psychology Bulletin, 17,* 283–288.

Dixon, M., & Laurence, J. (1992). Two hundred years of hypnosis research: Questions resolved? Questions unanswered! In E. Fromm & M. Nash (Eds.), *Contemporary hypnosis research* (pp. 34–66). New York: Guilford Press.

DuBreuil, S., & Spanos, N. P. (1993). Psychological treatment of warts. In J. W. Rhue, S. J. Lynn, & I. Kirsch (Eds.), *Handbook of clinical hypnosis* (pp. 623–648). Washington, DC: American Psychological Association.

Edmonston, W. E. (1981). *Hypnosis and relaxation: Modern verification of an old equation.* New York: Wiley.

Edmonston, W. E. (1991). Anesis. In S. J. Lynn & J. W. Rhue (Eds.), *Theories of hypnosis: Current models and perspectives* (pp. 197–240). New York: Guilford Press.

Edwards, S. D., & van der Spuy, H. (1985). Hypnotherapy as a treatment for enuresis. *Journal of Child Clinical Psychology, Psychiatry and Allied Health Disciplines, 26,* 161–170.

Ellenberger, H. F. (1970). *The discovery of the unconscious.* New York: Basic Books.

Ellis, A. (1962). *Reason and emotion in psychotherapy.* Secaucus, NJ: Lyle Stuart.

Ellis, A., & Dryden, W. (1997). *The practice of rational–emotive behavior therapy* (2nd ed.). Secaucus, NJ: Birscj Lane.

Enqvist, B., Bjorklund, C., Engman, M., & Jakobsson, J. (1997). Preoperative hypnosis reduces postoperative vomiting after surgery of the breasts. A prospective, randomized and blinded study. *Acta Anaesthiologica Scandinavica, 41,* 1028–1032.

Enqvist, B., von Konow, L., & Bystedt, H. (1995). Pre- and perioperative suggestion in maxillofacial surgery: Effects on blood loss and recovery. *International Journal of Clinical and Experimental Hypnosis, 43,* 284–294.

Erdelyi, M. (1994). Hypnotic hypermnesia: The empty set of hypermnesia. *International Journal of Clinical and Experimental Hypnosis, 42,* 379–390.

Erickson, M. H., Rossi, E. L., & Rossi, S. I. (1976). *Hypnotic realities: The induction of clinical hypnosis and forms of indirect suggestion.* New York: Irvington.

Ewer, T. C., & Stewart, D. E. (1986). Improvement in bronchial hyper-responsiveness in patients with moderate asthma after treatment with a hypnotic technique: a randomised controlled trial. *British Medical Journal (Clinical Research)*, *293*, 1129–1132.

Fairburn, C. G. (1985). Cognitive–behavioral treatment for bulimia. In D. M. Garner & P. E. Garfinkel (Eds.), *Handbook of treatment for eating disorders* (pp. 160–192). New York: Guilford Press.

Fairburn, C. G. (1997). Interpersonal psychotherapy for bulimia nervosa. In D. M. Garner & P. E. Garfinkel (Eds.), *Handbook of treatment for eating disorders* (2nd ed., pp. 278–294). New York: Guilford Press.

Fairburn, C. G., & Beglin, S. J. (1990). Studies of the epidemiology of bulimia nervosa. *American Journal of Psychiatry*, *147*, 401–408.

Fairburn, C. G., Jones, R., Peveler, R. C., Hope, R. A., & O'Connor, M. (1993). Psychotherapy and bulimia nervosa: The longer-term effects of interpersonal psychotherapy, behavior therapy, and cognitive behavior therapy. *Archives of General Psychiatry*, *50*, 419–428.

Fairburn, C. G., Marcus, M. D., & Wilson, G. T. (1993). Cognitive behavior therapy for binge eating and bulimia nervosa: A comprehensive treatment manual. In C. G. Fairburn & G. T. Wilson (Eds.), *Binge eating: Nature, assessment, and treatment* (pp. 361–404). New York: Guilford Press.

Fairburn, C. G., Norman, P. A., Welch, S. L., O'Connor, M. E., Doll, H. A., & Peveler, R. C. (1995). A prospective study of outcome in bulimia nervosa and the long-term effects of three psychological treatments. *Archives of General Psychiatry*, *52*, 304–312.

Fairburn, C. G., & Wilson, T. (1993). *Binge eating: Nature and assessment*. London: Guilford Press.

Farvolden, P., & Woody, E. Z. (2004). Hypnosis, memory, and frontal executive functioning. *International Journal of Clinical and Experimental Hypnosis*, *52*, 3–26.

Faymonville, M. E., Laureys, S., Degueldre, C., Del Fiore, G., Luxen, A., Franck, G., et al. (2000). Neural mechanisms of antinociceptive effects of hypnosis. *Anesthesiology*, *92*, 1257–1265.

Faymonville, M. E., Mambourg, P. H., Joris, J., Vrijens, B., Fissette, J., Albert, A., & Lamy, M. (1997). Psychological approaches during conscious sedation. Hypnosis versus stress reducing strategies: A prospective randomized study. *Pain*, *73*, 361–367.

Federoff, I. C., & Taylor, S. (2001). Psychological and pharmacological treatments of social phobia: A meta-analysis. *Journal of Clinical Psychopharmacology*, *21*, 311–324.

Fellows, B. J. (1995). Critical issues arising from the APA definition and description of hypnosis. *Contemporary Hypnosis*, *12*, 74–81.

Feske, U., & Chambless, D. L. (1995). Cognitive–behavioral versus exposure only treatment for social phobia: A meta-analysis. *Behavior Therapy*, *26*, 695–720.

Finkelstein, S. (2003). Rapid hypnotic inductions and therapeutic suggestions in the dental setting. *International Journal of Clinical and Experimental Hypnosis*, *51*, 77–85.

First, M. B., Spitzer, R. L., Gibbon, M., & Williams, J. B. W. (1996). *User's guide for the Structured Clinical Interview for DSM–IV Axis I Disorders: SCI–1 Clinical Version*. Washington, DC: American Psychiatric Association.

Fish, J. M. (1996). Prevention, solution focused therapy, and the illusion of mental disorders. *Applied and Preventive Psychology*, *5*, 37–40.

Foa, E., & Kozak, M. J. (1986). Emotional processing of fear: Exposure to corrective information. *Psychological Bulletin*, *99*, 20–35.

Foa, E., & Rothbaum, B. O. (1998). *Treating the trauma of rape: Cognitive–behavioral therapy for PTSD*. New York: Guilford Press.

Foa, E., Steketee, G., & Rothbaum, B. O. (1989). Behavioral/cognitive conceptualizations of post-traumatic stress disorder. *Behavior Therapy*, *20*, 155–176.

Frankel, F. H. (1994). Dissociation in hysteria and hypnosis: A concept aggrandized. In S. J. Lynn & J. W. Rhue (Eds.), *Theories of hypnosis: Current models and perspectives* (pp. 80–93). New York: Guilford Press.

Frankel, F. H., & Orne, M. T. (1976). Hypnotizability and phobic behavior. *Archives of General Psychiatry*, *33*, 1259–1261.

Franklin, B., Majault, S., LeRoy, J. B., Sallin, B., Bailly, J. S., D'Arcet, J., et al. (1970). Report on animal magnetism. In M. M. Tinterow (Ed.), *Foundations of hypnosis: From Mesmer to Freud* (pp. 82–128). Springfield, IL: Charles C. Thomas. (Original work published 1785)

Frauman, D., & Lynn, S. J. (1985). Rapport factors in hypnosis: A literature review. In G. Guantieri (Ed.), *Hypnosis in psychotherapy and psychosomatic medicine*. Verona, Italy: Post-Universitarie Verona.

Frauman, D., Lynn, S. J., Hardaway, R., & Molteni, A. (1984). Effects of subliminal symbiotic activation on hypnotic rapport and susceptibility. *Journal of Abnormal Psychology*, *93*, 481–483.

Freud, S. (1961). The unconscious. In J. Strachey (Ed. & Trans.), *The standard edition of the complete psychological works of Sigmund Freud* (Vol. 14, pp. 166–204). London: Hogarth Press. (Original work published 1915)

Fried, R. L. (1999). *Breathe well, be well: A program to relieve stress, anxiety, asthma, hypertension, migraine, and other disorders for better health*. New York: Wiley.

Friedman, H., & Taub, H. A. (1984). Brief psychological training procedures in migraine treatment. *American Journal of Clinical Hypnosis*, *26*, 187–200.

Friedman, M. A., & Wishman, M. A. (1998). Sociotrophy, autonomy, and bulimic symptomatology. *International Journal of Eating Disorders*, *23*, 439–442.

Friedman, M. J., Davidson, J. R., Mellman, T. A., & Southwick, S. M. (2000). Pharmacotherapy. In E. B. Foa, T. M. Keane, & M. J. Friedman (Eds.), *Effective treatments for PTSD* (pp. 84–105). New York: Guilford Press.

Fromm, E. (1979). The nature of hypnosis and other altered states of consciousness: An ego–psychological theory. In E. Fromm & R. Shor (Eds.), *Hypnosis: Developments in research and new perspectives* (2nd ed., pp. 81–103). Chicago: Aldine.

Fromm, E., & Nash, M. R. (1992). *Contemporary hypnosis research.* New York: Guilford Press.

Fromm, E., & Nash, M. R. (1997). *Mental Health Library Series: No. 5. Hypnosis and psychoanalysis.* Guilford, CT: International Universities Press.

Garner, D. M. (1991). *Eating Disorder Inventory—2 professional manual.* Odessa, FL: Psychological Assessment Resources.

Garner, D. M., & Bemis, K. M. (1982). A cognitive–behavioral approach to anorexia nervosa. *Cognitive Therapy and Research, 6,* 123–150.

Garner, D. M., & Garfinkel, P. E. (1979). The Eating Attitudes Test: An index of the symptoms of anorexia nervosa. *Psychological Medicine, 9,* 273–279.

Garry, M., & Polaschek, D. L. L. (2000). Imagination and memory. *Current Directions in Psychological Science, 9,* 6–10.

Garske, J. P. (1991). Clinical hypnosis and anorexia nervosa: Is therapeutic convergence feasible? *Contemporary Hypnosis, 8,* 86–94.

Gauld, A. (1996). *A history of hypnotism.* Cambridge, England: Cambridge University Press.

Geisser, M. E., Roth, R. S., Bachman, J. E., & Eckert, T. A. (1996). The relationship between symptoms of post-traumatic stress disorder and pain, affective disturbance and disability among patients with accident and non-accident related pain. *Pain, 66,* 207–214.

Gelfand, S., Ullman, L. P., & Krasner, L. (1963). The placebo response: An experimental approach. *Journal of Nervous and Mental Disease, 136,* 379–387.

Gevertz, L. (1996). Mirror, mirror, on the wall. *Contemporary Hypnosis, 13,* 80–83.

Gfeller, J. D. (1993). Enhancing hypnotizability and treatment responsiveness. In J. W. Rhue, S. J. Lynn, & I. Kirsch (Eds.), *Handbook of clinical hypnosis* (pp. 235–250). Washington, DC: American Psychological Association.

Gfeller, J., Lynn, S. J., & Pribble, W. (1987). Enhancing hypnotic susceptibility: Interpersonal and rapport factors. *Journal of Personality and Social Psychology, 52,* 586–595.

Gill, M. M., & Brenman, M. (1959). *Hypnosis and related states: Psychoanalytic studies in regression.* New York: International Universities Press.

Gillett, P., & Coe, W. C. (1984). The effects of rapid induction analgesia (RIA), hypnotic susceptibility and the severity of discomfort on reducing dental pain. *American Journal of Clinical Hypnosis, 27,* 81–90.

Goldstein, A. J., & Chambless, D. L. (1978). A reanalysis of agoraphobia. *Behavior Therapy, 9,* 47–59.

Gonsalkorale, W., Miller, V., Afzal, A., & Whorwell, P. J. (2003). Long-term benefits of hypnotherapy for irritable bowel syndrome. *Gut, 52,* 1623–1629.

Gorassini, D. R., & Spanos, N. P. (1986). A social–cognitive skills approach to the successful modification of hypnotic susceptibility. *Journal of Personality and Social Psychology, 50*, 1004–1012.

Gorassini, D. R., & Spanos, N. P. (1999). The Carleton Skill Training Program. In I. Kirsch, A. Capafons, E. Cardeña, & S. Amigó (Eds.), *Clinical hypnosis and self-regulation: Cognitive–behavioral perspectives* (pp. 141–177). Washington, DC: American Psychological Association.

Gould, R. A., Buckminster, S., Pollack, M. H., Otto, M. W., & Yap, L. (1997). Cognitive–behavioral and pharmacological treatment for social phobia: A meta-analysis. *Clinical Psychology Review, 8*, 819–844.

Gould, R. A., Otto, M. W., Pollack, M. H., & Yap, L. (1977). Cognitive–behavioral and pharmacological treatment of generalized anxiety disorder: A preliminary meta-analysis. *Behavior Therapy, 28*, 285–305.

Gravitz, M. A. (1991). Early theories of hypnosis: A clinical perspective. In S. J. Lynn & J. W. Rhue (Eds.), *Theories of hypnosis: Current models and perspectives* (pp. 19–42). New York: Guilford Press.

Green, J. P. (1996). Cognitive–behavioral hypnotherapy for smoking cessation: A case study in a group setting. In S. J. Lynn, I. Kirsch, & J. W. Rhue (Eds.), *Casebook of clinical hypnosis* (pp. 223–248). Washington, DC: American Psychological Association.

Green, J. P. (2000). Treating women who smoke: The benefits of using hypnosis. In L. Hornyak & J. P. Green (Eds.), *Healing from within: The use of hypnosis in women's health care* (pp. 91–118). Washington, DC: American Psychological Association.

Green, J. P., Barabasz, A., Barrett, D., & Montgomery, G. H. (2005). Forging ahead: The 2003 APA Division 30 definition of hypnosis. *International Journal of Clinical and Experimental Hypnosis, 53*, 259–264.

Green, J. P., & Lynn, S. J. (2000). Hypnosis and suggestion-based approaches to smoking cessation: An examination of the evidence. *International Journal of Clinical and Experimental Hypnosis, 48*, 195–224.

Green, J. P., Lynn, S. J., Weekes, J. R., Carlson, B., Brentar, J., Latham, L., & Kurzhals, R. (1990). Literalism as a marker of hypnotic "trance": Disconfirming evidence. *Journal of Abnormal Psychology, 99*, 16–21.

Greenwald, A. G., Draine, S. C., & Abrams, R. L. (1996, September 20). Three cognitive markers of unconscious semantic activation. *Science, 273*, 1699–1702.

Griffiths, R. A. (1984). Hypnosis in the treatment of bulimia nervosa: A case study. *Australian Journal of Clinical and Experimental Hypnosis, 12*, 105–112.

Griffiths, R. A. (1989). Hypnobehavioral treatment for bulimia nervosa: Preliminary findings. *Australian Journal of Clinical and Experimental Hypnosis, 17*(1), 79–87.

Griffiths, R. A. (1995). Hypnobehavioral treatment for bulimia nervosa: A treatment manual. *Australian Journal of Clinical and Experimental Hypnosis, 23*, 25–40.

Griffiths, R. A. (1997). Hypnosis as an adjunct in the treatment of bulimia nervosa. In B. J. Evans, G. J. Coman, & G. D. Burrows (Eds.), *Hypnosis for weight management and eating disorders* (pp. 164–178). Victoria, Australia: The Australian Journal of Clinical and Experimental Hypnosis.

Griffiths, R. A., & Channon-Little, L. (1993). The hypnotizability of patients with bulimia nervosa and partial syndromes participating in a controlled treatment outcome study. *Contemporary Hypnosis, 10,* 81–87.

Gross, M. (1983). Hypnosis in the therapy of anorexia hysteria. *American Journal of Clinical Hypnosis, 14,* 1–8.

Gruzelier, J. (1996). The state of hypnosis: Evidence and applications. *Quarterly Journal of Medicine, 89,* 313–317.

Haanen, H. C., Hoenderdos, H. T., van Romunde, L. K., Hop, W. C., Mallee, C., Terwiel, J. P., & Hekster, G. B. (1991). Controlled trial of hypnotherapy in the treatment of refractory fibromyalgia. *Journal of Rheumatology, 18,* 72–75.

Hammond, D. C. (1990). *Handbook of hypnotic suggestions and metaphors.* New York: Norton.

Hammond, D. C. (1992). *Manual for self-hypnosis.* Des Plaines, IL: American Society of Clinical Hypnosis.

Hammond, D. C., Garver, R. B., Mutter, C. B., Crasilneck, H. B., Frischolz, E., Gravitz, M. A., et al. (1995). *Clinical hypnosis and memory: Guidelines for clinicians and for forensic hypnosis.* Des Plaines, IL: American Society of Clinical Hypnosis.

Harmon, T. M., Hynan, M. T., & Tyre, T. E. (1990). Improved obstetric outcomes using hypnotic analgesia and skill mastery combined with childbirth education. *Journal of Consulting and Clinical Psychology, 58,* 525–530.

Hasegawa, H., & Jamieson, G. A. (2002). Conceptual issues in hypnosis research: Explanations, definitions and the state/non-state debate. *Contemporary Hypnosis, 19,* 103–117.

Haxby, D. G. (1995). Treatment of nicotine dependence. *American Journal of Health-System Pharmacy, 52,* 265–281.

Hayes, S. C. (2002). Buddhism and acceptance and commitment therapy. *Cognitive and Behavioral Practice, 9,* 58–66.

Hayes, S. C., & Gifford, E. V. (1997). The trouble with language: Experiential avoidance, rules, and the nature of verbal events. *Psychological Science, 8,* 170–174.

Hayes, S. C., Strosahl, K., & Wilson, K. G. (1999). *Acceptance and commitment therapy.* New York: Guilford Press.

Healy, D. (2003). Lines of evidence on the risks of suicide with selective serotonin reuptake inhibitors. *Psychotherapy and Psychosomatics, 72*(2), 71–79.

Healy, D., & Whitaker, C. (2003). Antidepressants and suicide: Risk–benefit conundrums. *Journal of Psychiatry and Neuroscience, 28,* 331–337.

Heide, F. J., & Borkovec, T. D. (1983). Relaxation induced anxiety: Paradoxical anxiety enhancement due to relaxation training. *Journal of Consulting and Clinical Psychology, 51*, 171–182.

Heimberg, R. G., & Juster, H. R. (1995). Cognitive–behavioral treatments: Literature review. In R. G. Heimberg, M. R. Liebowitz, D. A. Hope, & F. R. Schneier (Eds.), *Social phobia. Diagnosis, assessment, and treatment* (pp. 261–309). New York: Guilford Press.

Henry, D. (1985). *Subjects' expectancies and subjective experience of hypnosis.* Unpublished doctoral dissertation, University of Connecticut, Storrs.

Hilgard, E. R. (1965). *Hypnotic susceptibility.* New York: Harcourt, Brace & World.

Hilgard, E. R. (1973). The domain of hypnosis: With some comments on alternate paradigms. *American Psychologist, 28*, 972–982.

Hilgard, E. R. (1977). *Divided consciousness: Multiple controls in human thought and action.* New York: Wiley.

Hilgard, E. R. (1986). *Divided consciousness: Multiple controls in human thought and action* (Expanded ed.). New York: Wiley.

Hilgard, E. R. (1991). A neodissociation interpretation of hypnosis. In S. J. Lynn & J. W. Rhue (Eds.), *Theories of hypnosis* (pp. 83–104). New York: Guilford Press.

Hilgard, E. R. (1994). Neodissociation theory. In S. J. Lynn & J. W. Rhue (Eds.), *Dissociation: Clinical, theoretical and research perspectives* (pp. 32–51). New York: Guilford Press.

Hilgard, E. R., Crawford, H. J., Bowers, K., & Kihlstrom, J. (1979). A tailored SHSS:C, permitting user modification for special purposes. *International Journal of Clinical and Experimental Hypnosis, 27*, 125–133.

Hoek, H. W. (1991). The incidence and prevalence of anorexia nervosa and bulimia nervosa in primary care. *Psychological Medicine, 21*, 455–460.

Hofbauer, R. K., Rainville, P., Duncan, G. H., & Bushnell, M. C. (2001). Cortical representation of the sensory dimension of pain. *Journal of Neurophysiology, 86*, 402–411.

Hollon, S. D., Shelton, R. C., & Loosen, P. T. (1991). Cognitive therapy and pharmacotherapy for depression. *Journal of Consulting and Clinical Psychology, 59*, 88–99.

Holroyd, J. D. (1980). Hypnosis treatment for smoking: An evaluation review. *International Journal of Clinical and Experimental Hypnosis, 4*, 241–357.

Holroyd, J. D. (1996). Hypnotic treatment of clinical pain: Understanding why hypnosis is useful. *International Journal of Clinical and Experimental Hypnosis, 44*, 33–51.

Hornyak, L. M. (1996). Hypnosis in the treatment of anorexia nervosa. In S. J. Lynn, I. Kirsch, & J. W. Rhue (Eds.), *Casebook of clinical hypnosis* (pp. 51–73). Washington, DC: American Psychological Association.

Horvath, A. O., & Bedi, R. P. (2002). The alliance. In J. C. Norcross (Ed.), *Psychotherapy relationships that work.* New York: Oxford University Press.

Hull, C. L. (1933). *Hypnosis and suggestibility: An experimental approach.* New York: Appleton-Century-Crofts.

Hunt, W., & Bespalec, D. (1974). An evaluation of current methods of modifying smoking behaviors. *Journal of Clinical Psychology, 30,* 431–438.

Hyman, I. E., Jr., Husband, T. H., & Billings, F. J. (1995). False memories of childhood experiences. *Applied Cognitive Psychology, 9,* 181–197.

Hyman, I. E., Jr., & Pentland, J. (1996). The role of mental imagery in the creation of false childhood memories. *Journal of Memory and Language, 35,* 101–117.

Institute of Medicine. (2004). *Improving medical education: Enhancing the behavioral and social science content of medical school.* Washington, DC: National Academies Press.

Jacka, B. T. (1997). Weight management: A cognitive–behavioral approach, using hypnosis as a treatment strategy. In B. J. Evans, G. J. Coman, & G. D. Burrows (Eds.), *Hypnosis for weight management and eating disorders* (pp. 104–113). Victoria, Australia: The Australian Journal of Clinical and Experimental Hypnosis.

Jacknow, D. S., Tschann, J. M., Link, M. P., & Boyce, W. T. (1994). Hypnosis in the prevention of chemotherapy-related nausea and vomiting in children: A prospective study. *Journal of Developmental and Behavioral Pediatrics, 15,* 258–264.

Janet, P. (1973). *L'automatisme psychologique* [Psychological automatism]. Paris: Societé Pierre Janet. (Original work published 1889)

Jeffrey, L. K., & Jeffrey, T. B. (1988). Exclusion therapy in smoking cessation. *International Journal of Clinical and Experimental Hypnosis, 37,* 70–74.

Jeffrey, T. B., Jeffrey, L. K., Grueling, J. W., & Gentry, W. R. (1985). Evaluation of a brief group treatment package including hypnotic induction for maintenance of smoking cessation: A brief communication. *International Journal of Clinical and Experimental Hypnosis, 33,* 95–98.

Johnston, E., & Donoghue, J. (1971). Hypnosis and smoking: A review of the literature. *American Journal of Clinical Hypnosis, 13,* 265–272.

Joiner, T. E., Heatherton, T. F., Rudd, M. D., & Schmidt, N. B. (1997). Perfectionism, perceived weight status, and bulimic symptoms: Two studies testing a diathesis stress model. *Journal of Abnormal Psychology, 106,* 145–153.

Jones, J. C., & Barlow, D. H. (1990). The etiology of posttraumatic stress disorder. *Clinical Psychology Review, 10,* 299–328.

Kabat-Zinn, J. (2003). Mindfulness-based interventions in context: Past, present, and future. *Clinical Psychology: Science and Practice, 10,* 144–156.

Kallio, S., & Revonsuo, A. (2003). Hypnotic phenomena and altered states of consciousness: A multilevel framework of description and explanation. *Contemporary Hypnosis, 20,* 111–164.

Kallio, S., Revonsuo, A., Hamalainen, H., Markela, J., & Gruzelier, J. (2001). Anterior brain functions and hypnosis: A test of the frontal hypothesis. *International Journal of Clinical and Experimental Hypnosis, 49,* 95–108.

Kanfer, F. H., & Grimm, L. G. (1978). Freedom of choice and behavioral change. *Journal of Consulting and Clinical Psychology, 46,* 873–878.

Keane, T. M., Solomon, S., & Maser, J. (1996, November). *NIMH–National Center for PTSD assessment standardization conference.* Paper presented at the 12th annual meeting of the International Society for Traumatic Stress Studies, San Francisco, CA.

Keefe, F. J., Brown, G. K., Wallston, K. A., & Caldwell, D. S. (1989). Coping with rheumatoid arthritis pain: Catastrophizing as a maladaptive strategy. *Pain, 37,* 51–56.

Keefe, F. J., Caldwell, D. S., Baucom, D., Salley, A., Robinson, E., Timmons, K., et al. (1999). Spouse-assisted coping skills training in the management of knee pain in osteoarthritis: Long-term followup results. *Arthritis Care and Research, 12*(2), 101–111.

Kessler, R. C., McGonagale, K. A., Zhao, S., Nelson, C. B., Hughes, M., Eshleman, S., et al. (1994). Lifetime and 12-month prevalence of DSM–III–R psychiatric disorders in the United States: Results from the National Comorbidity Survey. *Archives of General Psychiatry, 51,* 8–19.

Kessler, R., Sonnega, A., Bromet, E., Hughes, M., & Nelson, C. (1995). Post-traumatic stress disorder in the National Comorbidity Survey. *Archives of General Psychiatry, 52,* 1048–1060.

Kihlstrom, J. F. (1992). Hypnosis: A sesquicentennial essay. *International Journal of Clinical and Experimental Hypnosis, 50,* 301–314.

Kihlstrom, J. F. (1997). Convergence in understanding hypnosis? Perhaps, but perhaps not quite so fast. *International Journal of Clinical and Experimental Hypnosis, 45,* 324–332.

Kihlstrom, J. F. (1998a). Dissociations and dissociation theory in hypnosis: Comment on Kirsch and Lynn (1998). *Psychological Bulletin, 123,* 186–191.

Kihlstrom, J. F. (1998b). Hypnosis and the psychological unconscious. In H. J. Friedman (Ed.), *Encyclopedia of mental health* (Vol. 2, pp. 467–477). San Diego: Academic Press.

Kihlstrom, J. F. (2003). The fox, the hedgehog, and hypnosis. *International Journal of Clinical and Experimental Hypnosis, 51,* 166–189.

Kihlstrom, J. F. (2005). Is hypnosis an altered state of consciousness *or what?* [Commentary on "Hypnotic Phenomena and Altered States of Consciousness: A Multilevel Framework of Description and Explanation" by S. Kallio & A. Revonsuo]. *Contemporary Hypnosis, 22,* 34–38.

Kileen, P. R., & Nash, M. R. (2003). The four causes of hypnosis. *International Journal of Clinical and Experimental Hypnosis, 51,* 195–231.

Kilpatrick, D. G. (1983). Rape victims: Detection, assessment, and treatment. *The Clinical Psychologist, 36,* 92–95.

Kirsch, I. (1978). Demonology and the rise of science: An example of the misperception of historical data. *Journal of the History of the Behavioral Sciences, 14,* 149–157.

Kirsch, I. (1980). Demonology and science during the scientific revolution. *Journal of the History of the Behavioral Sciences, 16,* 359–368.

Kirsch, I. (1985). Response expectancy as a determinant of experience and behavior. *American Psychologist, 40,* 1189–1202.

Kirsch, I. (1990). *Changing expectations: A key to effective psychotherapy*. Pacific Grove, CA: Brooks/Cole.

Kirsch, I. (1991). The social learning theory of hypnosis. In S. J. Lynn & J. Rhue (Eds.), *Theories of hypnosis: Current models and perspectives* (pp. 439–466). New York: Guilford Press.

Kirsch, I. (1994a). Defining hypnosis for the public. *Contemporary Hypnosis, 11*, 142–143.

Kirsch, I. (1994b). Clinical hypnosis as a nondeceptive placebo: Empirically derived techniques. *American Journal of Clinical Hypnosis, 37*, 95–106.

Kirsch, I. (1997a). Response expectancy theory and application: A decennial review. *Applied and Preventive Psychology, 6*, 69–79.

Kirsch, I. (1997b). Suggestibility or hypnosis: What do our scales really measure? *International Journal of Clinical and Experimental Hypnosis, 45*, 212–225.

Kirsch, I., & Braffman, W. (2001). Imaginative suggestibility and hypnotizability. *Current Directions in Psychological Science, 10*, 57–61.

Kirsch, I., & Council, J. R. (1992). Situational and personality correlates of suggestibility. In E. Fromm & M. Nash (Eds.), *Contemporary hypnosis research* (pp. 267–292). New York: Guilford Press.

Kirsch, I., Council, J. R., & Mobayed, C. (1987). Imagery and response expectancy as determinants of hypnotic behavior. *British Journal of Experimental and Clinical Hypnosis, 4*, 25–31.

Kirsch, I., & Lynn, S. J. (1995). The altered state of hypnosis: Changes in the theoretical landscape. *American Psychologist, 50*, 846–858.

Kirsch, I., & Lynn, S. J. (1998). Dissociation theories of hypnosis. *Psychological Bulletin, 123*, 100–115.

Kirsch, I., & Lynn, S. J. (1999). The automaticity of behavior in clinical psychology. *American Psychologist, 54*, 504–575.

Kirsch, I., Mobayed, C. P., Council, J. R., & Kenny, D. A. (1992). Expert judgments of hypnosis from subjective state reports. *Journal of Abnormal Psychology, 101*, 657–662.

Kirsch, I., Montgomery, G., & Sapirstein, G. (1995). Hypnosis as an adjunct to cognitive behavioral psychotherapy: A meta-analysis. *Journal of Consulting and Clinical Psychology, 63*, 214–220.

Kirsch, I., Moore, T. J., Scoboria, A., & Nicholls, S. S. (2002). The emperor's new drugs: An analysis of antidepressant medication data submitted to the U.S. Food and Drug Administration. *Prevention and Treatment, 5*, Article 23. Retrieved April 5, 2004, from http://www.journals.apa.org/prevention/volume5/pre0050023a.html

Kirsch, I., & Sapirstein, G. (1998). Listening to Prozac but hearing placebo: A meta-analysis of antidepressant medication. *Prevention and Treatment, 1*, 0002a. Retrieved April 5, 2004, from http://www.journals.apa.org/prevention/volume1/pre0010002a.html

Kirsch, I., Silva, C. E., Carone, J. E., Johnston, J. D., & Simon, B. (1989). The surreptitious observation design: An experimental paradigm for distinguishing artifact from essence in hypnosis. *Journal of Abnormal Psychology, 98*(2), 132–136.

Kirsch, I., Silva, C. E., Comey, G., & Reed, S. (1995). A spectral analysis of cognitive and personality variables in hypnosis: Empirical disconfirmation of the two-factor model of hypnotic responding. *Journal of Personality and Social Psychology, 69*, 167–175.

Klerman, G. L., Weissman, M. M., Rounsaville, B. J., & Chevron, E. S. (1984). *Interpersonal psychotherapy of depression*. New York: Basic Books.

Klopfer, B. (1957). Psychological variables in human cancer. *Journal of Projective Techniques, 21*, 331–340.

Kohen, D. P., & Olness, K. (1993). Hypnotherapy with children. In J. W. Rhue, S. J. Lynn, & I. Kirsch (Eds.), *Handbook of clinical hypnosis* (pp. 357–382). Washington, DC: American Psychological Association.

Kosslyn, S. M., Thompson, W. L., Costantini-Ferrando, M. F., Alpert, N. M., & Spiegel, D. (2000). Hypnotic visual illusion alters color processing in the brain. *American Journal of Psychiatry, 157*, 1279–1284.

Krakauer, S. Y. (2001). *Treating dissociative identity disorder: The power of the collective heart*. Philadelphia, PA: Brunner-Routledge.

Kramer, H., & Sprenger, J. (1971). *The Malleus Maleficarum of Kramer and Sprenger* (M. Summers, Trans.). Mineola, NY: Dover. (Original work published 1484)

Kroger, W. S. (1977). *Clinical and experimental hypnosis in medicine, dentistry, and psychology* (2nd ed.). Philadelphia: Lippincott.

Kroger, W. S., & Fezler, W. D. (1976). *Hypnosis and behavior modification imagery conditioning*. Philadelphia: Lippincott.

Kropotov, J. D., Crawford, H. J., & Polyakov, Y. I. (1997). Somatosensory event-related potential changes to painful stimuli during hypnotic analgesia: Anterior cingulate cortex and anterior temporal cortex intracranial recordings. *International Journal of Psychophysiology, 27*, 1–8.

Kuhn, T. S. (1971). *The structure of scientific revolutions* (2nd ed.). Chicago: University of Chicago Press.

Kulka, R. A., Fairbank, J. A., Jordan, B. K., Weiss, W., & Cranston, A. (1990). *Trauma and the Vietnam war generation: Report on the Vietnam Veterans Readjustment Study*. New York: Brunner-Routledge.

Kuttner, L. (1988). Favorite stories: A hypnotic pain-reduction technique for children in acute pain. *American Journal of Clinical Hypnosis, 30*, 289–295.

Labelle, L., Dixon, M., & Laurence, J. R. (1996). A multivariate approach to the prediction of hypnotic susceptibility. *International Journal of Clinical and Experimental Hypnosis, 44*, 250–264.

Lambert, S. A. (1996). The effects of hypnosis/guided imagery on the postoperative course of children. *Developmental and Behavioral Pediatrics, 17*, 307–310.

Lambert, S. (1999). Distraction, imagery, and hypnosis techniques for management of children's pain. *Journal of Child and Family Nursing, 2*, 5–15.

Lang, E. V., Benotsch, E. G., Fick, L. J., Lutgendorf, S., Berbaum, M. L., Berbaum, K. S., et al. (2000). Adjunctive non-pharmacological analgesia for invasive medical procedures: A randomised trial. *Lancet, 355*, 1486–1490.

Lang, E. V., Joyce, J. S., Spiegel, D., Hamilton, D., & Lee, K. K. (1996). Self-hypnotic relaxation during interventional radiological procedures: Effects on pain perception and intravenous drug use. *International Journal of Clinical and Experimental Hypnosis, 44*, 106–119.

Laurence, J.-R. (1997). Hypnotic theorizing: Spring cleaning is long overdue. *International Journal of Clinical and Experimental Hypnosis, 45*, 280–290.

Laurence, J.-R., & Perry, C. (1983a). Forensic use of hypnosis in the late nineteenth century. *International Journal of Clinical and Experimental Hypnosis, 31*, 266–283.

Laurence, J.-R., & Perry, C. (1983b, November 4). Hypnotically created memory among highly hypnotizable subjects. *Science, 222*, 523–524.

Laurence, J.-R., & Perry, C. (1988). *Hypnosis, will and memory: A psycho-legal history.* New York: Guilford Press.

Law, M., & Tang, J. L. (1995). An analysis of the effectiveness of interventions intended to help people stop smoking. *Archives of Internal Medicine, 155*, 1933–1941.

Lazarus, A. A. (1973). "Hypnosis" as a facilitator in behavior therapy. *International Journal of Clinical and Experimental Hypnosis, 21*, 25–31.

Levitt, E. E. (1993). Hypnosis in the treatment of obesity. In J. W. Rhue, S. J. Lynn, & I. Kirsch (Eds.), *Handbook of clinical hypnosis* (pp. 533–554). Washington, DC: American Psychological Association.

Lewinsohn, P. M., Striegel-Moore, R. H., & Seeley, J. R. (2000). Epidemiology and natural course of eating disorders in young women from adolescence to young adulthood. *Journal of the American Academy of Child and Adolescent Psychology, 13*, 1284–1292.

Liberman, R. (1964). An experimental study of the placebo response under three different situations of pain. *Journal of Psychiatric Research, 2*(4), 223–246.

Linehan, M. M. (1994). Acceptance and change: The central dialectic in psychotherapy. In S. C. Hayes, N. S. Jacobson, V. M. Follette, & M. J. Dougher (Eds.), *Acceptance and change: Content and context in psychotherapy* (pp. 73–86). Reno, NV: Context Press.

Liossi, C., & Hatira, P. (1999). Clinical hypnosis versus cognitive behavioral training for pain management with pediatric cancer patients undergoing bone marrow aspirations. *International Journal of Clinical and Experimental Hypnosis, 47*, 104–116.

Litz, B. T., Blake, D. D., Gerardi, R. G., & Keane, T. M. (1990). Decision making guidelines for the use of direct therapeutic exposure in the treatment of post-traumatic stress disorder. *Behavior Therapy, 13*, 91–93.

Loftus, E. F., & Pickrell, J. E. (1995). The formation of false memories. *Psychiatric Annals, 25*, 720–725.

Lynn, S. J. (1997). Automaticity and hypnosis: A sociocognitive account. *International Journal of Clinical and Experimental Hypnosis, 45,* 239–250.

Lynn, S. J. (2000). Hypnosis, the hidden observer, and not-so-hidden informed consent. *American Journal of Clinical Hypnosis, 43,* 105–106.

Lynn, S. J., Brentar, J., Carlson, B., Kurzhals, R., & Green, J. (1992). Posthypnotic experiences: A controlled investigation. In W. Bongartz (Ed.), *Hypnosis theory and research.* Konstanz, Germany: University of Konstanz Press.

Lynn, S. J., & Fite, R. (1998). Will the false memory debate increase acceptance of the sociocognitive model of hypnosis? *Contemporary Hypnosis, 15,* 171–174.

Lynn, S. J., & Garske, J. (Eds.). (1985). *Contemporary psychotherapies: Models and methods.* Columbus, OH: Charles E. Merrill.

Lynn, S. J., Green, J. P., Jacquith, L., & Gasior, D. (2003). Hypnosis and performance standards. *International Journal of Clinical and Experimental Hypnosis, 51,* 51–65.

Lynn, S. J., & Hallquist, M. (2004). Toward a scientific understanding of Milton Erickson's strategies and tactics: Hypnosis, response sets and common factors. *Contemporary Hypnosis, 21,* 63–78.

Lynn, S. J., Kirsch, I., Barabasz, A., Cardena, E., & Patterson, D. (2000). Hypnosis as an empirically supported adjunctive technique: The state of the evidence. *International Journal of Clinical and Experimental Hypnosis, 48,* 343–361.

Lynn, S. J., Kirsch, I., Neufeld, V., & Rhue, J. (1996). Clinical hypnosis: Assessment, applications, and treatment considerations. In S. J. Lynn, I. Kirsch, & J. W. Rhue (Eds.), *Casebook of clinical hypnosis* (pp. 3–30). Washington, DC: American Psychological Association.

Lynn, S. J., Kirsch, I., & Rhue, J. W. (1996). Maximizing treatment gains: Recommendations for the practice of clinical hypnosis. In S. J. Lynn, I. Kirsch, & J. W. Rhue (Eds.), *Casebook of clinical hypnosis* (pp. 395–406). Washington, DC: American Psychological Association.

Lynn, S. J., & Kvaal, S. (2004). *A comparison of three different hypnotic inductions.* Unpublished manuscript, Binghamton University, Binghamton, NY.

Lynn, S. J., & Lilienfeld, S. (2002). A critique of the "Franklin Report:" Hypnosis, belief, and suggestion. *International Journal of Clinical and Experimental Hypnosis, 50,* 369–386.

Lynn, S. J., Lock, T., Loftus, E. B., Lilienfeld, S. O., & Krackow, E. (2003). The remembrance of things past: Problematic memory recovery techniques in psychotherapy. In S. O. Lilienfeld, S. J. Lynn, & J. Lohr (Eds.), *Science and pseudoscience in clinical psychology* (pp. 205–239). New York: Guilford Press.

Lynn, S. J., Lock, T., Myers, B., & Payne, D. (1997). Recalling the unrecallable: Should hypnosis be used for memory recovery in psychotherapy? *Current Directions in Psychological Science, 6,* 79–83.

Lynn, S. J., Mare, C., Kvaal, S., Segal, D. A., & Sivec, H. (1994). The hidden observer, hypnotic dreams, and hypnotic age regression: Clinical implications. *American Journal of Clinical Hypnosis, 37,* 130–142.

Lynn, S. J., Martin, D., & Frauman, D. C. (1996). Does hypnosis pose special risks for negative effects? *International Journal of Clinical and Experimental Hypnosis, 44*, 7–19.

Lynn, S. J., Martin, D., & Hallquist, M. (2004). *Searching for the essence of hypnosis: Research using the real-simulator design*. Unpublished manuscript.

Lynn, S. J., & McConkey, K. M. (1998). *Truth in memory*. New York: Guilford Press.

Lynn, S. J., Myers, B., & Malinoski, P. (1997). Hypnosis, pseudomemories, and clinical guidelines: A sociocognitive perspective. In D. Read & S. Lindsay (Eds.), *Recollections of trauma: Scientific research and clinical practice* (pp. 305–331). New York: Plenum Press.

Lynn, S. J., & Nash, M. R. (1994). Truth in memory: Ramifications for psychotherapy and hypnotherapy. *American Journal of Clinical Hypnosis, 36*, 194–208.

Lynn, S. J., Nash, M. R., Rhue, J. W., Frauman, D. C., & Sweeney, C. A. (1984). Nonvolition, expectancies, and hypnotic rapport. *Journal of Abnormal Psychology, 93*, 295–303.

Lynn, S. J., Neufeld, V. R., & Mare, C. (1993). Direct versus indirect suggestions: A conceptual and methodological review. *International Journal of Clinical and Experimental Hypnosis, 41*, 124–152.

Lynn, S. J., Neufeld, V., & Matyi, C. L. (1987). Hypnotic inductions versus suggestions: The effects of direct and indirect wording. *Journal of Abnormal Psychology, 96*, 76–80.

Lynn, S. J., Neufeld, V., Rhue, J. W., & Matorin, A. (1993). Hypnosis and smoking cessation: A cognitive–behavioral treatment. In J. W. Rhue, S. J. Lynn, & I. Kirsch (Eds.), *Handbook of clinical hypnosis* (pp. 555–586). Washington, DC: American Psychological Association.

Lynn, S. J., & Rhue, J. W. (1991a). An integrative model of hypnosis. In S. J. Lynn & J. W. Rhue (Eds.), *Theories of hypnosis: Current models and perspectives* (pp. 397–438). New York: Guilford Press.

Lynn, S. J., & Rhue, J. W. (Eds.). (1991b). *Theories of hypnosis: Current models and perspectives*. New York: Guilford Press.

Lynn, S. J., Rhue, J. W., Kvaal, S., & Mare, C. (1993). The treatment of anorexia nervosa: A hypnosuggestive framework. *Contemporary Hypnosis, 10*, 73–80.

Lynn, S. J., Rhue, J. W., & Weekes, J. R. (1990). Hypnotic involuntariness: A social–cognitive analysis. *Psychological Review, 97*, 169–184.

Lynn, S. J., & Sherman, S. J. (2000). Clinical implications of sociocognitive models of hypnosis: Response set theory and Milton Erickson's strategic interventions. *American Journal of Clinical Hypnosis, 42*, 294–315.

Lynn, S. J., Shindler, K., & Meyer, E. (2003). Hypnotic suggestibility, psychopathology, and treatment outcome. *Sleep and Hypnosis, 3*, 2–12.

Lynn, S. J., & Sivec, H. (1992). The hypnotizable subject as creative problem solving agent. In E. Fromm & M. Nash (Eds.), *Contemporary perspectives in hypnosis research*. New York: Guilford Press.

Lynn, S. J., Snodgrass, M. J., Rhue, J., Nash, M., & Frauman, D. (1987). Attributions, involuntariness, and hypnotic rapport. *American Journal of Clinical Hypnosis, 30*, 36–43.

Lynn, S. J., Vanderhoff, H., Shindler, K., & Stafford, J. (2002). The effects of an induction and defining hypnosis as a "trance" vs. cooperation: Hypnotic suggestibility and performance standards. *American Journal of Clinical Hypnosis, 44*, 231–240.

Lynn, S. J., Weekes, J., Brentar, J., Neufeld, V., Zivney, O., & Weiss, F. (1991). Interpersonal climate and hypnotizability level: Effects on hypnotic performance, rapport, and archaic involvement. *Journal of Personality and Social Psychology, 60*, 739–743.

MacHovec, F. (1986). *Hypnosis complications: Prevention and risk management.* Springfield, IL: Thomas Books.

MacHovec, F. J., & Man, S. C. (1978). Acupuncture and hypnosis compared: Fifty-eight cases. *American Journal of Clinical Hypnosis, 88*, 129–130.

Mare, C., Lynn, S. J., Kvaal, S., Segal, D., & Sivec, H. (1994). Hypnosis and the dream hidden observer: Primary process and demand characteristics. *Journal of Abnormal Psychology, 103*, 316–332.

Marlatt, G. A. (2002). Buddhist philosophy and the treatment of addictive behavior. *Cognitive and Behavioral Practice, 9*, 42–50.

Martin, M. Y., Bradley, L. A., Alexander, R. W., & Alarcon, G. (1996). Coping strategies predict disability in patients with primary fibromyalgia. *Pain, 68*, 45–53.

Matthews, W. J., Kirsch, I., & Mosher, D. (1985). The "double" hypnotic induction: An initial empirical test. *Journal of Abnormal Psychology, 94*, 92–95.

Matthews, W. J., Lankton, S., & Lankton, C. (1993). An Ericksonian model of hypnotherapy. In J. W. Rhue, S. J. Lynn, & I. Kirsch (Eds.), *Handbook of clinical hypnosis* (pp. 187–214). Washington, DC: American Psychological Association.

Mattick, R. P., & Clarke, J. C. (1998). Development and validation of measures of social phobia scrutiny fear and social interaction anxiety. *Behaviour Research and Therapy, 6*, 455–470.

Mazzoni, G., & Kirsch, I. (2002). Autobiographical memories and beliefs. A preliminary metacognitive model. In B. L. Schwartz & T. J. Perfect (Eds.), *Applied metacognition* (pp. 121–145). New York: Cambridge University Press.

Mazzoni, G. A., Loftus, E. F., Seitz, A., & Lynn, S. J. (1999). Creating a new childhood: Changing beliefs and memories through dream interpretation. *Applied Cognitive Psychology, 13*, 125–144.

McBride, P. E. (1992). The health consequences of smoking: Cardiovascular diseases. *Medical Clinics of North America, 76*, 333–353.

McConkey, K. M. (1986). Opinions about hypnosis and self-hypnosis before and after hypnotic testing. *International Journal of Clinical and Experimental Hypnosis, 34*, 311–319.

McConkey, K. M. (1991). The construction and resolution of experience and behavior in hypnosis. In S. J. Lynn & J. W. Rhue (Eds.), *Theories of hypnosis: Current models and perspectives* (pp. 542–563). New York: Guilford Press.

McConkey, K. M., Barnier, A. J., & Sheehan, P. W. (1998). Hypnosis and pseudomemory: Understanding the findings and their implications. In S. J. Lynn & K. M. McConkey (Eds.), *Truth in memory* (pp. 227–259). New York: Guilford Press.

McGlashan, T. M., Evans, F. J., & Orne, M. T. (1969). The nature of hypnotic analgesia and placebo response to experimental pain. *Psychosomatic Medicine, 31*, 227–246.

Meares, A. (1961). An evaluation of the dangers of medical hypnosis. *American Journal of Clinical Hypnosis, 4*, 90–97.

Meichenbaum, D. (1994). *A clinical handbook/practical therapist manual for assessing and treating adults with post-traumatic stress disorder (PTSD)*. Clearwater, FL: Institute Press.

Meichenbaum, D., & Fong, G. T. (1993). How individuals control their own minds: A constructive narrative perspective. In D. M. Wegner & J. W. Pennebaker (Eds.), *Handbook of mental control* (pp. 473–490). New York: Prentice Hall.

Mellinger, D. I., & Lynn, S. J. (2003). *The monster in the cave: How to face your fear and anxiety and live your life*. New York: Berkley Books.

Merikle, P. M., & Joordens, S. (1997). Measuring unconscious influences. In J. D. Cohen & J. W. Schooler (Eds.), *Scientific approaches to consciousness* (pp. 109–123). Mahwah, NJ: Erlbaum.

Mesmer, F. A. (1779). *Memoire sur la decouverte du magnetisme animal, par M. Mesmer, docteur en medecine de la faculte do Vienne* [Memoir on the discovery of animal magnetism by Mr. Mesmer, doctor of medicine from the faculty of Vienna]. Geneva, Switzerland, and Paris: Didiot.

Meyer, E., & Lynn, S. J. (2004). *The impact of hypnotic inductions, imaginative suggestibility, response expectancies, and performance standards on hypnotic suggestibility and experiences*. Unpublished manuscript, Binghamton University, Binghamton, NY.

Meyer, E. C., & Lynn, S. J. (2005). *The determinants of hypnotic and nonhypnotic suggestibility*. Unpublished manuscript, Binghamton University, Binghamton, NY.

Meyer, T. J., Miller, M. L., Metzger, R. L., & Borkovec, T. D. (1990). Development and validation of the Penn State Worry Questionnaire. *Behaviour Research and Therapy, 28*, 487–495.

Miller, M. E., & Bowers, K. S. (1986). Hypnotic analgesia and stress inoculation in the reduction of pain. *Journal of Abnormal Psychology, 95*, 6–14.

Miller, M. E., & Bowers, K. S. (1993). Hypnotic analgesia: Dissociated experience or dissociated control? *Journal of Abnormal Psychology, 102*, 29–38.

Milling, L. S., & Costantino, C. A. (2000). Clinical hypnosis with children: First steps toward empirical support. *International Journal of Clinical and Experimental Hypnosis, 48*, 113–137.

Milling, L. S., Kirsch, I., Allen, G. J., & Reutenauer, E. L. (2005). The effects of hypnotic and nonhypnotic imaginative suggestion on pain. *Annals of Behavioral Medicine, 29,* 116–127.

Milling, L. S., Kirsch, I., Meunier, S. A., & Levine, M. R. (2002). Hypnotic analgesia and stress inoculation training: Individual and combined effects in analog treatment of experimental pain. *Cognitive Therapy and Research, 26,* 355–371.

Mills, A., & Lynn, S. J. (2000). Past-life experiences. In E. Cardena, S. J. Lynn, & S. Krippner (Eds.), *The varieties of anomalous experience* (pp. 283–314). New York: Guilford Press.

Mitchell, C. M., & Drossman, D. A. (1987). Survey of the AGA membership relating to patients with functional gastrointestinal disorders. *Gastroenterology, 92,* 1282–1284.

Mitchell, J. E., Halmi, K. A., Wilson, G. T., Agras, W. S., Kraemer, H. C., & Crow, S. (2002). A randomized secondary treatment study of women with bulimia nervosa who fail to respond to CBT. *International Journal of Eating Disorders, 32,* 271–281.

Moene, F. C., Spinhoven, P., Hoogduin, K. A. L., & Van Dyck, R. (2003). A randomized controlled trial of a hypnosis-based treatment for patients with conversion disorder, motor type. *International Journal of Clinical and Experimental Hypnosis, 51,* 29–50.

Montgomery, G. H., David, D., Winkel, G., Silverstein, J., & Bovbjerg, D. (2002). The effectiveness of adjunctive hypnosis with surgical patients: A meta-analysis. *Anesthesia and Analgesia, 94,* 1639–1645.

Montgomery, G. H., DuHamel, K. N., & Redd, W. H. (2000). A meta-analysis of hypnotically induced analgesia: How effective is hypnosis? *International Journal of Clinical and Experimental Hypnosis, 48,* 138–153.

Mowrer, O. H. (1960). *Learning theory and behavior.* New York: Wiley.

Myers, S. (2000). Empathic listening: Reports on the experience of being heard. *Journal of Humanistic Psychology, 40*(2), 148–173.

Nadon, R., & Laurence, J.-R. (1994). Ideographic approaches to hypnosis research: Or how therapeutic practice can inform science. *American Journal of Clinical Hypnosis, 37,* 85–94.

Nadon, R., Laurence, J.-R., & Perry, C. (1991). The two disciplines of scientific hypnosis: A synergistic model. In S. J. Lynn & J. W. Rhue (Eds.), *Theories of hypnosis: Current models and perspectives* (pp. 485–519). New York: Guilford Press.

Narrow, W. E., Rae, D. S., & Regier, D. A. (1998). *NIMH epidemiology note: Prevalence of anxiety disorders.* Retrieved April 5, 2004, from http://www.nimh.nih.gov/publicat/numbers.cfm

Nash, M. R. (1987). What, if anything, is regressed about hypnotic age regression? A review of the empirical literature. *Psychological Bulletin, 102,* 42–52.

Nash, M. R. (1991). Hypnosis as a special case of psychological regression. In S. J. Lynn & J. W. Rhue (Eds.), *Theories of hypnosis: Current models and perspectives* (pp. 171–194). New York: Guilford Press.

Nash, M. R. (1997). Why scientific hypnosis needs psychoanalysis (or something like it). *International Journal of Clinical and Experimental Hypnosis, 45*, 291–300.

Nash, M. R. (2001). The truth and hype of hypnosis. *Scientific American, 285*, 46–55.

Nash, M. R. (2002). Mesmer, Franklin, and The Royal Commission. *International Journal of Clinical and Experimental Hypnosis, 50*, 291–422.

Nash, M. R., & Baker, E. L. (1993). Hypnosis in the treatment of anorexia nervosa. In J. W. Rhue, S. J. Lynn, & I. Kirsch (Eds.), *Handbook of clinical hypnosis* (pp. 383–394). Washington, DC: American Psychological Association.

Nash, M. J., Drake, M., Wiley, R., Khalsa, S., & Lynn, S. J. (1986). The accuracy of recall of hypnotically age regressed subjects. *Journal of Abnormal Psychology, 95*, 298–300.

Nash, M. R., & Spinler, D. (1989). Hypnosis and transference: A measure of archaic involvement with the hypnotist. *International Journal of Clinical and Experimental Hypnosis, 37*, 129–144.

National Institute of Mental Health. (2001). *Best estimate 1-year prevalence rates based on ECA and NCS, ages 18–54.* Retrieved April 4, 2004, from www.niaa.nih.gov.gallery

National Institute of Mental Health. (2002). *Mental health: A report of the surgeon general—epidemiology of mental illness.* Retrieved April 3, 2004, from www.nimh.nih.gov

Neufeld, V., & Lynn, S. J. (1988). A single-session group self-hypnosis smoking cessation: A brief communication. *International Journal of Clinical and Experimental Hypnosis, 36*, 75–79.

Newman, M. G., Castonguay, L. G., Borkovec, T. D., & Molnar, C. (2004). Integrative psychotherapy for anxiety disorders. In R. Heimberg, D. S. Mennin, & C. L. Turk (Eds.), *Generalized anxiety disorder: Advances in research and practice* (pp. 320–350). New York: Guilford Press.

Nolen-Hoeksema, S. (1990). *Sex differences in depression.* Stanford, CA: Stanford University Press.

O'Brien, T. (1990). *The things they carried.* New York: Broadway.

Olness, K., & Gardner, G. G. (1988). *Hypnosis and hypnotherapy with children* (2nd ed). New York: Grune & Stratton.

Orne, M. T. (1959). The nature of hypnosis: Artifact and essence. *Journal of Abnormal Psychology, 58*, 277–299.

Orne, M. T. (1965). Undesirable effects of hypnosis: The determinants and management. *International Journal of Clinical and Experimental Hypnosis, 13*, 226–237.

Orne, M. T. (1979). On the simulating subject as a quasi-control group in hypnosis research: What, why and how? In E. Fromm & R. Shor (Eds.), *Hypnosis: Developments in research and new perspectives* (2nd ed., pp. 519–565). Chicago: Aldine.

Orne, M. T., & McConkey, K. M. (1981). Toward convergent inquiry into self-hypnosis. *International Journal of Clinical and Experimental Hypnosis, 29,* 313–323.

Page, R. A., & Green, J. P. (2002). Are recommendations to avoid hypnotic aftereffects being implemented? *Contemporary Hypnosis, 19,* 167–171.

Palace, E. M. (1995). A cognitive–physiological process model of sexual arousal and response. *Clinical Psychology Science and Practice, 2,* 370–384.

Patterson, D. R., Everett, J. J., Burns, G. L., & Marvin, J. A. (1992). Hypnosis for the treatment of burn pain. *Journal of Consulting and Clinical Psychology, 60,* 713–717.

Patterson, D. R., & Jensen, M. P. (2003). Hypnosis and clinical pain. *Psychological Bulletin, 129*(4), 495–521.

Patterson, D. R., Questad, K. A., & DeLateur, B. J. (1989). Hypnotherapy as an adjunct to pharmacologies for the treatment of pain from burn debridement. *American Journal of Clinical Hypnosis, 31,* 156–163.

Pedersen, L. L., Scrimgeour, W. G., & Lefcoe, N. M. (1975). Comparison of hypnosis plus counseling, counseling alone, and hypnosis alone in a community service smoking withdrawal program. *Journal of Consulting and Clinical Psychology, 43,* 920.

Perkins, K. A., Epstein, L. H., & Pastor, S. (1990). Changes in energy balance following smoking cessation and resumption of smoking in women. *Journal of Consulting and Clinical Psychology, 58,* 121–125.

Perry, C., Gelfand, R., & Marcovitch, P. (1979). The relevance of hypnotic susceptibility in the clinical content. *Journal of Abnormal Psychology, 89,* 598–603.

Perry, C., & Laurence, J.-R. (1986). Social and psychological influences on hypnotic behavior. *Behavioral and Brain Sciences, 9,* 478–479.

Perry, C., & Mullen, G. (1975). The effects of hypnotic susceptibility on reducing smoking behavior treated by an hypnotic technique. *Journal of Clinical Psychology, 31,* 498–505.

Pettinati, H. M., Horne, R. J., & Staats, J. M. (1985). Hypnotizability in patients with anorexia nervosa and bulimia. *Archives of General Psychiatry, 42,* 1014–1016.

Pettinati, H. M., Kogan, L. G., Margolis, C., Shrier, L., & Wade, J. J. (1989). Hypnosis, hypnotizability, and the bulimic patient. In L. M. Hornyak & E. K. Baker (Eds.), *Experiential therapies for eating disorders* (pp. 34–59). New York: Guilford Press.

Piccione, C., Hilgard, E. R., & Zimbardo, P. G. (1989). On the degree of stability of measured hypnotizability over a 25-year period. *Journal of Personality and Social Psychology, 56,* 289–295.

Pinnell, C. A., & Covino, N. A. (2000). Empirical findings on the use of hypnosis in medicine: A critical review. *International Journal of Clinical and Experimental Hypnosis, 48,* 170–194.

Pittman, R. K., Altman, B., Greenwald, E., Longpre, R. E., Macklin, M. L., Poire, R. E., & Steketee, G. S. (1991). Psychiatric complications during flooding therapy for post-traumatic stress disorder. *Journal of Clinical Psychiatry, 52,* 17–20.

Polivy, J., & Herman, C. P. (1985). Dieting and bingeing: A causal analysis. *American Psychologist, 40,* 193–201.

Poole, D., Lindsay, D., Memon, A., & Bull, R. (1995). Psychotherapy and the recovery of memories of childhood sexual abuse: U.S. and British practitioners' opinions, practices, and experiences. *Journal of Consulting and Clinical Psychology, 63,* 426–437.

Porter, S., Yuille, J. C., & Lehman, D. R. (1999). The nature of real, implanted, and fabricated childhood emotional events: Implications for the recovered memory debate. *Law and Human Behavior, 23,* 517–537.

Rainville, P., Duncan, G. H., Price, D. D., Carrier, B., & Bushnell, M. C. (1997, August 15). Pain affect encoded in human anterior cingulate but not somatosensory cortex. *Science, 277,* 968–971.

Rainville, P., & Price, D. D. (2003). Hypnosis phenomenology and the neurobiology of consciousness. *International Journal of Clinical and Experimental Hypnosis, 51,* 105–129.

Rapee, R. M. (1998). *Social phobia: Clinical application of evidence-based psychotherapy.* Northvale, NJ: Jason Aronson.

Ray, W. J., & Oathies, D. (2003). Brain imaging techniques. *International Journal of Clinical and Experimental Hypnosis, 51,* 97–104.

Reason, J. T. (1992). Cognitive underspecification: Its variety and consequences. In B. J. Baars (Ed.), *Experimental slips and human error* (pp. 71–91). New York: Plenum.

Reiss, S., & McNally, R. J. (1985). The expectancy model of fear. In S. Reiss & R. R. Bootzin (Eds.), *Theoretical issues in behavior therapy* (pp. 107–121). New York: Academic Press.

Reiss, S., Peterson, R. A., Gursky, D. M., & McNally, R. J. (1986). Anxiety sensitivity, anxiety frequency, and the prediction of fearfulness. *Behavior Research and Therapy, 24,* 1–8.

Research Committee of the British Tuberculosis Association. (1968). A report. *British Medical Journal, 3,* 774–777.

Resick, P. A. (1992). Cognitive treatment of crime-related post-traumatic stress disorder. In R. Peters, R. McMahon, & V. Quinsey (Eds.), *Aggression and violence throughout the life span* (pp. 171–191). Newbury Park, CA: Sage.

Resick, P. A., & Schnicke, M. K. (1992). Cognitive processing therapy for sexual assault victims. *Journal of Consulting and Clinical Psychology, 60,* 748–756.

Resnick, H. S., Kilpatrick, D. G., Dansky, B. S., Saunders, B. E., & Best, C. L. (1993). Prevalence of civilian trauma and posttraumatic stress disorder in a representative national sample of women. *Journal of Consulting and Clinical Psychology, 61,* 984–991.

Rhue, J. W., & Lynn, S. J. (1993). *Hypnosis and storytelling in the treatment of child sexual abuse: Strategies and procedures.* In J. W. Rhue, S. J. Lynn, & I. Kirsch (Eds.), *Handbook of clinical hypnosis* (pp. 455–478). Washington, DC: American Psychological Association.

Rhue, J. W., Lynn, S. J., & Kirsch, I. (1993). *Handbook of clinical hypnosis.* Washington, DC: American Psychological Association.

Rhue, J., Lynn, S., & Pintar, J. (1996). Narrative and imaginative storytelling: Treatment of a sexually abused child. In S. J. Lynn, I. Kirsch, & J. W. Rhue (Eds.), *Casebook of clinical hypnosis* (pp. 251–270). Washington, DC: American Psychological Association.

Rimpoche, B. (1981). The Mahamudra: Eliminating the darkness of ignorance, by Wang-Ch'ug Dorje (Commentary). Dharamsala, India: Library of Tibetan Works and Archives.

Roemer, L., Borkovec, M., Posa, S., & Borkovec, T. D. (1995). A self-report diagnostic measure of generalized anxiety disorder. *Journal of Behavior Therapy and Experimental Psychiatry, 4,* 345–350.

Roemer, L., Molina, S., & Borkovec, T. D. (1997). An investigation of worry content among generally anxious individuals. *The Journal of Nervous and Mental Disease, 185,* 314–319.

Rosen, S. (1982). *My voice will go with you: The teaching tales of Milton H. Erickson.* New York: Norton.

Rothbaum, B. O., Meadows, E. A., Resnick, P., & Foy, D. (2000). Cognitive–behavioral therapy. In E. B. Foa, T. M. Keane, & M. J. Friedman (Eds.), *Effective treatments for PTSD* (pp. 60–83). New York: Guilford Press.

Sanders, S. (1991). *Clinical self-hypnosis: The power of words and images.* New York: Guilford Press.

Sarbin, T. R. (1950). Contributions to role-taking theory: I. Hypnotic behavior. *Psychological Review, 57,* 225–270.

Sarbin, T. R. (1989). The construction and reconstruction of hypnosis. In N. P. Spanos & J. F. Chaves (Eds.), *Hypnosis: The cognitive–behavioral perspective* (pp. 400–416). Buffalo, NY: Prometheus Books.

Sarbin, T. R. (1991). Hypnosis: A fifty-year perspective. *Contemporary Hypnosis, 8,* 1–16.

Sarbin, T. R. (1997). Hypnosis as conversation: Believed-in imaginings revisited. *Contemporary Hypnosis, 14,* 203–215.

Sarbin, T. R. (1999). Whither hypnosis? A rhetorical analysis. In I. Kirsch, A. Capafons, E. Cardena-Buelna, & S. A. Borras (Eds.), *Clinical hypnosis and self-regulation: Cognitive–behavioral perspectives* (pp. 105–116). Washington, DC: American Psychological Association.

Sarbin, T. R., & Coe, W. C. (1972). *Hypnosis: A social psychological analysis of influence communication.* New York: Holt, Rinehart & Winston.

Sarbin, T. R., & Slagle, R. W. (1979). Hypnosis and psychophysiological outcomes. In E. Fromm & R. E. Shor (Eds.), *Hypnosis: Developments in research and new perspectives* (2nd ed., pp. 273–303). New York: Aldine.

Schlutter, L. C., Golden, C. J., & Blume, H. G. (1980). A comparison of treatments for prefrontal muscle contraction headache. *British Journal of Medical Psychology*, 53, 47–52.

Schoenberger, N. E. (1996). Cognitive–behavioral hypnotherapy for phobic anxiety. In S. J. Lynn, I. Kirsch, & J. W. Rhue (Eds.), *Casebook of clinical hypnosis* (pp. 33–49). Washington, DC: American Psychological Association.

Schoenberger, N. E. (2000). Research on hypnosis as an adjunct to cognitive–behavioral psychotherapy. *International Journal of Clinical and Experimental Hypnosis*, 48, 154–169.

Schoenberger, N. E., Kirsch, I., Gearan, P., Montgomery, G., & Pastyrnak, S. L. (1997). Hypnotic enhancement of a cognitive–behavioral treatment for public speaking anxiety. *Behavior Therapy*, 28, 127–140.

Schubert, D. K. (1983). Comparison of hypnotherapy with systematic relaxation in the treatment of cigarette habituation. *Journal of Clinical Psychology*, 39, 198–202.

Scoboria, A., Mazzoni, G., Kirsch, I., & Milling, L. (2002). Immediate and persisting effects of misleading questions and hypnosis on memory reports. *Journal of Experimental Psychology: Applied*, 8, 26–32.

Segal, Z. V., Williams, J. M. G., & Teasdale, J. D. (2002). *Mindfulness-based cognitive therapy for depression: A new approach for preventing relapse.* New York: Guilford Press.

Sheehan, P. W. (1991). Hypnosis, context, and commitment. In S. J. Lynn & J. W. Rhue (Eds.), *Theories of hypnosis: Current models and perspectives* (pp. 520–541). New York: Guilford Press.

Sheehan, P. W., & Perry, C. W. (1976). *Methodologies of hypnosis.* Hillsdale, NJ: Erlbaum.

Sheinin, J. C. (1988). Pathophysiologic and clinical aspects of medical, endocrine, and nutritional abnormalities and adaptations in eating disorders. In B. Blinder, B. Chaitin, & R. Goldstein (Eds.), *The eating disorders: Medical and psychological bases of diagnosis and treatment* (pp. 227–234). New York: PMA Publishing.

Sherman, S. J., & Lynn, S. J. (1990). Social–psychological principles in Milton Erickson's psychotherapy. *British Journal of Experimental and Clinical Hypnosis*, 7, 37–46.

Sherman, S. J., Skov, R. B., Hervitz, E. F., & Stock, C. B. (1981). The effects of explaining hypothetical future events: From possibility to probability to actuality and beyond. *Journal of Experimental Social Psychology*, 17, 142–157.

Shor, R. E. (1979). The fundamental problem in hypnosis research as viewed from historic perspectives. In E. Fromm & R. E. Shor (Eds.), *Hypnosis: Developments in research and new perspectives* (Rev. 2nd ed., pp. 15–41). Chicago: Aldine.

Silva, C. E., & Kirsch, I. (1987). Breaching hypnotic amnesia by manipulating expectancy. *Journal of Abnormal Psychology, 96,* 325–329.

Silva, C., & Kirsch, I. (1992). Interpretive sets, expectancy, fantasy proneness, and dissociation as predictors of hypnotic response. *Journal of Personality and Social Psychology, 63,* 847–856.

Simon, M. J., & Salzberg, H. C. (1985). The effect of manipulated expectancies on posthypnotic amnesia. *International Journal of Clinical and Experimental Hypnosis, 33,* 40–51.

Sivec, H. J., Lynn, S. J., & Malinoski, P. T. (1997). *Early memory reports as a function of hypnotic and nonhypnotic age regression.* Unpublished manuscript, State University of New York at Binghamton.

Smith, S. D., Rosen, D., Trueworthy, R. C., & Lowman, J. T. (1979). A reliable method for evaluating drug compliance in children with cancer. *Cancer, 43,* 169–173.

Southworth, S., & Kirsch, I. (1988). The role of expectancy in exposure-generated fear reduction in agoraphobia. *Behaviour Research & Therapy, 26,* 113–120.

Spanos, N. P. (1971). Goal-directed fantasy and the performance of hypnotic test suggestions. *Psychiatry, 34,* 86–96.

Spanos, N. P. (1986). Hypnotic behavior: A social–psychological interpretation of amnesia, analgesia, and "trance logic." *The Behavioral and Brain Sciences, 9,* 499–502.

Spanos, N. P. (1991). A sociocognitive approach to hypnosis. In S. J. Lynn & J. W. Rhue (Eds.), *Theories of hypnosis: Current models and perspectives* (pp. 324–361). New York: Guilford Press.

Spanos, N. P. (1996). *Multiple identities and false memories: A sociocognitive perspective.* Washington, DC: American Psychological Association.

Spanos, N. P., & Barber, T. X. (1974). Toward a convergence in hypnosis research. *American Psychologist, 29,* 500–511.

Spanos, N. P., Burgess, C. A., Roncon, V., Wallace-Capretta, S., & Cross, W. (1993). Surreptitiously observed hypnotic responding in simulators and skill-trained and untrained high hypnotizables. *Journal of Personality and Social Psychology, 65,* 391–398.

Spanos, N. P., & Chaves, J. F. (1989). *Hypnosis: The cognitive–behavioral perspective.* Buffalo, NY: Prometheus Books.

Spanos, N. P., & Chaves, J. F. (1991). History and historiography of hypnosis. In S. J. Lynn & J. W. Rhue (Eds.), *Theories of hypnosis: Current models and perspectives* (pp. 43–82). New York: Guilford Press.

Spanos, N. P., Cobb, P. C., & Gorassini, D. (1985). Failing to resist hypnotic test suggestions: A strategy for self-presenting as deeply hypnotized. *Psychiatry, 48,* 282–292.

Spanos, N. P., & Hewitt, E. C. (1980). The hidden observer in hypnotic analgesia: Discovery or experimental creation? *Journal of Personality and Social Psychology, 39,* 1201–1214.

Spanos, N. P., Menary, E., Gabora, M. J., DuBreuil, S. C., & Dewhirst, B. (1991). Secondary identity enactments during hypnotic past-life regression: A socio-cognitive perspective. *Journal of Personality and Social Psychology, 61,* 308–320.

Spanos, N. P., Radtke, H. L., & Bertrand, L. D. (1984). Hypnotic amnesia as strategic enactment: Breaching amnesia in highly susceptible subjects. *Journal of Personality and Social Psychology, 47,* 1155–1169.

Spanos, N. P., Rivers, S. M., & Ross, S. (1977). Experienced involuntariness and response to hypnotic suggestions. In W. E. Edmonston Jr. (Ed.), *Conceptual and investigative approaches to hypnosis and hypnotic phenomena* (Vol. 296, pp. 208–221). New York: New York Academy of Sciences.

Spanos, N. P., Stenstrom, R. J., & Johnston, J. C. (1988). Hypnosis, placebo, and suggestion in the treatment of warts. *Psychosomatic Medicine, 50,* 245–260.

Spanos, N. P., Williams, V., & Gwynn, M. (1990). Effects of hypnotic, placebo, and salicylic acid treatments on wart regression. *Psychosomatic Medicine, 52,* 109–114.

Spiegel, D. (1981). Vietnam grief work using hypnosis. *American Journal of Clinical Hypnosis, 24,* 33–40.

Spiegel, D. (1992). The use of hypnosis in the treatment of PTSD. *Psychiatric Medicine, 10,* 21–30.

Spiegel, D. (1998). Using our heads: Effects of mental state and social influence on hypnosis. *Contemporary Hypnosis, 15,* 175–177.

Spiegel, D., & Bloom, J. R. (1983). Group therapy and hypnosis reduce metastatic breast carcinoma pain. *Psychosomatic Medicine, 45,* 333–339.

Spiegel, D., Frischholz, E. J., Fleiss, J. L., & Spiegel, H. (1993). Predictors of smoking abstinence following a single-session restructuring intervention with self-hypnosis. *American Journal of Psychiatry, 150,* 1090–1097.

Spiegel, D., Hunt, T., & Dondershine, H. E. (1988). Dissociation and hypnotizability in post-traumatic stress disorder. *American Journal of Psychiatry, 145,* 301–305.

Spiegel, H. (1989). Should therapists test for hypnotizability? *American Journal of Clinical Hypnosis, 32,* 15–16.

Spiegel, H., & Spiegel, D. (1978). *Trance and treatment: Clinical uses of hypnosis.* New York: Basic Books.

Spinhoven, P., Van Dyck, R., Hoogduin, K., & Schaap, C. (1991). Differences in hypnotizability of Dutch psychiatric outpatients according to two different scales. *Australian Journal of Clinical and Experimental Hypnosis, 19,* 107–116.

Spitzer, R. L., Devlin, M., Walsch, B. T., Hasin, K. D., Wing, R. R., Marcus, M. D., et al. (1992). Binge eating disorder: A multisite field trial of the diagnostic criteria. *International Journal of Eating Disorders, 11,* 191–203.

Steblay, N. M., & Bothwell, R. K. (1994). Evidence for hypnotically refreshed testimony: The view from the laboratory. *Law and Human Behavior, 18,* 635–651.

Stroud, M. W., Thorn, B. E., Jensen, M. P., & Boothby, J. L. (2000). The relation between pain beliefs, negative thoughts, and psychosocial functioning in chronic pain patients. *Pain, 84,* 347–352.

Strupp, H. H. (1998). Negative process: Its impact on research, training, and practice. In R. F. Bornstein & J. M. Masling (Eds.), *Empirical studies of the therapeutic hour: Vol. 8. Empirical studies of psychoanalytic theories* (pp. 1–26). Washington, DC: American Psychological Association.

Stutman, R. K., & Bliss, E. L. (1985). Posttraumatic stress disorder, hypnotizability, and imagery. *American Journal of Psychiatry, 142,* 741–743.

Sullivan, M. J., & Neish, N. (1998). Catastrophizing, anxiety and pain during dental hygiene treatment. *Community Dentistry & Oral Epidemiology, 37,* 243–250.

Sullivan, M. J., & Neish, N. (1999). The effects of disclosure on pain during dental hygiene treatment: The moderating role of catastrophizing. *Pain, 79,* 155–163.

Sullivan, M. J., Rodgers, W. M., & Kirsch, I. (2001). Catastrophizing, depression and expectancies for pain and emotional distress. *Pain, 91,* 147–154.

Sullivan, P. F. (1995). Mortality in anorexia nervosa. *American Journal of Psychiatry, 152,* 1053–1054.

Sutcliffe, J. P. (1960). "Credulous" and "skeptical" views of hypnotic phenomena: A review of certain evidence and methodology. *International Journal of Clinical and Experimental Hypnosis, 8,* 73–101.

Syrjala, K. L., Cummings, C., & Donaldson, G. W. (1992). Hypnosis or cognitive behavioral training for the reduction of pain and nausea during cancer treatment: A controlled clinical trial. *Pain, 48,* 137–146.

Szechtman, H., Woody, E., Bowers, K. S., & Nahmias, C. (1998). Where the imaginal appears real: A positron emission tomography study of auditory hallucinations. *Proceedings of the National Academy of Sciences, 95,* 1956–1960.

Tart, C. T. (1983). Altered states of consciousness. In R. Harré & R. Lamb (Eds.), *The encyclopedic dictionary of psychology* (pp. 19–20). Cambridge, MA: MIT Press.

Taylor, S. (1996). Meta-analysis of cognitive–behavioral treatments for social phobia. *Journal of Behavior Therapy and Experimental Psychiatry, 27,* 1–9.

Teasdale, J. D. (1985). Psychological treatments for depression: How do they work? *Behaviour Research and Therapy, 23,* 157–165.

Teasdale, J. D., Segal, Z. V., & Williams, J. M. G. (2003). Mindfulness training and problem formulation. *Clinical Psychology: Science and Practice, 10,* 157–160.

Telch, C. F., Agras, W. S., Rossiter, E. M., Wilfley, D., & Kenardy, J. (1990). Group cognitive–behavioral treatment for the non-purging bulimic: An initial evaluation. *Journal of Consulting and Clinical Psychology, 58,* 629–635.

Thakur, K. (1980). Treatment of anorexia nervosa with hypnotherapy. In H. Wain (Ed.), *Clinical hypnosis in medicine* (pp. 446–493). Chicago: Yearbook.

Thompson-Brenner, H., Glass, S., & Westen, D. (2003). A multidimensional meta-analysis of psychotherapy for bulimia nervosa. *Clinical Psychology: Science and Practice, 10,* 269–287.

Tloczynski, J., Malinonowski, A., & LaMorte, R. (1997). Rediscovering and re-applying contingent informal meditation. *Psychologia, 40,* 14–21.

Tobin, D. L., Reynolds, R. V. C., Holroyd, K. A., & Creer, T. L. (1986). Self-management and social learning theory. In K. A. Holroyd & T. L. Creer (Eds.), *Self-management of chronic disease: Handbook of clinical interventions and research.* Orlando, FL: Academic Press.

Torem, M. (1992). The use of hypnosis with eating disorders. *Psychiatric Medicine, 10,* 105–117.

Turk, D. C., & Rudy, T. E. (1992). Classification logic and strategies in chronic pain. In D. C. Turk & R. Melzack (Eds.), *Handbook of pain assessment* (pp. 409–428). New York: Guilford Press.

U.S. Department of Health, Education, and Welfare. (1990). *Smoking and health: A report of the surgeon general* (DHEW Publication No. PHS79-50066). Washington, DC: Author.

U.S. Department of Health and Human Services. (1990). *The health benefits of smoking cessation: A report of the Surgeon General* (DHHS publication No. CDC 90–8416). Rockville, MD: Author.

Vanderlinden, J., & Vandereycken, W. (1988). The use of hypnotherapy in the treatment of eating disorders. *International Journal of Eating Disorders, 18,* 145–150.

Van Etten, M., & Taylor, S. (1998). Comparative efficacy of treatments for posttraumatic stress disorder: A meta-analysis. *Clinical Psychology and Psychotherapy, 5,* 126–145.

Vijselaar, J., & Van der Hart, O. (1992). The first report of hypnotic treatment of traumatic grief: A brief communication. *International Journal of Clinical and Experimental Hypnosis, 40,* 1–6.

Viswesvaran, C., & Schmidt, F. (1992). A meta-analytic comparison of the effectiveness of smoking cessation methods. *Journal of Applied Psychology, 77,* 554–561.

Von Dedenroth, T. (1964). The use of hypnosis with "tobaccomaniacs." *American Journal of Clinical Hypnosis, 6,* 326.

Vrana, S., & Lauterbach, D. (1994). Prevalence of traumatic events and post-traumatic stress psychological symptoms in a nonclinical sample of college students. *Journal of Traumatic Stress, 7,* 289–302.

Wadden, T. A., & Anderton, C. H. (1982). The clinical use of hypnosis. *Psychological Bulletin, 91,* 215–243.

Wade, K. A., Garry, M., Read, J. D., & Lindsay, D. S. (2002). A picture is worth a thousand lies: Using false photographs to create false childhood memories. *Psychonomic Bulletin and Review, 9,* 597–603.

Wagstaff, G. F. (1991). Compliance, belief, and semantics in hypnosis: A nonstate sociocognitive perspective. In S. J. Lynn & J. W. Rhue (Eds.), *Theories of hypnosis: Current models and perspectives* (pp. 362–396). New York: Guilford Press.

Wagstaff, G. (1998). The semantics and physiology of hypnosis as an altered state: Towards a definition of hypnosis. *Contemporary Hypnosis, 15,* 149–165.

Wakeman, J. R., & Kaplan, J. Z. (1978). An experimental study of hypnosis in painful burns. *American Journal of Clinical Hypnosis, 21,* 3–12.

Walsh, R. (1999). Asian contemplative disciplines: Common practices, clinical applications, and research findings. *Journal of Transpersonal Psychology, 31*(2), 83–107.

Wampold, B. (2001). *The great psychotherapy debate: Models and findings.* Mahwah, NJ: Erlbaum.

Watkins, H. H. (1980). The silent abreaction. *International Journal of Clinical and Experimental Hypnosis, 28,* 101–113.

Wegner, D. M. (1994). Ironic processes of mental control. *Psychological Review, 101,* 34–52.

Wegner, D. M. (1997). When the antidote is the poison: Ironic mental control processes. *Psychological Science, 8,* 148–151.

Weinstein, E. J., & Au, P. K. (1991). Use of hypnosis before and during angioplasty. *American Journal of Clinical Hypnosis, 34,* 29–37.

Weiss, B. L. (1988). *Many lives, many masters.* New York: Simon & Schuster.

Weiss, D. S., & Marmar, C. R. (1997). The Impact of Event Scale—Revised. In J. P. Wilson & T. M. Keane (Eds.), *Assessing psychological trauma and PTSD* (pp. 399–428). New York: Guilford Press.

Weitzenhoffer, A. M. (1985). In search of hypnosis. In D. Waxman, P. C. Misra, M. Gibson, & M. A. Basker (Eds.), *Modern trends in hypnosis* (pp. 67–88). New York: Plenum.

Weitzenhoffer, A. M., & Hilgard, E. (1962). *Stanford Hypnotic Susceptibility Scale: Form C.* Palo Alto, CA: Consulting Psychologists Press.

Weston, D., & Morrison, K. (2001). A multidimensional meta-analysis of treatments for depression, panic, and generalized anxiety disorder: An empirical examination of the status of empirically supported therapies. *Journal of Consulting and Clinical Psychology, 69,* 875–899.

White, R. W. (1941). A preface to a theory of hypnotism. *Journal of Abnormal and Social Psychology, 36,* 477–505.

Whitehouse, W. G., Dinges, D. F., Orne, E. C., & Orne, M. T. (1988). Hypnotic hypermnesia: Enhanced memory accessibility or report bias? *Journal of Abnormal Psychology, 97,* 289–295.

Whorwell, P. J., Prior, A., & Colgan, S. M. (1987). Hypnotherapy in severe irritable bowel syndrome: Further experience. *Gut, 28,* 423–425.

Whorwell, P. J., Prior, A., & Faragher, E. B. (1984). Controlled trial of hypnotherapy in the treatment of severe, refractory irritable bowel syndrome. *Lancet, 2,* 1232–1234.

Wickless, C., & Kirsch, I. (1989). The effects of verbal and experiential expectancy manipulations on hypnotic susceptibility. *Journal of Personality and Social Psychology, 57,* 762–768.

Wilfley, D. E., Agras, W. S., Telch, C. F., Rossiter, E. M., Schneider, J. A., Cole, A. G., et al. (1993). Group cognitive–behavioral therapy and interpersonal psychotherapy for the nonpurging bulimic: A controlled comparison. *Journal of Consulting and Clinical Psychology, 61,* 296–305.

Williamson, D. A., Gleaves, D., & Lawson, O. J. (1991). Biased perception of overeating in bulimia nervosa and compulsive binge eaters. *Journal of Psychopathology and Behavioral Assessment, 13,* 257–268.

Wilson, G. T., & Fairburn, C. G. (1993). Cognitive treatments for eating disorders. *Journal of Consulting and Clinical Psychology, 61,* 261–269.

Wilson, G. T., & Fairburn, C. G. (2002). Treatments for eating disorders. In P. E. Nathan & J. M. Gorman (Eds.), *Treatments that work* (pp. 559–592). New York: Oxford University Press.

Wilson, G. T., & Pike, K. M. (2001). Eating disorders. In D. H. Barlow (Ed.), *Clinical handbook of psychological disorders* (pp. 332–375). New York: Guilford Press.

Wilson, S. C., & Barber, T. X. (1981). Vivid fantasy and hallucinatory abilities in the life histories of excellent hypnotic subjects ("somnabules"): Preliminary report with female subjects. In E. Klinger (Ed.), *Imagery: Vol. 2. Concepts, results, and applications* (pp. 133–152). New York: Plenum Press.

Wilson, S. C., & Barber, T. X. (1983). The fantasy-prone personality: Implications for understanding imagery, hypnosis, and parapsychological phenomena. In A. A. Sheikh (Ed.), *Imagery: Current theory, research, and application* (pp. 340–387). New York: Wiley.

Wilson, T. D., & Capitman, J. A. (1982). Effects of script availability on social behavior. *Personality and Social Psychology Bulletin, 8,* 11–20.

Wonderlich, S. A., & Mitchell, J. E. (1997). Eating disorders and comorbidity: Empirical, conceptual, and clinical implications. *Psychopharmacology Bulletin, 33,* 381–390.

Woody, E. Z., & Bowers, K. S. (1994). A frontal assault on dissociated control. In S. J. Lynn & J. W. Rhue (Eds.), *Dissociation: Clinical and theoretical perspectives* (pp. 52–79). New York: Guilford Press.

Woody, E., & Farvolden, P. (1998). Dissociation in hypnosis and frontal executive function. *American Journal of Clinical Hypnosis, 40,* 206–216.

Woody, E., & Sadler, P. (1998). On reintegrating dissociated theories: Comment on Kirsch and Lynn (1998). *Psychological Bulletin, 123,* 192–197.

Wright, B. R., & Drummond, P. D. (2000). Rapid induction analgesia for the alleviation of procedural pain during burn care. *Burns, 26,* 275–282.

Yapko, M. D. (1986). Hypnosis and strategic interventions in the treatment of anorexia nervosa. *American Journal of Clinical Hypnosis, 28,* 224–232.

Yapko, M. D. (1989). Disturbances of temporal orientation as a feature of depression. In M. D. Yapko (Ed.), *Brief therapy approaches to treating anxiety and depression* (pp. 106–118). New York: Brunner/Mazel.

Yapko, M. D. (1992). *Hypnosis and the treatment of depression: Strategies for change.* New York: Brunner/Mazel.

Yapko, M. D. (1993). Hypnosis and depression. In J. W. Rhue, S. J. Lynn, & I. Kirsch (Eds.), *Handbook of clinical hypnosis* (pp. 339–355). Washington, DC: American Psychological Association.

Yapko, M. D. (2002). *Treating depression with hypnosis: Integrating cognitive–behavioral and strategic approaches.* Philadelphia: Brunner-Routledge.

Yapko, M. D. (2003). *Trancework: An introduction to the practice of clinical hypnosis* (2nd ed.). New York: Brunner-Routledge.

Yehuda, R., Resnick, H., Kahana, B., & Giller, E. L. (1993). Long-lasting hormonal alterations in extreme stress in humans: Normative or maladaptive? *Psychosomatic Medicine, 55,* 287–297.

Young, D. (1995). The use of hypnotherapy in the treatment of eating disorders. *Contemporary Hypnosis, 12,* 148–153.

Young, J., & Cooper, L. M. (1972). Hypnotic recall amnesia as a function of manipulated expectancy. *Proceedings of the 80th Annual Convention of the American Psychological Association, 7,* 857–858.

Young, P. C. (1926). An experimental study of mental and physical functions in the normal and hypnotic states: Additional results. *American Journal of Psychology, 37,* 345–356.

Zeltzer, L. K., Dolgin, M. J., LeBaron, S., & LeBaron, C. (1991). A randomized, controlled study of behavioral intervention for chemotherapy distress in children with cancer. *Pediatrics, 88,* 34–42.

Zeltzer, L. K., & LeBaron, S. M. (1982). Hypnosis and nonhypnotic techniques for reduction of pain and anxiety during painful procedures in children and adolescents with cancer. *Journal of Pediatrics, 101,* 1032–1035.

Ziedonis, D., & Williams, J. (2003). Management of smoking in people with psychiatric disorders. *Current Opinion in Psychiatry, 16,* 305–315.

Zitman, F. G., Van Dyck, R., Spinhoven, P., & Linssen, A. C. (1992). Hypnosis and autogenic training in the treatment of tension headaches: A two-phase constructive design study with follow-up. *Journal of Psychosomatic Research, 36,* 219–228.

AUTHOR INDEX

Hollon, S. D., 81, 122, 133
Holroyd, J. D., 32, 36, 39, 80
Holroyd, K. A., 82–83
Hoogduin, K. A. L., 37, 209
Hope, R. A., 102
Horne, R. J., 99
Hornyak, L. M., 103
Horvath, A. O., 42
Hughes, M., 159
Hull, C. L., 15
Hunt, T., 161
Hunt, W., 80
Husband, T. H., 201
Hyman, I. E., Jr., 201, 204
Hynan, M. T., 176

Institute of Medicine, 175

Jacka, B. T., 104
Jacknow, D. S., 193
Jackson, T. L., 80
Jacquith, L., 24
Jakobsson, J., 193
Jamieson, G. A., 5, 198, 199, 199–200, 200
Janet, P., 14
Jeffrey, L. K., 81
Jeffrey, T. B., 81
Jensen, M. P., 178
Jimerson, D. C., 99
Johnston, E., 80
Johnston, J. C., 192
Johnston, J. D., 26
Joiner, T. C., 105
Jones, J. C., 160
Jones, R., 102
Joordens, S., 45
Jordan, B. K., 159
Joris, J., 176
Joyce, J. S., 176
Juster, H. R., 137

Kabat-Zinn, J., 133
Kahana, B., 159
Kallio, S., 5, 20, 198
Kanfer, F. H., 32
Kaplan, J. Z., 176, 177
Kattan, M., 191

Keane, T. M., 161, 163
Keefe, F. J., 178
Kenardy, J., 117
Kenny, D. A., 4
Kessler, R. C., 121, 136, 159
Khalsa, S., 203
Kihlstrom, J. F., 20, 198, 208
Kileen, P. R., 5
Kilpatrick, D. G., 159, 161
Kirsch, I., 3, 4, 5, 8, 14, 19, 22, 24, 25, 26, 32, 33, 36, 38, 39, 40, 41, 42, 43, 44, 46, 51, 53, 61, 67, 72, 122, 124, 130, 137, 138, 139, 177, 178, 198, 199, 202, 206, 207, 211
Kleber, R. J., 160
Klerman, G. L., 101
Klopfer, B., 38
Kogan, L. G., 99
Kohen, D. P., 76, 77
Kosslyn, S. M., 199
Kozak, M. J., 155, 162
Krackow, E., 202
Kraemer, H. C., 102
Krakauer, S. Y., 76
Kramer, H., 9
Krasner, L., 177
Kroger, W. S., 103
Kropotov, J. D., 200
Kuhn, T. S., 198
Kulka, R. A., 159
Kurzhals, R., 18
Kuttner, L., 176
Kvaal, S., 18, 29, 53, 103

Labelle, L., 28
LaJoy, R., 32
Lambert, S., 78, 192
Lamy, M., 176
Lang, E. V., 176, 180, 192
Lankton, C., 15, 41
Lankton, S., 15, 41
Laurence, J.-R., 26, 28, 199, 200, 201, 208
Lauterbach, D., 159
Law, M., 81
Lawson, O. J., 97
Lazarus, A. A., 32, 150
LeBaron, C., 78
LeBaron, S. M., 78

Nelson, C., 159
Neufeld, V. R., 33, 42, 80, 82, 104, 194
Newman, M. G., 155
Nicholls, S. S., 39
Nolen-Hoeksema, S., 160

Oathies, D., 200
O'Brien, T., 160
O'Connor, M., 102
Ollendick, T. H., 139
Olness, K., 76, 77
Orne, E. C., 201
Orne, M. T., 15, 27, 37, 40, 61, 178,
    198, 201, 208
Otto, M. W., 139

Page, R. A., 210
Palace, E. M., 38
Pastor, S., 83
Pastyrnak, S. L., 139
Patterson, D., 3, 32, 176
Payne, D., 33
Payne, T. J., 83
Pederson, L. L., 80
Pentland, J., 204
Perkins, K. A., 83
Perry, C., 26, 28, 82, 198, 200, 201
Peterson, R. A., 140
Pettinati, H. M., 99
Peveler, R. C., 102
Piccione, C., 23
Pickrell, J. E., 201
Pike, K. M., 102
Pinnell, C. A., 175, 176
Pintar, J., 76
Pittman, R. K., 163
Polaschek, D. L. L., 204
Polivy, J., 106
Pollack, M. H., 139
Polyakov, Y. I., 200
Poole, D., 200
Porter, S., 201
Posa, S., 140
Pribble, W., 42
Price, D. D., 177, 198
Prior, A., 191

Questad, K. A., 176

Radtke, H. L., 19
Rae, D. S., 135
Rainville, P., 177, 198, 200
Rapee, R. M., 137
Ray, W. J., 200
Read, J. D., 201
Reason, J. T., 45
Reed, S., 32, 40
Regier, D. A., 135
Reiss, S., 38, 137, 138, 140
Research Committee of the
    British Tuberculosis Society,
    191
Resick, P. A., 170
Resnick, H., 159
Resnick, H. S., 159
Resnick, P., 161
Reutenauer, E. L., 178
Revonsuo, A., 5, 20, 198
Reynolds, R. V. C., 82–83
Rhue, J., 33
Rhue, J. W., 3, 18, 24, 26, 33, 38, 40, 51,
    53, 61, 67, 76, 77, 80, 103, 198,
    206, 211
Rimpoche, 134
Rivers, S. M., 23
Rodgers, W. M., 178
Roemer, L., 140, 155
Roncon, V., 26
Rosen, D., 78
Rosen, S., 72
Ross, S., 23
Rossi, E. L., 51
Rossi, S. I., 51
Rossiter, E. M., 117
Roth, R. S., 178
Rothbaum, B. O., 161, 162, 166
Rounsaville, B. J., 101
Rudd, M. D., 105
Rudy, T. E., 178
Rush, A. J., 122
Ryken, K., 18, 209

Sadler, P., 20
Salzberg, H. C., 33
Sanders, S., 61
Sapirstein, G., 3, 36, 39, 122, 130
Sarbin, T. R., 21, 26, 198, 199
Sarles, H., 177
Saunders, B. E., 159

SUBJECT INDEX

Automatic activation, and response sets, 25
Automatic thoughts
    making note of, 148
    as self-suggestions, 123–126
Avoidance, and anxiety disorders, 138, 155

Baquet, 11
Barber, Theodore X., 21–22, 61
Beck Depression Inventory, 105
Beck's cognitive therapy, for depression, 122–123, 124
Behavioral medicine, 175
    hypnosis in, 175–176, 191–193
Behavioral or real-life exposure, 151–152
Belief in reality of event, in McConkey's model, 28
Believed-in imaginings, 21
Benivieni, Antonio, 8, 9
Bernheim, Hippolyte, 14–15
Binet, Alfred, 3, 14
Binge eating
    vs. addiction, 118
    avoiding of, 97–98
        in example, 110
    deferring of, 111
    dieting as temptation toward, 107
    education about, 106–107
    identification of causes of, 114–115
    and obesity, 117
    understanding of, 107–108
    value placed on, 109
    See also Eating disorders
Black-or-white thinking, 128
Body image, and eating disorders, 116
Body scan
    in anchoring technique, 65
    in closed-fist technique, 75
    in eating-disorder treatment, 111
    and relaxation exercises, 54–56, 57, 183–185
    in self-control relaxation training, 144
    for worry, 154
Borderline character structure, as hypnosis contraindication, 37
Boulder model, vii
Boundaries, security of (bubble), 69–70
Braid, James, 6, 13, 14

Brain functioning, and hypnotic suggestion, 20, 199–200
Breathing
    in dentistry, 195
    in hypnotic treatment of surgical patients, 192
    in pain management, 182–183, 189
    panic, 142
    in relaxation example, 56–57
    in self-control relaxation training, 143–146
Bubble (induction technique), 69–70
    and age regression, 73
Bulimia nervosa (BN), 99, 100, 101
    and body image technique, 116
    cognitive restructuring techniques for, 112
    dysfunctional thoughts in, 112
    See also Eating disorders

Canadian Psychiatric Association (CPA), on memory recovery, 205
Catalepsy
    as hypnosis sign, 205
    spontaneous arm, 40
    as staged in Charcot's conception of hypnosis, 13–14
Catastrophic thinking
    and anxiety, 136–137
    in management of acute pain, 186
    modifying of, 146–150
    reduction of (pain management), 178
Charcot, Jean Martin, 13–15, 40
Chevreul pendulum illusion, 46–47, 50, 51
    in example, 49–50
    and suggestibility, 207
Child abuse
    and age regression, 74
    and recovered memories, 200
    and storytelling, 77
Childbirth, hypnosis with, 176, 177
Children
    clinical hypnosis with, 76–78
    pain management for (distraction example), 190
Clinical considerations, in smoking cessation program, 96

Depression, *continued*
    building positive expectations,
        130–133
    and self-esteem, 129
    relapse prevention (mindfulness
        training), 133–134
*Diagnostic and Statistical Manual of Mental
    Disorders* (3rd ed.; *DSM–III*), 7, 36
Disqualification, as cognitive distortion,
    127
Dissociated-control theory, 20
Dissociated personalities, creation of
    through hypnosis, 200
Dissociation, in Barber's position, 22
Dissociative disorders, 7, 10, 36–37
    and age regression, 169
    and Charcot, 14
    and Comfort the Child technique,
        172
    as contraindication to use of
        hypnosis (unstabilized), 37
    and experience of safety and
        security, 67
    hypnosis in treatment of, 15
Distraction, in pain management,
    189–190

Eating Attitudes Test, 105
Eating disorders
    and experience of safety and
        security, 67
    hypnosis in treatment of, 103–105
        assessment for, 105–106
        with cognitive–behavioral
            therapy, 106–117
    prevalence of, 100–101
    research on treatment of, 101–103
    subclinical, 101
Eating Disorders Examination, 105
Eating Disorders Inventory—2, 105
Education, in smoking cessation program,
    82
Egypt, history of hysteria in, 7
Elevator exercise, 165
Emergency response, 141
Emotional processing, of interpersonal
    feelings, 155–156
Emotional thinking, 128–129
Empty-chair technique, 129
Erickson, Milton H., 15

Esdaile, James, 12
Everyday life, in anchoring techniques,
    65–66
Executive control, 19
Expectancy(ies), and expectations, 24,
    38–42
    anxiety, 137–138
    in Barber's view of therapy, 22
    and behavior of hypnotized
        individuals, 13
    in depression treatment, 130
    Franklin Commission's recognition
        of, 12
    and hypnotic pain control, 179
    in Kirsch's theory, 24
    in memory recovery, 202
    and pain, 177
    in past-life regressions, 204
    positive
        in depression treatment, 130–133
        in pain management, 180
        in PTSD treatment, 164
        and waking suggestions, 207
    and response set theory, 25
    self-fulfilling response, 38
    and sociocognitive theorists, 26
    in Spanos model, 22
    and suggestibility, 40
    and therapeutic alliance, 43
    therapist's creation of, 29
    and wart loss, 192
Expectancy building, 130–133
Expectancy control procedures, by
    Franklin Commission, 12
Expectancy modification
    and hypnotic inductions, 39–40
    and responsiveness, 41
Exposure-based cognitive–behavioral
    treatments, 74
Exposure therapy
    conditions for avoidance of, 166
    knowledge of family dynamics
        necessary for, 173
    for PTSD, 161, 162–167
    research needed on, 173
Eye closure relaxation technique, 59–60
Eye-roll induction, in dentistry, 195

Facilitative information, for patients,
    45–46

and strong emotions, 74
and wart loss, 192
Imaginal exposure, 150–151, 153
Imagination, and Franklin Commission's findings, 12
Imagination inflation, 204
Imaginative (imaginal) rehearsal, 72, 115, 116
Impact of Event Scale—Revised, 161
Induction techniques, 53–54
    arm levitation, 51–52, 60–61
    and children, 76–77
    for deepening, 62–64
    patient's collaboration in, 44–45, 78
    posthypnotic suggestion, 64–66 (see also Posthypnotic suggestion)
    relaxation-based, 54–57
        eye closure, 59–60
        staircase, 57–59, 63
        (see also Relaxation training)
    self-hypnosis, 61–62 (see also Self-hypnosis)
    for smoking cessation, 89 (see also Smoking cessation program)
    termination, 66
    See also Hypnotic inductions
Informed consent or choice, 32, 205, 211
Inner advisor, 29, 70
Inner observer, 29, 168
Integrative model of Lynn, 24–25
Interactional models, 26–28
Internal dialogue of patient, 29
International Journal of Clinical and Experimental Hypnosis, 3
Interpersonal feelings, emotional processing of, 155–156
Interpersonal therapy (IPT)
    for depression, 122–123
    for eating disorders, 101–102
Interpretations, 35
Intrusive imagery. See Flashbacks
In vivo exposure, for PTSD, 167
Irritable bowel syndrome, hypnotic treatment of, 191

James, William, 3
Janet, Pierre, 14

Kihlstrom, J. F., 20
Kirsch's response expectancy theory, 24

Lavoisier, Antoine, 11
Lethargy, as staged in Charcot's conception of hypnosis, 13–14
Liebeault, August, 14–15
Lynn's integrative model, 24–25

Magnetism, replaced by "hypnosis," 13. See also Animal magnetism
Magnification and minimization, 127–128
McConkey's model, 28
Meanings, 35
    of pain, 178–179
    placed on hypnotist's communications, 28
    and PTSD reactions, 169
Meditation, patient's experience with, 43–44
Memory(ies)
    in PTSD treatment, 168
    as reconstructive, 124, 201
Memory recovery through hypnosis, 28, 200–206
    as point of controversy, 197
    and reliability of memory, 33
Mesmer, Franz Anton, 9–10
Mesmerism and mesmerists, 6, 10, 11, 12
    cultural expectations about, 204–205
    misconceptions of, 44
Metaphors
    in expectation building, 131
    as priming, 71–72
Middle Ages, and hysteria, 7
Mindfulness training
    for depression, 133–134
    for GAD, 155
    and PTSD, 168
Mind reading, 126–127
Misconceptions, correcting of (in patient), 44–45, 210–211
Monoideism, 13
Motivated cognitive commitment, 28
Motivation
    in smoking cessation program, 82, 96
        in program description, 85
Movies, and dissociative identity disorder, 36
Multiple cues, 66
Multiple personalities, creation of through hypnosis, 200
Myths, correcting of (in patient), 44–45

age progression and regression, 169
assessment, 161–162
cognitive restructuring, 169–173
exposure therapy, 162–167
and flashback periods, 163, 167–168, 172
and memories, 168
mindfulness, 168
research needed on, 173
Preparing the patient, 42–47, 210–212
example of, 47–51
and fail-safe induction, 51–52
and gradual change or setbacks, 52
for subsequent sessions, 64
Primary process, 18, 28
Priming, 45, 71, 72
Prior experience with hypnosis (of patient), assessment of, 43
Problem solving
in eating-disorder treatment, 115
facilitating of, 70–76
Professional societies, on memory recovery, 205–206
Pseudomemories, 200, 209
Psychoanalytic theory, 17–18
clinical implications of, 28
Psychotherapy, for depression, 122, 133
Psychotic decompensation, as hypnosis contraindication, 37
Puysegur, Marquis de, 10–11, 12

Race, Victor, 11
Rapport, hypnotic, 27–28, 29
Real-simulator design, 27
Recall, as reconstructive, 124. *See also* Memory recovery through hypnosis
Reestimation, in modification of catastrophic thoughts, 147–150
Reframing, 15
Regression
age, 18, 28, 43
topographic, 18
Rehearsal, imaginative (imaginal), 72, 115, 116
Reinterpretation, in pain management, 189
Relapse
in eating-disorder program, 115

in smoking cessation program, 89
Relapse prevention
in depression treatment, 133–134
in obesity treatment, 119
in smoking cessation, 83
Relaxation-based techniques, 54–57
eye closure, 59–60
staircase, 57–59
Relaxation training
in dentistry, 194
and hypnosis, 32, 35
in pain management, 182–183, 186
patient's experience with, 43–44
and primary process, 18
in smoking cessation program, 90–92
Renaissance, and demonic possession, 8
Repetition, in hypnotic inductions, 129
Research
on eating-disorder treatment, 101–103
needed on addition of hypnosis to CBT, 120
in hypnosis, vii, 5
needed on hypnosis and PTSD, 173
on neurophysiological concomitants, 200
on self-help protocol for depression, 133
on smoking cessation program, 95–96
Response expectancy, and pain-catastrophizing relation, 178
Response expectancy theory of Kirsch, 24
Response set theory, 25
Responsiveness, individual differences in, 40–41
Role theory of hypnosis, 21

Safety and security, promoting feelings of, 67–68
Sarbin, Theodore, 21
Secret Window (movie), 36
Self-control relaxation training (SCRT), 143–146
Self-efficacy, in smoking cessation program, 82
Self-esteem, and depression, 129
Self-fulfilling prophecies, in Barber's view of therapy, 22

Weight gain
    and set-point weight, 109
    and smoking cessation, 83, 87, 96–
        97, 97–98
Weiss, Brian, 203
White, Robert W., 197–198
Witchcraft trials, 9

Wording of suggestions, 22–23
Worry, treatment of, 153–156. *See also*
    Anxiety disorders
Wundt, Wilhelm, 3

Young, P. C., 15

ABOUT THE AUTHORS

Steven Jay Lynn, PhD, is a professor of psychology at the State University of New York at Binghamton and a diplomate (American Board of Professional Psychology) in clinical and forensic psychology. A former president of the American Psychological Association (APA) Division 30 (Society of Psychological Hypnosis), Dr. Lynn is the author or editor of 14 books and more than 230 articles on hypnosis, abnormal psychology, psychotherapy, dissociation, anomalous experiences, and memory. He is a recent recipient of the APA Division 30 Award for Distinguished Contributions to Scientific Hypnosis and the Chancellor's Award from the State University of New York for Excellence in Scholarship, Creativity, and Professional Activities. Dr. Lynn serves on 11 editorial boards, including the *Journal of Abnormal Psychology*, and he is an editor of *Contemporary Hypnosis*. His Laboratory of Consciousness and Cognition is funded by the National Institute of Mental Health.

Irving Kirsch, PhD, of the University of Plymouth, has published 7 books, 37 book chapters, and more than 150 scientific journal articles on placebo effects, antidepressant medication, hypnosis, and suggestion. His work has been extensively covered in the media, with feature articles in *The New York Times*, *Newsweek*, *Science*, *Lancet*, *Scientific American*, *Smithsonian*, *Science News*, *The Washington Post*, and many other newspapers and magazines around the world. He has appeared on television documentaries and news programs broadcast on ABC, HBO, NPR, the Discovery Channel, and the BBC.